Conceptualising Public Health

In Germanic and Nordic languages, the term for 'public health' literally translates to 'people's health', for example *Volksgesundheit* in German, *folkhälsa* in Swedish and *kansanterveys* in Finnish. Covering a period stretching from the late nineteenth century to the present day, this book discusses how understandings and meanings of public health have developed in their political and social context, identifying ruptures and redefinitions in its conceptualisation. It analyses the multifaceted and interactive rhetorical play through which key concepts have been used as political tools, on the one hand, and shaped the understanding and operating environment of public health, on the other.

Focusing on the blurred boundaries between the social and the medico-scientific realms, from social hygiene to population policy, *Conceptualising Public Health* explores the sometimes contradictory and paradoxical normative aims associated with the promotion of public health. Providing examples from Northern Europe and the Nordic countries, whilst situating them in a larger European and international context, it addresses questions such as:

- How have public health concepts been used in government and associated administrative practices from the early twentieth century up to the present?
- How has health citizenship been constructed over time?
- How has the collective entity of 'the people' been associated with and reflected in public health concepts?

Drawn from a range of disciplinary backgrounds, the authors collected here each examine a particular way of understanding public health and assess how key actors or phenomena have challenged, altered or confirmed past and present meanings of the concept. *Conceptualising Public Health* is of interest to students and scholars of health and welfare state development from diverse backgrounds, including public health, sociology of health and illness, and social policy as well as medical, conceptual and intellectual history.

Johannes Kananen is Adjunct Professor of Social Policy and works currently as Senior Lecturer at the Swedish School of Social Science, University of Helsinki, Finland.

Sophy Bergenheim is a PhD Candidate in political history at the University of Helsinki, Finland.

Merle Wessel is Lecturer in Nordic history at the University of Greifswald, Germany.

Routledge Studies in Public Health

www.routledge.com/Routledge-Studies-in-Public-Health/book-series/RSPH

Conceptualising Public Health

Historical and Contemporary Struggles over Key Concepts

**Edited by
Johannes Kananen,
Sophy Bergenheim and
Merle Wessel**

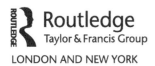

Routledge
Taylor & Francis Group

LONDON AND NEW YORK

First published 2018
by Routledge
4 Park Square, Milton Park, Abingdon, Oxon OX14 4RN
605 Third Avenue, New York, NY 10017

First issued in paperback 2023

Routledge is an imprint of the Taylor & Francis Group, an informa business

British Library Cataloguing-in-Publication Data
A catalogue record for this book is available from the British Library

Library of Congress Cataloging-in-Publication Data
A catalog record for this book has been requested

ISBN: 978-1-03-257001-3 (pbk)
ISBN: 978-1-138-03683-3 (hbk)
ISBN: 978-1-315-17827-1 (ebk)

DOI: 10.4324/9781315178271

Typeset in Times New Roman
by Keystroke, Neville Lodge, Tettenhall, Wolverhampton

Contents

List of figures

Contributors

Annika Berg has a PhD in the history of science and ideas (Uppsala University 2009) and is a Senior Lecturer in the history of ideas at the Department of Culture and Aesthetics, Stockholm University. Her research concentrates largely on the social, cultural and political history of medicine and healthcare, in relation to which she takes a special interest in questions of gender and intersectionality, power and governance, knowledge transfer and postcolonial perspectives.

Sophy Bergenheim is a PhD Candidate in political history at the Faculty of Social Sciences of the University of Helsinki. Her historical research interests include the Nordic welfare states, medical history, housing policy and urban history, gender history and the history of knowledge as well as conceptual and intellectual history. In her dissertation, Bergenheim studies Finnish social and health policy NGOs as policy actors and experts in the 1930s–1960s.

Johan Edman is Adjunct Professor of History and Senior Lecturer at the Department of Criminology at Stockholm University. Edman has mainly conducted research on social exclusion, the treatment of vagrants and substance misusers from the nineteenth century onwards, and alcohol and drug policy in the twentieth century. He has recently finished two research projects: on transnational alcohol conferences and on the medicalisation of excessive behaviours. Currently he is working on a project on the knowledge-base of Swedish alcohol policy during the years 1911–2009.

Ainur Elmgren is a historian. She defended her doctoral thesis on stereotypes of Swedishness in the Finnish press 1918–1939 at Lund University in 2008. Since 2010, she has participated in several international research projects at the University of Helsinki, publishing on topics ranging from openness, political identities or the driving forces of democracy in Finland and Sweden, to the conceptual history of -isms such as populism and 'Jesuitism'. She is also interested in the graphic arts, and draws historical comics. She is currently working on a biography of the Finnish journalist Erkki Vala.

Outi Hakola works as a senior researcher (Academy of Finland Research Fellow) in area and cultural studies, University of Helsinki. Her background is in media studies, and her research concentrates on questions of emotions in fictive films, television drama and social media. Her major publications are *Rhetoric of Modern Death in American Living Dead Films* (Intellect/University of Chicago Press, 2015); *Death and Mortality: From Individual to Communal Perspectives* (co-edited with Sara Heinämaa and Sami Pihlström, University of Helsinki, 2015); and *Death in Literature* (co-edited with Sari Kivistö, Cambridge Scholars, 2014).

Minna Harjula is a researcher at the Faculty of Social Sciences, University of Tampere, Finland. Her research interests focus on the history of welfare policies from the point of view of health and citizenship. Harjula currently works at the Finnish Centre of Excellence in Historical Research. She will continue her research on lived welfare state at the new Centre of Excellence in the History of Experiences, University of Tampere in 2018.

Matilda Hellman, PhD, is Adjunct Professor of Sociology. Hellman is a senior sociologist whose work has focused specifically on lifestyles and addictions, and the ways in which idea world setups are embedded in habits, politics and governance. She is director of the University of Helsinki Centre for Research on Addiction Control and Governance (CEACG). She is also a guest researcher at the National Institute for Health and Welfare (THL), and editor of the journal *Nordic Studies on Alcohol and Drugs*.

Johannes Kananen is Adjunct Professor of Social Policy, and currently works as Senior Lecturer at the Swedish School of Social Science, University of Helsinki. His research interests include the historical and contemporary transformations of the Nordic welfare state model. He has focused on topics such as power and political change in the areas of work, labour markets and unemployment policy, and, more recently, in the field of public health.

Norma Montesino is an Adjunct Professor in the School of Social Work, Lund University, Sweden, where her current main research interest is migration in social work, and social history. Her research focuses on the treatment of groups perceived as poor aliens in the Swedish context. In her dissertation (*The Gypsy Question: Intervention and Romanticism*, 2002) she studied Swedish policies towards Roma groups during the twentieth century. More recent studies include the emergence and development of the institutionalised reception of refugees in the Swedish welfare services. A current research project focuses on ethnical relationships in social work education.

Ida Ohlsson Al Fakir has a PhD in history and works as a postdoctoral research fellow at the Hugo Valentin Centre, Uppsala University, Sweden. Her areas of research include Swedish Roma policies and the history of the Swedish welfare state, the history of medicine and science, and social citizenship studies. The current research project concerns Christian problematisations of migration and the Church of Sweden's social work with migrants and minorities at the beginning of the twentieth century.

Teemu Ryymin is a Professor of Modern Political History in the Department of Archaeology, History, Cultural Studies and Religion, University of Bergen in Norway. His fields of expertise include the use of history, history of health and medicine, and history of minorities in Northern Scandinavia, as well as historiography and methodology in historical research. His most current publication (as editor) is *Historie og politikk. Historiebruk i norsk politikkutforming etter 1945* (Oslo: Universitetsforlaget, 2017).

Helena Tolvhed is an Adjunct Professor in the Department of History, Stockholm University. Her research interests are cultural and gender history in the twentieth century, and have centred on sport and health as empirical fields. The book *På damsidan* (2015, English: *On the Ladies' Side: Femininity, Agency and Power in Swedish Sport 1920–1990*) examines sport as a historical arena for subordination and struggle, but also as community, pleasure and emancipation for women. Tolvhed is presently working on the project 'From People's Health to "Healthism"? New Femininities and Masculinities in Health and Fitness from 1970'.

Paul Weindling is Research Professor in History of Medicine at Oxford Brookes University. In 1999–2004, he was a member of the Max-Planck-Gesellschaft President's Committee for the History of the Kaiser-Wilhelm-Gesellschaft under National Socialism, and was on the advisory boards of the AHRC project on German-Jewish refugees, and on the history of the Robert Koch-Institute. He is currently on the advisory board of the German Society for Psychiatry project on psychiatrists in Nazi Germany, and is a member of the project on the history of the German Foundation for Memory, Responsibility and the Future. He is a Trustee of the Council for Assisting Refugee Academics (CARA).

Merle Wessel is Lecturer in Nordic history at the University of Greifswald, Germany. Her forthcoming thesis – *An Unholy Union? Eugenic Feminism in the Nordic Countries, ca. 1890–1940* – deals with the use of eugenic rhetoric by Nordic feminists in emancipation discourses. Her main research interests are gender and medical history in Northern Europe.

Acknowledgements

In November 2015, the Centre for Nordic Studies (CENS) at the University of Helsinki, Finland organised a conference entitled Conceptualising Public Health. It gathered scholars from various fields – including historians, sociologists and media researchers – who were interested in a critical assessment of public health concepts and discourses. The conference served as a mobilising thrust for a concrete endeavour to fill a research void in medical history, public health history, medical sociology and conceptual history.

Directed by Professor Peter Stadius, CENS is an important hub for conceptual history research, and we are really grateful for the crucial support it has given us. CENS has supported the production of this book by hosting conferences and workshops, and facilitated contacts between scholars across Northern Europe working in fields related to public health. Commenting on earlier drafts of the book's chapters, Johan Strang at CENS has also provided important stimuli for the work on this book. Most importantly, the perspective on public health adopted in the book draws on the tradition of conceptual history, which is fostered and developed at CENS in an excellent intellectual atmosphere.

Teemu Ryymin has read an earlier version of the entire manuscript and provided helpful comments and feedback. We would like to thank Teemu for devoting his time, in addition to contributing to the book as a co-author. We are grateful to Elianne Riska for reading and commenting on parts of the manuscript, and for valuable feedback and insights. We also wish to thank the anthology's contributors, Ida Ohlsson Al Fakir, Annika Berg and Norma Montesino, for their helpful comments on the introductory chapter.

The Swedish School of Social Science has supported the book by funding the efficient editorial assistance work of Irene Henriksson at the final stages of preparing the manuscript. We are also grateful to Café Espresso Edge for the nice atmosphere we have benefited from at our numerous editorial meetings over the years.

Most importantly, we wish to thank all the contributors to this volume. The project has led to the establishment of an inspiring network of scholars, and the anthology has been a collaborative effort.

Helsinki, 31 August 2017
Johannes Kananen, Sophy Bergenheim, Merle Wessel

1 Conceptualising public health

An introduction

Sophy Bergenheim, Johan Edman,
Johannes Kananen and Merle Wessel

Studying key concepts of public health: The aim of this book

This book has grown out of an insight that the concept of public health has been important in the historical development of modern societies. While connotations and associations have varied with time and place, the language around public health has expressed a concern for the health and well-being of the citizens of a nation state. It has served as a tool for constructing, developing and establishing practices, goals and discourses for health policy at a national and international level. It should therefore be given further academic attention.

Public health is conceptualised slightly differently in the English language and in other Germanic languages, such as German and Swedish. In English, the key concept is *public health*, accompanied by other interrelated concepts such as *national health* and *population health* (the latter often used in studies in public health, e.g., in the *Scandinavian Journal of Public Health*). The Nordic and German concepts share a similar etymological basis; namely, the word for public health translates literally to 'people's health' (Swedish: *folkhälsa*, Norwegian: *folkehelse*, Finnish: *kansanterveys*, Danish: *folkesundhed*, Icelandic: *lýðheilsa*, German: *Volksgesundheit*). The Nordic and German concepts thus have a markedly different connotation compared to the English counterparts: they contain a stronger association with a (culturally) unified people.

The title of our book is *Conceptualising Public Health: Historical and Contemporary Struggles over Key Concepts*. As the title reveals, we are not focusing on one single term, e.g., 'public health', but on key concepts in plural. The time period of this volume encompasses the late nineteenth and the twentieth century. During this period, the medical and social discourse has been dominated and contested by various crucial concepts, and we thus extend our analytical gaze to a broader group of concepts. In addition to public health, key concepts discussed in this book include, among others: hygiene, social hygiene and social medicine; racial hygiene and eugenics; and social disability and health management. We also discuss Nordic and English variations of public health concepts, which have not necessarily always been synonymous.

A clear-cut distinction between these concepts and their various uses is sometimes demanding, or outright futile. This fuzziness, however, is not regarded as inherently problematic in this book, but, rather, as an intriguing study subject. Our aim is not to provide rigid and simplified definitions for key concepts. We do not take concepts at face value, as something possessing an essential or timeless and ahistorical nature. Instead, we approach concepts and their discourses as contingent and historical phenomena; we analyse how the uses of different key concepts and the meanings attributed to them have varied with time, place and actor. Moreover, we study the interplay of concepts and discourses. An important focus of this volume is the overlapping boundary between the social realm and the medical or scientific sphere.

The concepts related to the development of medicine and health policy can serve as a lens for understanding the historical transformations of the welfare states in general, and for analysing the changing relationship between the state and the individual, in particular. More specifically, the book aims at identifying ruptures and redefinitions in the conceptualisations of medicine and health policy in the twentieth century in the Nordic countries and elsewhere in Europe.

The objective of this volume is to provide an analytical account of the historicity, contingency and political nature of key concepts related to health and health policy. We perceive and analyse concepts as normative tools and weapons of debate that shape the understanding of contemporary realities. In this mission, we dedicate special attention to the differentiation between historical or empirical concepts and analytical terms. By this, we mean the difference between the use of, for example, 'public health' by contemporary actors in its original context, and an analytical reading of the actors' understanding and use of the concepts. By being aware of and making this distinction, we seek to avoid taking concepts (be they analytical or empirical) for granted, and to thereby be wary of slipping into anachronic interpretations and labelling.

Historical development in the nineteenth and twentieth centuries

Disease prevention in the collective

George Rosen, author of the classic *A History of Public Health*,[1] argues that from the seventeenth century onwards, a mercantilist approach perceived the population as a resource, which helped to legitimise health on a collective level as an economic necessity.[2] It should be noted, however, that mercantilism was a markedly different political system centred on the (absolute) ruler. The economy or the health of the population did not, in other words, serve a larger collective or entity like the nation state, but the political elite. In contrast, in the postlude to the French Revolution, individual and population health was elevated to a universal human right. These two perspectives create an interesting tension that seems to reappear time and again in the conceptual history of public health.

Existing research on the history of public health has identified a medical, scientific and social reform movement in the nineteenth century which had the aim of eliminating the pathogenic conditions identified in poor housing, inadequate sanitation, dangerous workplaces and poverty.[3] Industrialisation has been identified as the driving force of the process that, on the one hand, contributed to urbanisation with a concentration of sources of infection and, on the other hand, required a large and healthy workforce.[4] Efforts to reach these aims included a focus on social structures, social activism and a determination to improve the living conditions of the population in general.

Whereas nineteenth-century public health focused on the environment as a source of illness, in the early twentieth century it was complemented by a pro-phylactic approach. It placed the focus on the individual, in order to prevent disease in the collective as well as in the individual. Political opposition (in the US) to the progressive ambitions of older public health, new insurance statistics with a focus on lifestyle factors and an actual reduction of contagious diseases in the industrialised urban communities around the turn of the century contributed to a shift in perspective.[5]

The first half of the twentieth century was also in other ways a turning point in Western public health discourse. Many Western former imperial states, particularly in Europe, embraced democracy, communism, authoritarianism or fascism. This was not only a big political change, but resulted in social transformations as well. As nations struggled for hegemony in a spirit of rising nationalism, they intensified their focus on the national and social body, i.e., the population. The First World War was a peak of this development, when a war dominated by technology and modern forces of destruction hit the Western world, and left not only the national body but also the physical body of the individual with deep wounds. Eric Hobsbawm calls this time the "Age of Catastrophe".[6] This stimulated an increasing interest in health, the individual and the health of the entire population, as well as the development of new medical knowledge about the human body.

Technological and scientific progress was manifested in new ways of detecting disease and new treatments. Albert Calmette and Camille Guérin first created a vaccine against widespread tuberculosis (TB) in 1906. From the 1920s onwards, medical scientists started developing vaccines further (the first successful vaccine, against smallpox, had been introduced in the late eighteenth century). The development of penicillin by Sir Alexander Fleming in 1928 and its first use in the Second World War on soldiers constituted a turning point in health care. After the Second World War, both treatments – vaccination and penicillin – became widely available to the public in the Western world.

In our effort to understand how conceptualisations of public health and medicine have changed through history, in this book, we have sought to identify characterising developments. Clear-cut periodisations are often anachronistic in that, firstly, they mask how change in ideas, concepts and practices is gradual and even slow – and not necessarily even recognised by contemporaries. Secondly, they overlook how concepts and notions are built on past concepts and notions; i.e., how new ideas and concepts carry their history with them. In this book, we study how public health, health policy and medicine have been conceptualised at different times, and how these conceptualisations have evolved. Furthermore, we see them as interrelated, each creating their own layer on which later actors build new concepts. Therefore, rather than seeking to identify or label breaking points or distinct periods, we look at transition periods during which ideas, concepts and practices gradually take on new forms.

Since we are, in a sense, chasing a moving target, we need to focus on selected aspects of public health in order to make sense of conceptual change. In the early twentieth century, conceptualisations and notions included the concept of hygiene in its various forms[7] and eugenics (or 'racial hygiene', as it was called in German and the Nordic languages), as well as a focus on the individual as part of the collective (population, people, race, etc.).

Eugenics was one of many ways to conceptualise public health in the early twentieth century. Eugenicists drew upon Darwinian ideas of natural selection and their applications, such as those of Darwin's cousin, Francis Galton. The idea was to shape and improve the quality of the population (or 'race'). Galton saw eugenics as a means to manipulate natural selection in humankind.[8] In his book *Memories of My Life* (1908), Galton described eugenics as follows:

> Its first object is to check the birth-rate of the Unfit, instead of allowing them to come into being, though doomed in large numbers to perish prematurely. The second object is the improvement of the race by furthering the productivity of the Fit by early marriages and healthful rearing of their children. Natural selection rests upon excessive production and wholesale destruction; Eugenics on bringing no more individuals into the world than can be properly cared for, and those only of the best stock.[9]

Galton spoke as if from a position above the rest of the society. From this perspective, Galton and his followers were able to divide people into "Fit" and "Unfit" groups. The "Fit" were those whose offspring were thought to be beneficial for the future of the "race".

Positive eugenics (i.e., encouraging the reproduction of individuals with desired qualities) and negative eugenics (restricting the reproduction of individuals with undesired qualities) became government policy throughout the Western world in the early twentieth century. In the late 1920s and early 1930s, many countries enacted marriage and sterilisation laws that included marriage impediments or allowed forced sterilisation on eugenic and social grounds such as epilepsy, schizophrenia, feeble-mindedness or deaf-muteness. The most well-known case is probably Germany, but the United States, France, Great Britain and the Nordic countries, for example, also had legislation with eugenic features. Social and health policies in most Western countries were influenced by eugenic ideas during the period before the Second World War.

Class and gender were important social categories in health-related discourses and practices. Women have been actors as well as recipients of health policies and socio-medical measures. Eugenics, health policy and pronatalist population policy intertwined, and many measures and policies were targeted at ('fit' or potentially 'fit') families, mothers and children in order to encourage procreation and reduce infant mortality and health risks related to pregnancy and childbirth. Furthermore, women played an important role as physicians and nurses, providing these health care measures that were partly developed by women in political and expert positions.

In addition, health regulations did not only target the ill or defective, but also the lower classes. Social and medical categories intersected in the notions of 'fit'. Typical problems of the poorer classes such as criminality, poor living conditions or immoral behaviour were medicalised. Problem definitions also implied choices of the kind of expert knowledge required for solving the problems. The Nordic countries largely followed these Western trends.

To reformulate the ideas of the early twentieth century, they can be characterised as focused on prevention, the collective and the long term (the cultivation of hereditary qualities). These notions also had their own rationale of inclusion and exclusion. Some individuals of the adult generations were seen as unfit and a source of degeneration of the population, and controlling them can be understood both in terms of inclusion and exclusion. Labelling them 'unfit' was, of course, excluding; but submitting to this control (e.g., sterilisation) was also framed as a channel for increased social acceptability and inclusion. Moreover, control over the procreation of 'unfit' individuals was seen as preventing the birth of new generations destined for poor hereditary and social disposition, and thereby exclusion.

Focus from prevention and the collective to the health of the individual

After the Second World War, the atrocities committed by Nazi Germany and the destruction brought by the war prompted efforts to begin social development anew and to break with the past. In 1948, two important international organisations were established: the World Health Organization (WHO) and the United Nations (UN). The creation of WHO added a global perspective to the prevailing public health discourse with a strong national focus. The vision of an open and liberal post-war world paved the way for a shift from contagionist, quarantine-based public health to sanitary disease control.[10] A new focus on chronic diseases and lifestyle diseases was central. As an example of this, historian Dorothy Porter has illustrated how the conceptual link between smoking and lung cancer in the 1950s resulted in awareness campaigns rather than a smoking ban.[11]

More generally, the UN Declaration of Human Rights (1948) asserted that "[a]ll human beings are born free and equal in dignity and rights. They are endowed with reason and conscience and should act towards one another in a spirit of brotherhood" (Article 1). The declaration sought to grant everyone equal rights and freedoms without distinction of any kind, such as race, colour, sex, language or religion (Article 2). It sought to grant everyone the right to life (Article 3) and the right to found a family and to marry (Article 16).[12]

The UN declaration may be interpreted as a reversal of Galton's ideas about improving the quality of the 'race' by encouraging reproduction of the 'fit'. However, while we have learned to take the Second World War as an almost obvious breaking point (denoted in common expressions like 'interwar' or 'post-war'), from the perspective of public health, it is difficult to say what kind of clear-cut breaking point the period after the Second World War actually constituted. Rather, as noted earlier, it would be more apt to talk about a transition period.

Granted, there were also deliberate efforts to break with the past, but the development was slow. In the course of the 1950s and 1960s, different hygiene concepts gradually disappeared from the vocabulary or began to refer primarily to a more specific, microbial level (e.g., oral hygiene, hand hygiene, etc.) rather than having strong social connotations (such as social hygiene or racial hygiene). Public health emerged as an academic discipline, replacing and encompassing the discipline of hygiene, sometimes also social medicine. Legislation and practices with eugenic features were gradually dismantled; by the 1970s, marriage and sterilisation laws had been reformed.

In line with this development, the old tension of population as a resource and health as a universal right acquired a new form. Whereas the early twentieth-century ideas can be characterised by a top-down and long-term approach as well as a focus on the collective and the prevention of disease, by the 1970s and 1980s, the focus had shifted to health (not just disease) and the current-generation individual. This post-war development has been labelled 'New Public Health' (NPH).[13]

In the 1970s, health was beginning to be perceived as an individual and social right of all to be promoted through primary health care. This idea was manifested in the 1978 Alma-Ata Declaration and WHO's Health for All programme.[14] Public services were founded on modern social and medical sciences that were divided into different subdisciplines. These new or developed fields also provided academic education for various professional groups working for and administering the welfare state.

This focus on the individual reflected the overall development in the Western countries. In the 1980s–1990s, the focus further intensified, and the previous collectivist order was renegotiated.[15] At the macro level, there was yet another shift of attention from society as a whole to the individual, this time emphasising not only individual responsibility but also liberty and autonomy. This approach was accompanied by a new economic rationale, which was derived from the Chicago School (neoclassical economics) and later complemented by business economics.[16] One of the most iconic expressions of this neoliberal logic is Margaret Thatcher's interview from 1987 in which she promptly announced that there exists no such thing as society. She questioned the justification of collectivism, according to which policies could be designed with the whole population or society in mind, and instead stressed individual responsibility and autonomy.[17]

Health policies or ideas did not take quite such an abrupt turn. However, a new concept or idea emphasising individualism was coined: health promotion. It was most notably manifested in the 1986 Ottawa Charter, which promoted increased opportunities for making healthy choices.[18]

In contrast to early twentieth-century ideas, this new perspective on health had a short-term focus in that it sought to affect the health of the current generation. Furthermore, rather than imposing an overt top-down approach, individuals themselves were given a central role in caring for their health. Following the thoughts of Alan Petersen and Deborah Lupton, as well as Nikolas Rose, in the spirit of neoliberalism, the so-called New Public Health emphasised individual freedom and choice. This emphasis, for its part, obscured the normative requirements of this type of self-governance and 'healthism', or the construction of a new kind of 'healthy citizen' as the ideal. These new ideals, for their part, contained a new form of intolerance towards individuals who do not fit these criteria.[19]

As we pointed out earlier, twentieth-century ideas should not be understood in dichotomous terms of inclusion or exclusion. The same applies to New Public Health. The (often left-leaning) promotion of health as well as primary health care was intended to reduce health inequality and further good health for all, thereby operating first and foremost on inclusive notions. Furthermore, an understanding of the individual as an autonomous actor was also an empowering counter-reaction to the previously mentioned expert-driven, top-down approach. However, the new focus on health and the individual has also brought along covertly exclusive and normative notions in its emphasis on individual responsibility and 'blindness' in regard to socio-economic and health-related abilities. Nevertheless, NPH is not to be understood merely as a neoliberal expansion of the medical and health care field, but (yet again) as a complex and nuanced phenomenon that cannot be unambiguously placed on a left–right axis.

In addition to the new operational environment created by the new economic rationale, which also opened up the provision of health care to private businesses, another layer of meaning that builds on old conceptualisations is discussed by scholars such as Adele Clark et al. In the period around 1985–1990, they identify a conceptual transformation driven by a shift of focus of the life sciences from the cellular level to the molecular level.[20] Thus, it is a transformation that has coincided with the renegotiation of the post-war collectivist order in the Nordic countries, individualisation of culture[21] and shifts of economic thinking (particularly the rise of neoclassical economic theory).

Considering these layers of meaning we detect around the 1970s and 1980s, we may think of the conceptualisations of (public) health, health policy and medicine as evolving at two levels: on the one hand, there is a scientific or technological dimension where the natural sciences and primarily biology and the medical sciences define the contents and boundaries of the concept of health. On the other hand, there is a political, social and administrative dimension whereby the scientific contents and forms of knowledge are translated into policy and practice. Neither dimension is fixed through time, and a multitude of developments affect the way each of these dimensions evolves.

The Nordic development

The Nordic welfare state model is known for its combination of social equality, a large public sector and economic efficiency. At the same time, the conceptualisations underlying Nordic welfare policy making reveal intriguing tensions. There was widespread rhetoric on universalism in the post-war period: every citizen should be included in society, and public services and social security should be available for all. However, eugenics continued to play a part in post-war conceptualisations of public health in the Nordic countries, raising the question of the limits of Nordic universalism.[22] Despite its name, universalism did not encompass all citizens, and it is interesting to examine the boundaries and distinctions made between groups of people in this respect.

Eugenics is an example of the tensions and conceptual ambiguity also in the Nordic welfare states. On the one hand, there was a spirit of managing the population from above by applying ideas developed by social engineers such as Gunnar and Alva Myrdal or K. K. Steincke. Also in the Nordic countries, the fear of population degeneration resulted in sterilisation laws that remained in force until the mid-1970s, albeit with moderating revisions (however, some post-war revisions, such as Finland's, were even stricter).[23] The sterilisation laws complemented earlier marriage laws (enacted in Sweden in 1915, followed by Norway in 1918, Denmark in 1922 and Finland in 1929) which, through the prevention of marriage, sought to regulate the procreation of individuals with hereditary defects. Similarly to the general Western development, health policy, family policy and population policy intertwined and included classist and gendered notions.

On the other hand, efforts to manage the quality of the population were combined with aims to include as many people as possible within the realm of active citizenship in the spirit of (social) democracy.[24] Previous research has pointed towards a collectivist tendency in Nordic welfare policy that increased equality on the one hand, but sought to define the roles of people from above, from the systemic level of society, on the other.[25] Collectivism was a legal principle that was reflected, for instance, in social security legislation.[26] Unemployed job seekers, for example, had an obligation to look for work in order to maintain eligibility to social security benefits.

In terms of health policy, the Nordic countries have followed Western trends. The first national health laws were implemented in the second half of the nineteenth century (Norway 1860, Sweden 1874, Finland 1879) with the aim of preventing epidemics and increasing housing and food hygiene.[27] The Nordic countries were not directly involved in the First World War – with the exception of Finland, which gained independence (1917) and underwent a civil war (1918) in connection with the Russian Revolution of 1917; but there was a shared sense of crisis with the rest of the Western world.

After the Second World War, the public health concept of 'people's health' (*folkhälsa*) started to gain hegemony in the Nordic countries. A key dimension in this shift of perspective was the changing relationship between the individual and society. As in the general development, in the 1950s–1970s there was, among key policy makers, still a strong focus on the collective level, and the individual was viewed as a part of the whole. Thus, connotations of pre-war conceptualisations, including the top-down approach associated with eugenics, remained in place. Gradually, the collectivist focus began to open up for more individualist notions, such as neoliberalism and New Public Health.

Neoclassical economic ideas began to influence also the Nordic countries around the 1990s, mainly through the authority of international organisations such as the European Union (EU) and the Organisation for Economic Co-operation and Development (OECD), and after the crisis of Social Democracy.[28] Organised business promoted new ideas of market efficiency and budgetary austerity.[29] Like elsewhere, these new ideas of the centrality of the market mechanism challenged previous collectivist ideas, such as 'people's health'. New ideas had yet again to be adapted to past traditions, which created room for conceptual innovations and local variations.

In this process of creating conceptual bridges from the old to the new, the interaction between medical science and politics has been central in the Nordic countries. Traditionally, Nordic policy making has relied strongly on experts and expert knowledge.[30]

Conceptual history

In our efforts to treat the meanings of concepts as contested rather than fixed, we are indebted to the academic tradition of conceptual history. As the name suggests, the study of conceptual history consists of concepts and their historical contexts. The field has traditionally been dominated by two distinct approaches: the German *Begriffsgeschichte*, after the work of Reinhart Koselleck; and the Anglo-American Cambridge School, associated with Quentin Skinner and J. G. A. Pocock. *Begriffsgeschichte* is focused on studying the use and development of individual, central concepts (*Grundbegriffe*, basic or key concepts). It is best known for the eight-volume lexicon of historical basic concepts, *Geschichtliche Grundbegriffe*, and the related methodological discussion. The Cambridge approach, on the other hand, is more focused on language, rhetoric and discourse rather than individual concepts. Skinner, for example, studies speech acts, linguistic conventions and rhetorical moves – i.e., language and concepts as political tools or games.

These two approaches have been perceived as separate or even incompatible. However, both Skinner and Koselleck share the fundamental understanding that concepts should be studied in their political and social context; as factors that shape the understanding of contemporary realities.[31] Koselleck notes that all concepts have two aspects: on the one hand, they point to something external, the context in which they are used; on the other, this context and reality are perceived through categories provided by language. Concepts are, therefore, both indicators of and factors in political and social life. Moreover, he sees history of concepts and history of discourse as inseparable. Analysing and understanding concepts – their content, meaning and importance – requires not only linguistic but also extra-linguistic context, which is provided, among others, by the analysis of discourse.[32] Skinner, for his part, seeks to understand how concepts can be used in argument – what, exactly, they are used for. He concludes that both he and Koselleck assume that normative concepts should not be treated as statements of the world, but as tools and weapons of debate.[33]

Both approaches, in other words, reject taking concepts and their meanings for granted, but see concepts and discourse as arenas and tools of political debate – as something that shapes as well as restricts the way reality is perceived. Following

Jussi Kurunmäki, *Begriffsgeschichte* and Cambridge approaches can thus be under-stood as complementary to each other rather than incommensurable. Furthermore, Kurunmäki describes conceptual history as a research strategy with which it is possible to reveal the historicity of concepts; to find political conflicts in processes that might otherwise seem uncontested and self-evident.[34]

Our contribution to existing literature

A conceptual history-orientated reading of the history of public health

The history of public health and health policy has been examined from different perspectives and in different academic fields – such as public health history, public health literature, medical history, medical sociology and health sociology. The lit-erature is extensive and, due to lack of space, we are unable to present all praise-worthy and relevant literature. In this section, we have instead selected works that have acted as inspiration and/or provide illustrating examples of how this book contributes to the existing discussion.

Many publications have sought to provide accounts of the history of public health with various perspectives and approaches. Susan Gross Solomon et al. have rejected the idea of public health as an issue first and foremost of the nation state, and instead focus on the tensions and interfaces between transnational, national and local issues and agencies, primarily in the 1920s–1940s.[35] Theodore H. Tulchinsky and Elena Varavikova deliver an extensive account of the development of medicine and the provision and organisation of health care in the twentieth and twenty-first centuries.[36] In a similar vein, in *Health, Civilization and the State*, Dorothy Porter has outlined a broad history of the provision and organisation of health services from ancient times to the twenty-first century.[37] In *The History of Public Health and the Modern State*, edited by Porter, a number of scholars offer an overall view of the history of public health on a geographically broad scale.[38]

With the exception of Tulchinsky and Varavikova and Karin Johannisson's article on Sweden in *The History of Public Health and the Modern State*,[39] the above-mentioned do not deal with the Nordic countries, despite discussing public health in the welfare states. The Nordic development has primarily been discussed in the context of individual countries, with some works providing com-parative perspectives. They deal with public health history from a social scientific or historical scientific perspective, noting the impact of socio-economic, institu-tional, political and geographic factors.[40] Other themes touched upon include the connection between nation-building and citizenship,[41] as well as the interface between the medical and scientific as well as social life.[42]

Michel Foucault's poststructuralist approach and his concepts of (bio)power and governmentality have inspired several studies within medical history and medical sociology, such as the well-known works of David Armstrong[43] and Nikolas Rose.[44] Scholars explicitly dealing with public health with a Foucauldian approach include Alan Petersen and Deborah Lupton, as well as Signild Vallgårda, who have studied NPH and Danish and Swedish public health policy, respectively, as political apparatuses whose language, discourse and strategies obscure power relations, the construction of new kinds of ideal citizens and (self-)governmentality imposed on individuals.[45]

Moreover, while the works presented above excel in their analysis and scope in many respects, their relationship with the concept of public health is problematic from the perspective adopted in this book (with some exceptions, however, such as Roger Qvarsell,[46] Johannisson and Vallgårda, as well as Petersen and Lupton). The concept is adopted as an analytical term without acknowledging, analysing or problematising its historicity; alternatively, the historical concept is taken at face value, without giving attention to the underlying and coexisting uses and meanings or other relevant historical concepts.

As an example, when Solomon et al. write about the 'shifting boundaries of public health', they recognise that public health may have different goals at different times; but they do not reflect the extent to which the very concept of 'public health' might be conceptualised differently at different times and in different languages. This creates an impression of 'public health' as being a fixed, unmovable entity, which it arguably is not.

Lene Koch, who has previously studied compulsory sterilisations in Denmark,[47] has taken a critical distance to such approaches. Instead, she has studied twentieth-century 'eugenics' from an explicitly conceptual history perspective, by applying a Koselleckian analysis. She reveals a transformation from a concept loaded with expectations for the scientific, technological and social development of the future, to 'eugenics' associated with dangerous threat and notions of compulsion, ethnic cleansing and crime.[48]

In the 2000s, not many studies have analysed public health concepts from an explicitly (or even implicitly) conceptual history perspective. The works of, e.g., Qvarsell and Johannisson date to the 1990s, whereas Vallgårda, despite her Foucauldian approach, explicitly delimits her study to a "pragmatic" approach – while, however, acknowledging how *folkhälsa/folkesundhed* could benefit from a conceptual historical analysis.[49] Of more recent works addressing this particular research void could be mentioned that of two contributors to this volume, Annika Berg and Minna Harjula. Berg has studied public health (*folkhälsa*) as an ideology in the Swedish welfare state development. In her dissertation, she contests the notion of public health as a uniform, coherent project; furthermore, she critically examines *folkhälsa* as well as *folk* as elastic, transformative concepts, as well as tracing the transnational dimensions and implications of *folkhälsa*.[50] In her comprehensive study of Finnish health policy in the twentieth century, Harjula includes an analysis of conceptual development. She traces the intertwined and overlapping developments of key concepts such as racial hygiene (*rotuhygienia*), public health (*kansanterveys*) and population policy (*väestöpolitiikka*), critically examining their uses and meanings.[51]

With this volume, we wish to continue on the road paved by these studies on public health and other key concepts in health policy and medicine.[52] In our conceptual historical endeavour, we dedicate our attention to the historicity, political nature, contingency and flexibility of a broad plethora of concepts and discourses in the history of health policy and medicine. We strive to analyse how language both constructs and delimits how the world and how contemporary realities are perceived and understood. In a Foucauldian streak, we also acknowledge how language, knowledge and power are intertwined with policies and governmentality, as well as factors such as gender and class. In addition, our book is focused on Northern Europe and provides comparative perspectives on the Nordic countries, which have been somewhat disregarded in the international discussion.

As mentioned earlier, in our endeavour, we emphasise the differentiation between analytical terms and empirical/historical concepts. This distinction is by no means always easy, and many interpretations could certainly be provided on a number of occasions. Nevertheless, to clarify our analytical thought processes and approaches to our readers, we have, as far as possible, tried to differentiate between historical/empirical concepts and analytical concepts by different use of language. When the chapters discuss historical and empirical concepts, the authors use concepts as the contemporary actors have used them in the original language, e.g. *folkhälsa* or *socialmedicin*; or, if the actors have conceptualised their terminology and discourse in English, the concepts are in English and italicised, e.g., *public health*. Whenever the authors themselves elaborate on their own analytical reading of historical concepts, they use English terms without italicisation, e.g., public health, social hygiene.

Below are a couple of illustrating examples from Chapter 8 of our book, by Norma Montesino and Ida Ohlsson Al Fakir:

> [S]ocialt handikapp [social disability] was related to diverse criteria such as age (children and the elderly poor), family situation (families with several children, single mothers), education (illiteracy), cultural belonging (minorities or non-European poor), etc.

> Social workers . . . defined their [Roma families'] alleged social disability in terms of dependence on welfare.

The examples illustrate how the authors place the Swedish term for 'social disability' and its use and meaning in its original historical context. They also provide their reading of how the concept was operated and understood by contemporary actors (the social workers).

The chapters

Chapter 2 by Paul Weindling deepens this introduction's discussion around the connection between racial hygiene/eugenics and public health. It compares German and British nineteenth-century notions of eugenics and hygiene, as well as providing a comprehensive overview of the history and development of eugenics as a science in early twentieth-century to post-war Britain, Germany and Europe. According to Weindling, eugenic ideals were embedded in twentieth-century public health concepts, structures and interventions.

In Chapter 3, Merle Wessel continues on the topic of eugenics, public health and medical expertise. Her focus is on the first female physicians in Sweden and Finland in the late nineteenth and early twentieth century. They were very engaged in providing prophylactic health care and disseminating health knowledge for women. Wessel analyses the feminist, class-related and eugenic notions in the female doctors' endeavours.

Chapter 4 by Ainur Elmgren shows that the narrative of the benefits of negative eugenic measures was not received unanimously unquestioned. By studying leftist cultural intellectuals in 1930s Finland and their campaign against the 1935 Sterilisation Act, she highlights how medical experts were not the sole participants in health policy discourses. Furthermore, even though the law was enforced, Elmgren shows how a pronounced discussion around civic and human rights was initiated already in the interwar era.

In Chapter 5, Minna Harjula traces the twentieth-century development of Finnish health-related key concepts. She argues that in national health policy, *kansanterveys* (public health) replaced *rotuhygienia* (racial hygiene) in post-war Finland. Furthermore, she explores the shifting inclusive and exclusive dimensions in health policy, and how they are reflected in notions and uses of key concepts.

In Chapter 6, Annika Berg and Teemu Ryymin highlight the similarities and differences in how two highly influential twentieth-century medical actors in Norway and Sweden, Karl Evang and Axel Höjer, understood the concepts *folkehelse* and *folkhälsa*, respectively. They also explore the transnational and global dimensions of Evang's and Höjer's works and conceptions, as well as comparing the Nordic concepts with 'public health'. The chapter illuminates how key concepts should always be analysed in their specific contexts, as their meanings may vary even in the vocabulary of one actor.

In Chapter 7, Sophy Bergenheim broadens the focus from governmental actors and medical experts to non-governmental organisations (NGOs). She examines the conceptions of 'people' and 'people's health' of two Finnish social and health policy organisations in the 1940s and 1950s, and compares them against notions of 'race' and 'racial hygiene' in the 1920s and 1930s. She concludes that the above-mentioned concepts were 'sister concepts', intertwined and coexisting still in the 1940s and 1950s.

Chapter 8 by Norma Montesino and Ida Ohlsson Al Fakir examines the transfer of public health concepts and categories into the realm of social policy. They analyse how social workers and medical experts have used *socialt handikapp* (social disability) in managing European refugees and a group of Roma people in post-war Sweden. Despite new policies and practices being legitimised by a rhetoric of social inclusion, they have, in contrast, contributed to marginalising structures.

In Chapter 9, Johan Edman studies how alcohol policy has been framed as a public health problem in international alcohol conferences. A long time frame, 1885–1992, reveals how the framing of alcohol as a problem has largely reflected racial hygienic and public health trends, with strong influences from NPH at the end of the research period.

Chapter 10 by Matilda Hellman continues on the theme of substance abuse. She focuses on international organisations and epistemic communities in the post-war era, and studies concepts, worldviews and epistemologies as gathering and main-streaming forces in global and international alcohol, drug and tobacco policies. In this, she identifies the idea and rubric of *dependency* as crucial for seeing and constructing a common aetiology.

In Chapter 11, Johannes Kananen focuses on an internationally renowned public health initiative – the North Karelia Project that took place in Finland in 1972–1997. Kananen argues that the project not only functioned within the frame of *kansanterveys*, but also contributed to new national and international conceptions of public health, partially through depoliticising and authoritative expert definitions of public health goals and measures.

In Chapter 12, Helena Tolvhed and Outi Hakola approach the topic of health from a media research approach. They study new, individualistic and commercial-ised representations of health in Swedish health and fitness magazines (1960–2010) and Finnish health journalism (2010–2016). Tolvhed and Hakola note the emergence of new norms in health and health management, which involve normative representations of femininity, class and ability, much in a neoliberal spirit of NPH.

In Chapter 13, the editors conclude the book with a brief summary of its core contributions, as well as implications for future research and discussion.

Notes

1 George Rosen, *A History of Public Health* (Baltimore: Johns Hopkins University Press, [1958] 2015).
2 Ibid.; George Rosen, *From Medical Police to Social Medicine: Essays on the History of Health Care* (New York: Science History Publications, 1974).
3 Peter Baldwin, *Contagion and the State in Europe, 1830–1930* (Cambridge: Cambridge University Press, 1999); Amy Fairchild et al., 'The exodus of public health: What history can tell us about the future', *American Journal of Public Health* 100, no. 1 (2010): 54–63.
4 Dorothy Porter, 'The social contract of health in the twentieth and twenty-first centuries: Individuals, corporations, and the state', in *Shifting Boundaries of Public Health: Europe in the Twentieth Century*, ed. Susan Gross Solomon et al. (Woodbridge: Boydell & Brewer, 2008), 45–60.
5 James A. Gillespie, 'Europe, America, and the space of international health', in *Shifting Boundaries of Public Health: Europe in the Twentieth Century*, ed. Susan Gross Solomon et al. (Woodbridge: Boydell & Brewer, 2008), 114–37.
6 Eric Hobsbawm, *The Age of Extremes: A History of the World, 1914–1991* (New York: Random House, 1996).
7 Eva Palmblad, *Medicinen som samhällslära* (Göteborg: Daidalos, 1990).
8 Philippa Levine and Alison Bashford, 'Introduction: Eugenics and the modern world', in *The Oxford Handbook of the History of Eugenics*, ed. Philippa Levine and Alison Bashford (Oxford: Oxford University Press, 2010), 3–24.
9 Francis Galton, *Memories of My Life* (London: Methuen, 1908), 232; Levine and Bashford, 'Introduction: Eugenics'.
10 Gillespie, 'Space of international health'.
11 Porter, 'Social contract of health'.

12 UN General Assembly, *Universal Declaration of Human Rights*, 10 December 1948, 217 A (III), www.refworld.org/docid/3ae6b3712c.html (accessed 6 June 2017).
13 E.g., Niyi Awofeso, 'What's new about the "New Public Health"?', *American Journal of Public Health* 94, no. 5 (2004): 705–9; Alan Petersen and Deborah Lupton, *The New Public Health: Health and Self in the Age of Risk* (London: Sage, 1996); Theodore H. Tulchinsky and Elena Varavikova, *The New Public Health: An Introduction for the 21st Century* (San Diego: Academic Press, 2000).
14 Awofeso, 'What's new?'
15 Johannes Kananen, *The Nordic Welfare State in Three Eras: From Emancipation to Discipline* (London: Routledge, 2014).
16 See, e.g., Anu Kantola and Hannele Seeck, 'Dissemination of management into politics: Michael Porter and the political uses of management consulting', *Management Learning* 42, no. 1 (2011): 25–47.
17 Margaret Thatcher, quoted in Douglas Keay, 'Aids, education and the year 2000', *Woman's Own*, 31 October 1987, 8–10.
18 Awofeso, 'What's new?'
19 Petersen and Lupton, *New Public Health*; Nikolas Rose, *Powers of Freedom: Reframing Political Thought* (Cambridge: Cambridge University Press, 1999).
20 Adele E. Clark et al., eds, *Biomedicalization: Technoscience, Health and Illness in the US* (Durham, NC and London: Duke University Press, 2010).
21 Ulrich Beck and E. Beck-Gernsheim, *Individualization. Institutionalized individualism and its Social and Political Consequences* (London: Sage, 2002); Anthony Giddens, *Modernity and Self-Identity: Self and Society in the Late Modern Age* (Stanford: Stanford University Press, 1991).
22 See also Pauli Kettunen and Klaus Petersen, eds, *Beyond Welfare State Models. Transnational Historical Perspectives on Social Policy* (Cheltenham: Edward Elgar, 2011); Nanna Kildal and Stein Kuhnle, eds, *Normative Foundations of the Welfare State. The Nordic Experience* (London: Routledge, 2005).
23 On sterilisation policies in the Nordic countries, see, e.g., Gunnar Broberg and Nils Roll-Hansen, eds, *Eugenics and the Welfare State: Sterilization Policy in Denmark, Sweden, Norway, and Finland* (East Lansing: Michigan State University Press, 2005); Gunnar Broberg and Mattias Tydén, *Oönskade i folkhemmet: Rashygien och sterilisering i Sverige* (Stockholm: Dialogos, 2005); Mattias Tydén, *Från politik till praktik: De svenska steriliseringslagarna 1935–1975* (Stockholm: Acta Universitatis Stockholmiensis, 2002); Lene Koch, *Tvangssterilisation i Danmark 1929–67* (Copenhagen: Gyldendal, 2000); Marjatta Hietala, 'From race hygiene to sterilization: The eugenics movement in Finland', in *Eugenics and the Welfare State: Sterilization Policy in Denmark, Sweden, Norway, and Finland*, ed. Gunnar Broberg and Nils Roll-Hansen (East Lansing: Michigan State University Press, 2005), 195–258; Maria Björkman, *Den anfrätta stammen: Nils von Hoftsen, eugeniken och steriliseringarna 1909–1963* (Stockholm: Arkiv Förlag, 2011).
24 See also Jussi Kurunmäki and Johan Strang, eds, *Rhetorics of Nordic Democracy* (Helsinki: Finnish Literature Society, 2010).
25 Kananen, *Nordic Welfare State*.
26 Patrick Glenn, *Legal Traditions of the World* (Oxford: Oxford University Press, 2007); Richard Sennett, *The Culture of the New Capitalism* (Cambridge: Polity Press, 2006).
27 Palmblad, *Medicinen som samhällslära*, 11; Marjatta Hietala, *Services and Urbanization at the Turn of the Century: The Diffusion of Innovations* (Helsinki: Suomen Historiallinen Seura, 1987).
28 Sami Outinen, *Sosiaalidemokraattien tie talouden ohjailusta markkinareaktioiden ennakointiin: Työllisyys sosiaalidemokraattien politiikassa Suomessa 1975–1998* (Helsinki: Into, 2015); cf. Jenny Andersson, *The Library and the Workshop: Social Democracy and Capitalism in the Knowledge Age* (Stanford: Stanford University Press, 2010).

29 Mark Blyth, *Great Transformations: Economic Ideas and Institutional Change in the Twentieth Century* (Cambridge: Cambridge University Press, 2002).
30 See also Johanna Rainio-Niemi, *Small State Cultures of Consensus. State Traditions and Consensus-Seeking in the Neo-Corporatist and Neutrality Policies in Post-1945 Austria and Finland* (Helsinki: University of Helsinki, 2008); Åsa Lundqvist and Klaus Petersen, eds, *In Experts We Trust: Knowledge, Politics and Bureaucracy in Nordic Welfare States* (Odense: University Press of Southern Denmark, 2010).
31 Quentin Skinner, 'Rhetoric and conceptual change', *Finnish Yearbook of Political Thought* 3, no. 1 (1999): 60–73; Reinhart Koselleck, 'A response to comments on the *Geschichtliche Grundbegriffe*', in *The Meanings of Historical Concepts. New Studies on Begriffsgeschichte*, ed. Hartmut Lehmann and Melvin Richter (Washington, DC: German Historical Institute, 1996), 59–70.
32 Koselleck, 'A response', 61–5.
33 Skinner, 'Rhetoric and conceptual change', 62.
34 Jussi Kurunmäki, 'Käsitehistoria: Näkökulma historian poliittisuuteen ja poliittisen kielen historiallisuuteen', *Politiikka* 43, no. 2 (2001): 142–55.
35 Solomon et al., *Shifting Boundaries of Public Health*.
36 Tulchinsky and Varavikova, *New Public Health*.
37 Dorothy Porter, *Health, Civilization and the State: A History of Public Health from Ancient to Modern Times* (London: Routledge, 1999).
38 Dorothy Porter, ed., *The History of Public Health and the Modern State* (Amsterdam: Rodopi, 1994).
39 Karin Johannisson, 'The people's health: Public health policies in Sweden', in *The History of Public Health and the Modern State*, ed. Dorothy Porter (Amsterdam: Rodopi, 1994), 165–82.
40 Gösta Carlsson and Ola Arvidsson, eds, *Kampen för folkhälsan: Prevention i historia och nutid* (Stockholm: Natur och Kultur, 1994); Ilpo Helén and Mikko Jauho, eds, *Kansalaisuus ja kansanterveys* (Helsinki: Gaudeamus, 2003); Helene Laurent, 'War and the emerging social state: Social policy, public health and citizenship in wartime Finland', in *Finland in World War II: History, Memory, Interpretations*, ed. Tiina Kinnunen and Ville Kivimäki (Leiden: Brill, 2012), 315–54.
41 E.g., Karin Johannisson, 'Folkhälsa: Det svenska projektet från 1900 till 2: a världskriget', in *Lychnos: Årsbok för idé- och lärdomshistoria*, by Lärdomshistoriska samfundet (Uppsala: Lärdomshistoriska samfundet, 1991), 139–95; Johannisson, 'People's health'; Helén and Jauho, *Kansalaisuus ja kansanterveys*; Signild Vallgårda, *Folkesundhed som politik: Danmark og Sverige fra 1930 til i dag* (Aarhus: Aarhus Universitetsforlag, 2004).
42 E.g., Johannisson, 'Folkhälsa'; Vallgårda, *Folkesundhed som politik*.
43 David Armstrong, *Political Anatomy of the Body: Medical Knowledge in Britain in the Twentieth Century* (Cambridge: Cambridge University Press, 1983).
44 E.g., Rose, *Powers of Freedom*; Nikolas Rose, *Politics of Life Itself: Biomedicine, Power and Subjectivity in the Twenty-first Century* (Princeton: Princeton University Press, 2007).
45 Petersen and Lupton, *New Public Health*; Vallgårda, *Folkesundhed som politik*; Signild Vallgårda, 'Det goda livet och det goda samhället: Styrning i folkhälsopolitiken eller hur välfärdsstaten söker forma människor', in *Frihed, lighed og tryghed: Velfaerdspolitik i Norden*, ed. Hilda Rømer Christensen et al. (Århus: Jysk Selskab for Historie, 2001), 90–107.
46 Roger Qvarsell, '"Ett sunt folk i ett sunt samhälle": Hälsoupplysning, hälsovård och hälsopolitik i ett idéhistoriskt perspektiv', in *Kampen för folkhälsan: Prevention i historia och nutid*, ed. Gösta Carlsson and Ola Arvidsson (Stockholm: Natur och Kultur, 1994), 76–108.
47 Koch, *Tvangssterilisation i Danmark 1929–67*.

48 Lene Koch, 'Past futures: On the conceptual history of eugenics: A social technology of the past', *Technology Analysis & Strategic Management* 18, no. 3 (2006): 329–44.

49 Vallgårda, *Folkesundhed som politik*, 21.

50 Annika Berg, *Den gränslösa hälsan: Signe och Axel Höjer, folkhälsan och expertisen* (Uppsala: Acta Universitatis Upsaliensis, 2009).

51 Minna Harjula, *Terveyden jäljillä: Suomalainen terveyspolitiikka 1900-luvulla* (Tampere: Tampere University Press, 2007).

52 Among other important themes to which this anthology's authors have contributed, and this volume seeks to contribute for its part, health citizenship should be mentioned. See, e.g., Minna Harjula, *Hoitoonpääsyn hierarkiat: Terveyskansalaisuus ja terveyspalvelut 1900-luvulla* (Tampere: Tampere University Press, 2015); Ida Ohlsson Al Fakir, *Nya rum för socialt medborgarskap: Om vetenskap och politik i "Zigenarundersökningen" – en socialmedicinsk studie av svenska romer 1962–1965* (Växjö: Linnaeus University Press, 2015); Teemu Ryymin, '"Health citizenship": A short introduction', in *Citizens, Courtrooms, Crossings*, ed. Astri Andresen et al. (Bergen: Stein Rokkan Centre for Social Studies, 2008), 7–13.

2 Conceptualising eugenics and racial hygiene as public health theory and practice

Paul Weindling

Linking race to hygiene

Eugenics arose at a crucial historical juncture in terms of demography (with the declining birth rate) and morbidity (with the shift to the greater prevalence of chronic diseases) in the early twentieth century. These epidemiological transitions, in turn, shaped public health measures and associated rationales. This chapter will examine eugenic concepts of population health, and how these entered public health in terms of concepts and practices, especially as deriving from the founders of eugenics – notably Francis Galton in Britain and Wilhelm Schallmayer and Alfred Ploetz in Germany. Their theoretical writings provided fundamental concepts of how population health could be sustained in an emergent welfare state. Eugenic ideas of eradicating physical and mental disabilities, and overall improvement of reproductive and population health, became norms embedded in public health concepts, structures and interventions, persisting until at least a new critical awareness from the mid-1960s which was less directive and more oriented to the person and his or her rights.

Historical interest in a critical history of eugenics and the associated ideology of Social Darwinism dates from the mid-1960s' era of civil rights protests in the USA. A new critical epistemology marked the ending of a positivistic and progressivist approach to the history of eugenics. The view of eugenics as a progressive science was typified by C.P. Blacker, the British eugenicist and psychiatrist. Blacker saw expert-driven eugenics as enlightened and necessary, although he was careful to separate eugenics from National Socialism in his chronicle *Eugenics: Galton and After*.[1] The alternative critical position was at first to critique eugenics and Social Darwinism as movements primarily concerning the racist ultra-right in a progression from Darwin to Hitler. Although such highly questionable interpretations survive, a range of challenging methodologies and historiographies uncovered far wider issues in eugenics, concerning coercive institutions and racially and genetically legitimated interventions in fertility. The insights of Michel Foucault and others on authoritarian strategies of experts, as well as the ground-breaking ideas of Donald MacKenzie on social constructions of statistical science as expressing conflicting professional interests, influenced historical reconstructions of German eugenics during the 1980s. They led to a critical assessment of eugenics as an expression of middle-class power strategies in a modernising state and society.[2] The history of eugenics, race and hygiene came to be recognised as having coercive implications, especially for public health issues as related to reproduction, heredity, ethnicity and gender.

The German concept of *Rassenhygiene* (in English *racial hygiene*; in Swedish *rashygien*) was a composite linking the idea of race with the German concept of *Hygiene* as the new science of disease control and cure. *Rassenhygiene* covered various approaches to public health and population during the upheavals of industrialisation and urbanisation of the later nineteenth century. The term *Rassenhygiene* made its first appearance in 1895 after the spectacular successes of the microbiologists Robert Koch and Louis Pasteur. *Rassenhygiene* as a hybrid concept implied that hereditary particles could be somehow cleansed from the inherited genetic material – just as the germs of infectious diseases such as cholera, diphtheria and tuberculosis (TB) could be identified and eradicated. The physician, biologist and utopian enthusiast Alfred Ploetz outlined how hereditary health problems could be 'humanely' solved by chromosomal engineering.[3] The vision was futuristic in that Ploetz had only a very limited evidence-basis for a hereditary component to disabilities and disease. How the pathogens in the germplasm could be 'humanely' eliminated was a matter of speculation.

Ploetz saw Scandinavia as the motherland of the *Germanen*: he admired the Nordic type to which he ascribed racial superiority in terms of psychology, physique and fitness. In any event, the term *Rassenhygiene* was projected to appeal to professionals and scientists inclined to social reform. A wider public was prepared to place its faith in scientifically based solutions to social problems of poverty, crime, insanity and disease.[4]

Since the successes of Max von Pettenkofer from the 1860s and Robert Koch in the later nineteenth century, *Hygiene* achieved immense success in Germany as a new academic discipline.[5] A contrast emerged with Anglo-American concepts of *hygiene*, which meant general cleansing and improved sanitation. Thus, the German sense of *Hygiene* had a laboratory basis, in contrast to the more public-oriented Anglo-American sense of the term as a general cleansing. This difference can be found in contrasting German and Anglo-American approaches to eugenics. Ploetz launched the periodical *Archiv für Rassen- und Gesellschaftsbiologie* (Archive for Racial and Societal Biology) in 1904 to cover inheritance of diseases and physical traits, as well as the declining birth rate among elite population groups. In 1905, Ploetz founded the *Gesellschaft für Rassenhygiene* (Racial Hygiene Society) in Berlin (the name was universal rather than specifically German). He regarded the Society as a breeding group, and encouraged not only professionals to join, but also their wives and children, and students – effectively as an elite breeding group – in the hope that those in the group would procreate mentally and physically superior offspring. The German Racial Hygiene Society had a larger number of biologists and medical specialists than its equivalent in Britain and its Empire – the Eugenic Education Society, launched in 1907.[6]

Ploetz was concerned about health conditions in Germany, and of the 'white races' more generally. He conceptualised how *Rassenhygiene* would become a new medical specialisation at a crucial juncture of demographic change with the declining birth rate and increasing life expectancy. Eugenicists recognised a 'modern' morbidity pattern with the shift to chronic diseases. Whereas Ploetz was a visionary, his scientific ally, Ernst Rüdin, applied genetics in researching the supposed hereditary component of 'schizophrenia', understood in a narrowly biologistic sense.[7] Rüdin took matters forward in terms of implementation by advising on German sterilisation legislation in 1933, which designated 'schizophrenics' as a target group. The proportions of 'schizophrenics' who were sterilised varied at each tribunal – for example nearly 30 per cent in Bremen and 7 per cent in Halle.[8]

The responses to fundamental shifts in mortality, morbidity and the changing population structure, in turn, shaped public health measures in the early twentieth century in looking to biology for technical 'solutions' to intractable problems of poverty and physical and mental illness. The approach was preventive, and required a directive from the scientific elite dictating biomedical regulations. Indicative of the collectivist implications of eugenics, there emerged social- ised models of annual health examinations linked to health passports, indicating that only the eugenically healthy could have full civic freedoms. The Bavarian psychiatrist Wilhelm Schallmayer pronounced that the physician had a primary responsibility to society, rather than to the sick individual.[9] Around 1890, Schallmayer outlined a collectivised system of public health in which eugenically trained physicians served the state as a biomedical entity, rather than caring for the individual sick person: indeed, keeping carriers of pathogenic genes alive could damage future generations. Schallmayer developed a scheme of corporate national racial service, and the purification of hereditary elements in the population by means of health passports. These had to be kept up to date with an annual medical inspection. This collectivist model opened the way to stigmatise a range of medical conditions, behaviours and identities as pathological threats to the body politic, or *Volkskörper*. This strategy represented a fundamental shift in terms of the social- isation of health within the emerging welfare state – welfare itself became, over time, regarded as a combined state and professional responsibility, rather than a private duty. The approach could be seen as the assertion of power by scientifically oriented professions armed with new diagnostic and preventive techniques within a variety of political frameworks.

German–British distinctions

The question arises whether a distinction can be drawn between the German models of Ploetz and Schallmayer and the British model of Francis Galton, who indeed coined the term *eugenics* in 1883. Galton, a statistician, was concerned with heredity and reproduction within a wider context of demography and epidemiology, as well as the psychology of behaviour and intelligence as determined by inheritance. Galton's starting point was a critique of his cousin Charles Darwin's ideas of natural and sexual selection. Galton objected to Darwin's speculative theory of circulating 'pangenes' transmitting environmentally acquired traits from one generation to another. Instead, Galton substituted a statistical scheme of gemmules transmitting hereditary traits. He argued that these would account for traits distributed according to a Gaussian or Bell curve. As there was reversion towards the mean (i.e., the average) from the low or high ends of the population distribution, each person in every generation required expert assessment to determine schooling and occupation. Galton's 'biometrical' approach correlated mental and physical traits. He stressed the need to limit the reproduction of less desirable physical and mental qualities, which he saw as proliferating with industrialisation. The distribution of biological traits went with concepts of population health. Galton (and, similarly, Darwin) was interested in *race* in the sense of a population with distinctive ethnic characteristics: Darwin was, in any case, inconsistent in the meanings he ascribed to the term *race*. Galton had geographical and anthropological interests, and drew a distinction between those he viewed as more 'primitive' races, such as the 'Negro', and more evolved, such as Chinese and Jews.[10]

In social terms, Galton offered a critique of liberal notions of individual self-improvement by positing a deterministic model of a 'natural' social order with inherited traits distributed on a Gaussian or Bell curve. The combining and distribution of traits varied over generations: what was necessary was to assess talent in each generation. Those more talented would be selected for elite education and take expert roles in directing society. Galton's utopia, *Kantsaywhere*, advocated a social model which was 'modern' with regard to the power accorded to scientifically expert social elites.[11] The new model of social order challenged aristocratic privilege and mass democracy as degenerative: Galton limited the proliferation of a social underclass whose 'excess' reproduction distorted the presumed natural balance of society. Implicit in this expert-administered model was a regulatory state with directive roles taken by selected technocrats.

A further fundamental difference between Britain and Germany was the organisation and financing of health care. Germany – with the introduction of sickness insurance in 1883 – initiated a durable model of medical provision. This strengthened the medical profession overall, while the sickness insurance funds were autonomous corporations, independent of the state. Sickness insurance was not eugenic in itself: it drew financial resources into medicine. Germany extended benefits to family dependants and maternity provision, and to treat sexually transmitted diseases: all this was 'ahead' of Britain. Eugenicists demanded that resources be focused on those deemed 'fit', and that those deemed 'unfit' should be excluded from resources. A paradox was that in order to exclude the presumed defective from procreation, social segregation incurred costs. The Mental Deficiency Act of 1913 established a system of life-long detention, affecting some 65,000 persons until its repeal in 1959. The trend in Britain was ultimately towards a unitary state-financed and state-regulated health service, although this was finally achieved only with the new National Health Service (NHS) in 1948. Medical institutions such as sanatoria and psychiatric hospitals proliferated throughout Europe and North America. Eugenicists were divided in their opinions regarding the benefits of custodial institutions that prevented those deemed unfit from reproducing; but, at the same time, eugenicists condemned the costs of these institutions as imposing burdens on the fit. One set of eugenicists advocated custodial detention for the feeble-minded, whereas others from around 1900 lobbied for sterilisation. Here a contrast emerged among British eugenicists who advocated 'colonies' for mental defectives, as opposed to German and US advocates of sterilisation, which rendered institutional containment superfluous.[12]

The Galtonian model required scientifically trained oversight, not just in medicine but also in psychology, statistics and the sciences. Ploetz, by comparison, had a more biological approach. Comparing the Eugenic Education Society (EES) to the Racial Hygiene Society, we find both include doctors; but the German society had more notable biologists (not least the leading Darwinists, Ernst Haeckel and August Weismann), and overall a higher proportion of medical professionals. Ploetz targeted academic recruits to validate his new science. By way of contrast, the EES was unable to recruit Karl Pearson, whose statistical approach continued Galton's legacy at the Francis Galton Eugenics Laboratory at University College London (UCL). Pearson certainly cultivated links to medical officers, as in *Eugenics and Public Health*, which originally was a lecture addressed to public health officers, delivered at the York congress of the Royal Sanitary Institute in 1912.[13] For their part, British medical officers were responsive to eugenics in 1912 in the build-up to the International Congress of Eugenics, which was held in London.[14] The initiative for a public association passed to the lay enthusiast and founder of the Eugenics Education Society, Mrs Sybil Gotto (later Neville-Rolfe), whose approach was more moralistic on reproductive morals than that of the often more pragmatic public health professionals. She was a formidable figure on international committees concerned with sexually transmitted diseases, but she was slow to eventually accept the medical benefits of contraception.[15] While there were prominent women among German racial hygienists (such as the biologist Agnes Bluhm), Sybil Gotto exemplifies how women achieved greater influence in British eugenics. It should also be noted that, by the early twentieth century, women in Britain advanced further than in Germany in terms of academic studies; Marie Stopes, a palaeobotanist before becoming a noted campaigner for contraception, exemplifies this. In Germany, a patriarchal public health establishment espoused eugenic views to curb birth control: figures like Hans Harmsen clashed with a libertarian movement for 'sexual reform'.[16]

Eugenics as public health

Eugenics became a norm embedded in public health concepts, structures and interventions. Around 1900 in Germany (but in the morally more censorious UK, only during the First World War) eugenicists became concerned with sexually transmitted diseases. The ever-inventive Galton had already devised practical eugenic measures – such as health examinations prior to marriage – to screen for sexually transmitted diseases and hereditary abnormalities. The implementation of health measures was designed to limit a range of 'racial poisons' such as alcohol, tuberculosis and sexually transmitted diseases, as well as 'mental deficiency' and 'feeble-mindedness'. In Germany, eugenic concerns with physical and mental degeneration resulted in high-profile campaigns against these 'racial poisons'. Only during the First World War did state authorities contemplate disease control from a reproductive perspective. During the war, eugenically minded experts acted as guardians of national health by serving on committees on the declining birth rate.

At one level, the idea of *Rassenhygiene* dealt with a population in the sense of a breeding group. It considered conflicting approaches to public health, notably the shift to chronic degenerative diseases, and the diminishing of infant mortality. German eugenics intertwined with the Nordic in several ways: as a physical and psychological model. The Secretary of the new Racial Hygiene Society, Ernst Rüdin, travelled to Norway and Sweden in 1907 and 1909 to recruit members. In the event, the Swedish Racial Hygiene Society was founded in 1910 as a branch affiliated to the German society.[17] It had high numbers of physicians and medical students among its members.

The idea of a 'hereditary constitution' allowed for a 'hereditarian', but not necessarily racist, form of eugenics. The term was introduced by Ferdinand Hueppe, a lapsed follower of Robert Koch concerned about the limitations of the causality of infectious bacteria, and was widely taken up. The idea was developed by Adolf Gottstein, who was the medical officer of Berlin-Charlottenburg and, from 1919 to 1924, director of the Prussian medical department. Other public health reformers who gravitated to eugenics include the university professors of hygiene Carl Flügge in Berlin and Max von Gruber in Munich. The social hygienist Alfred Grotjahn prioritised fertility control from a eugenic perspective, as did the Vienna anatomist and social reformer Julius Tandler. The idea of a 'constitution' allowed for combinations of hereditary and environmental factors whereby eugenics became mainstream.[18]

Race became an ambivalent term – on the one hand, meaning a population as a breeding group and, on the other, a mystic spirit. To a wider academic public, Ploetz spoke of race as a breeding group. In this sense, it was a collective concept of a population. In Germany, a lurking racist ideology became radicalised: Ploetz took note of which of the Society's members were Jewish, and he sought to curb Jewish influence. From 1912, Ploetz and Lenz developed an inner Nordic grouping known as *Der Bogen* (the Bow) centred on secret Nordic rituals (the bow was a fertility symbol); after the First World War, they formed a *Widar-Bund*, honouring Widar, the Norse god of light. There was thus a collectivist idea of population health and, at the same time, a racist model of eugenics in Germany. For a while, there were two eugenics societies in Weimar Germany: the Racial Hygiene Society and the *Bund für Volksaufartung* (League for Regeneration), which was more oriented to public health and welfare.[19]

German ideas of Scandinavia show a polarity between Nordic racism and Nordic eugenics. Until the 1980s, the historical focus was on Nordic racism – notably the writings of the anthropologist Hans F.K. Günther, who in 1922 idealised the Nordic race in his widely read *Rassenkunde des deutschen Volkes* (Racial Knowledge of the German People). The Nordic psychology ultimately fed into the writings of the SS and ideas of sustaining the German peasant. These ideas were certainly shared by racial hygienists Eugen Fischer and Fritz Lenz. For the Germans, Nordic values were linked to an idealising of rural populations, rather than to admiration for welfare initiatives.

A valued recruit was the *völkisch* publisher Julius Lehmann, who forged alliances among the racial ultra-right while developing racial hygiene as a science of preventive medicine and communicating it through his medical publications to the wider profession. In 1911, he published the catalogue of the section on racial hygiene at the International Hygiene Exhibition, held in Dresden. Ploetz encouraged liberal and left-wing advocates of social medicine to join in the imperialist agitation. Before the First World War, racial hygiene acquired support among ultra-nationalists. All members of the German Racial Hygiene Society had to have the German 'mother tongue' and belong to the 'white race'. The incorporation of Nordic members can be seen as part of a strategy to promote a Greater German approach to racial hygiene.

Jewish members were experts in the prevention of chronic degenerative diseases. Among them were dermatologist Alfred Blaschko; ophthalmologist Arthur Czellitzer, founder of the *Gesellschaft für jüdische Familienforschung* (Society for Jewish Family Research) and later killed at the Sobibor extermination camp in 1943; and Adolf Gottstein, epidemiologist and medical officer of Charlottenburg. Max Hirsch, the pioneer of 'social gynaecology' was concerned with the reproductive risks to women in hazardous situations, for example due to manual labour. Medical statistician Wilhelm Weinberg (who was 'half Jewish') dealt with statistics of maternal mortality, TB and haemophilia. He chaired the Stuttgart Racial Hygiene Society. The Jewish geneticists Richard Goldschmidt and Hermann Poll were genetic advocates of eugenics. The Jewish eugenicists were progressives in drawing attention to the new prevalence of chronic degenerative diseases. Political and racial tension over Jews and socialists resulted in the split of the welfare-orientated League for Regeneration from the Racial Hygiene Society in 1925. There was also a society for Jewish family research, developed by Czellitzer.

Nationalist fervour linked eugenics to the *völkisch* movement – the publisher Lehmann racialised eugenics by sponsoring Günther to write the *Rassenkunde des deutschen Volkes*. Hitler's library contained several of Günther's works. Lehmann published the journal *Volk und Rasse* (People and Race) from the mid-1920s, gaining support from the SS. Non-racist forms of eugenics permeated the Weimar welfare state, with measures to curb the propagation of the asocial and feeble-minded, and to curb the spread of so-called racial poisons. Lehmann secured control of the loss-making *Archiv für Rassen- und Gesellschaftsbiologie* in 1922. He added to this the *Zeitschrift für Rassenphysiologie* (Journal for Racial Physiology), which was focused on race and blood groups.[20]

After the First World War, German eugenicists feared that the German race, or *Volk*, was being exterminated by hunger and territorial loss. Hunger was linked to poor economic growth and disease. The welfare state in the Weimar Republic instituted a number of positive eugenic measures, such as marriage advisory clinics and family allowances. 'Red' Vienna under Julius Tandler, an anatomist and advocate of body type theories, launched major initiatives in housing, as well as the first birth control clinic. In 1927, a national eugenics institute was founded, the Kaiser Wilhelm Institute for Anthropology, which received funding from the state as well as private sources. Otmar von Verschuer carried out research on twins to see which traits were inherited and which acquired.[21]

In Britain, the Eugenics Society gained influential supporters such as biologist Julian Huxley and cell biologist John R. Baker, who researched chemical contraception. Known as 'Volpar', this was sponsored by the Society, although Marie Stopes was upset by competition to her 'Pro-Race' rubber cap.[22] There was sporadic sympathy at the level of Medical Officers of Health. A select few sought to implement a radical eugenics agenda of sterilisation. This can be seen in the unique and arguably exceptional case of Leicester, where the Medical Officer of Health, Killick Millard, arranged six sterilisation operations on children who were blind and presumed to be mentally subnormal. C.P. Blacker (Secretary of the Eugenics Society 1931–1961) reported that: "sterilisation on eugenic grounds has occasionally been performed in this country and without mishap".[23] At the same time, the Eugenics Society ran a campaign for voluntary sterilisation legislation, which, however, failed. In general, the labour movement was critical of sterilisation.[24]

During the Depression of 1929, there were demands for sterilisation as a means of 'curing' Germany of its social problem groups such as juvenile delinquents, habitual criminals and the feeble-minded. In 1928, the Swiss canton of Vaud legislated for sterilisation, and in certain German-speaking Swiss cantons, sterilisations were routine. Danish legislative models were influential for the Swiss, as well as precedents from US states, notably California, where coercive sterilisation was applied.

While eugenics pervaded state welfare in 1920s' Germany and Austria, it also shaped community-based initiatives beyond the state. This can be seen in colonial contexts and among the expatriate German communities. Austrian psychiatrists joined the Nazi Party illegally, and some left to work with the demographer and psychiatrist Ernst Rüdin. After the 1933 Nazi takeover, state-imposed eugenic monitoring of the population was implemented. Eugenicists launched national hereditary biological surveys and hereditary databanks, and advocated segregating 'racial deviants'.

The Nazi era

Hitler took up various eugenic themes, such as sterilisation and the damage to the nation's hereditary stock through sexually transmitted disease. He warned how German blood could be corrupted by mixing with Jews. The expectation that Hitler would pursue eugenic policies was initially confirmed in July 1933, when the Nazis passed a sterilisation law. Rüdin served as an advisor in drafting the law. He was influenced not only by US states with coercive sterilisation, but also by the Danish sterilisation law of 1929, as well as Swiss practices. The German law was targeted at a range of clinical conditions, most notably schizophrenia, muscular dystrophy, Huntington's chorea, epilepsy, severe mental defect, inherited deafness and chronic alcoholism. Sexual and mental abnormalities attracted especial interest. Geneticist, doctor and right-wing activist Otmar von Verschuer, based at the Frankfurt public health clinic, led the way in studies on twins.

In 1933, race and welfare were fused along with the rapid Nazification of the German welfare state. Public health was centralised so as to issue orders for sterilisation. Sterilisation was authorised by tribunals of two doctors and a lawyer. At least 375,000 individuals were sterilised by German authorities (including in annexed Austria and the Sudeten German-occupied territory), and there were an estimated 5,000 deaths from complications; 385 'mixed-race' children, aged 13–16, were sterilised in 1937. They were also subjected to psychological, anthropological and genetic evaluations.

In September 1935, the Reich Citizenship Law limited citizenship to those of 'German and related blood'. The Blood Protection Law forbade marriages and sexual relations between Germans, Jews and non-whites alike. These were the so-called Nuremberg Laws. They were based on the idea that blood could be infected by sexual relations with someone of another race.

The Marriage Law of 1935 required hereditary health examinations prior to marriage. Nazi health propaganda encouraged people deemed as good eugenic breeding stock to have at least three children. Health offices registered the birth of the unfit, and from mid-1939, this could have fatal consequences. Marriage certificates involved tests to make sure that no one with a sexually transmitted disease or carrying a genetic disease got married. Nazi racial experts set out to identify and research male homosexuals, many of whom were held in concentration camps, along with other racially stigmatised categories – notably Jews, Sinti and Roma, hereditary criminals, and the 'work-shy'.

In June 1936, a Central Office to 'Combat the Gypsy Nuisance' opened in Munich. This office became the headquarters of a national databank on so-called Gypsies. Robert Ritter, a medical anthropologist at the Reich Health Office, concluded that 90 per cent of the Gypsies were 'of mixed blood'. He described them as "the products of mating with the German criminal asocial sub-proletariat" and as "primitive" people "incapable of real social adaptation".[25]

The Kaiser Wilhelm Institute for Anthropology trained SS doctors in genetics. From 1935, a medical lobby around Hitler pressed for the introduction of killing the malformed and incurable, although the practice was not introduced until October 1939. Hitler saw the sick as an economic burden on the healthy, and wished to rid the German race of their 'polluting' effects on the nation's 'genetic treasury'.

The numbers of mentally ill and disabled killed with carbon monoxide in the initial phase – code-named 'T4' (after the administrative office at Tiergartenstrasse 4, Berlin) – amounted to 70,273 persons. The killings were based on medical records sent to the clandestine panel of psychiatrists in Berlin. In 1941, the Roman Catholic bishop of Münster, Clemens Galen, expressed his condemnation, and some opposition from distressed relatives was voiced as well. This resulted in a fake halt. 'Euthanasia' personnel, including physicians and technicians, were transferred to the *Aktion Reinhardt*, which ran the extermination camps of Bełżec,

Sobibor and Treblinka, to kill with carbon monoxide gas. Euthanasia continued in concentration camps where prisoners were selected for killing, so-called special children's wards, and in other clinical locations. Physicians, who were assisted by nurses, killed their victims by starvation, injection and by administering deadly drugs. Those killed included newborn babies, children, the mentally disturbed and the infirm. Sometimes victims were killed for merely challenging the staff in institutions, even though they were in good health, and others did not qualify as so-called incurables in accordance with the Nazi theory. Some physicians killed because of the scientific interest of the 'cases'. Austria had relatively high numbers of euthanasia killings, although numbers of sterilisation victims were lower. The rationales were to save costs of institutional care, to use institutions for other forms of medical care, and to purge genes deemed pathogenic from the racial 'genetic treasury'.

Carl Schneider, professor of psychiatry at Heidelberg University, was an adjudicator for euthanasia, and saw this as an opportunity for histo-pathological research. He wanted to determine the difference between inherited and acquired *idiocy* (a medical term for a severe form of mental disability): therefore, 52 children were examined, each for six weeks in the clinic. In the event, 21 of the children were killed so as to compare the diagnosis, made when they were alive, with the post-mortem pathological evidence.[26]

Robert Ritter directed measures of registration and psychological evaluation of Roma and Sinti. He was supported by psychologists and racial anthropologists. Their observations were followed by incarcerations of Roma and Sinti in concentration camps, notably Auschwitz, where the women and children were killed in July 1944.

The pressure increased to use imprisoned humans for experiments. Eugenic experiments included research on several hundred Jewish women held in Auschwitz for chemical sterilisation experiments, and the X-ray sterilisation experiments on Greek and Polish Jewish men in November 1942. The SS anthropologists Bruno Beger and Hans Fleischhacker selected 115 Jewish men and women to be killed for an anatomical skeleton collection (in the event, 86 were transported to Alsace and gassed; the largest group were Sephardic Greek Jews). The year 1944 marked a high point in unethical research in the basic medical sciences. Many younger researchers (like Josef Mengele) hoped for academic appointments on the basis of unique research findings.

Racial experts from various disciplines from anthropology to agriculture planned extermination of Jews and Slavs to make way for German farmsteads. The Kaiser Wilhelm Institute anthropologist Wolfgang Abel surveyed Nordic qualities of Russians, and Fritz Lenz reviewed the suitability of Ukraine for Nordic settlement.

Nazi demographers were assisted by census techniques and collected medical, health and welfare data. Data on diseases and crime were analysed, and states organised central registries. Hamburg Welfare was established in order to centralise and analyse the statistics. They used the new technology of Hollerith punch cards, using an IBM patent. These techniques assisted in calculations of the numbers of

Jews, how many had emigrated and the location of those remaining. They calculated how many full, half and quarter Jews still lived in the Reich. SS demographer Richard Korherr's calculations on the numbers of Jews in the occupied territories assisted Adolf Eichmann with the implementation of the Final Solution. In 1943, Korherr calculated for Himmler and Hitler how many Jews had been killed, country by country. Similar techniques were applied to identify social deviants and for the genocidal measures against the Roma. In the occupied territories, notably the Netherlands, census techniques were used in the deportation of Jews to the concentration and death camps of the east.

Josef Mengele worked as an assistant to Otmar von Verschuer, the expert on the genetics of twins. Mengele joined the Nazi Party and the SS in 1938, and from November 1940 worked with the SS Race and Settlement Office on ethnic German returnees from such locations as the Baltics. In June 1941, Mengele joined a combat unit, and in May 1943 he was sent to Auschwitz as a camp doctor. Scientific research was an informal, spare-time activity. As Mengele selected new arrivals at Auschwitz for poison gassing, he could exploit his position in the selection of twins and other subjects of genetic interest (notably, persons with growth anomalies). The implications for public health were never clearly indicated by Mengele or Verschuer to the German Research Fund: however, it would be reasonable to assume that an intention was the elimination of hereditary defects and growth anomalies from the hereditary stock of the German 'race'. Such medical experiments underpinned a system of differential health care, primarily for those deemed to belong to the racial elite, enhancing fertility (as can be seen in Clauberg's scheme for a City of Mothers) and exclusion (by elimination) of presumed racial undesirables, whether on grounds of ethnicity or of substandard genetic constitution.

Legacies

Post-war Britain set about instituting the National Health Service in 1948. Financed through state tax revenues, the ethos was inclusion and universality rather than selectivity. While the NHS represented an end to eugenic ideals of selection and exclusion, whether the physically and mentally disabled have always received their entitlements is an open question.

Post-war Germany often turned a blind eye to racial criminals. The German state ignored the financial support Mengele received from his family business in agricultural machinery; and other racial criminals, such as Horst Schumann (responsible for X-ray experiments in Auschwitz), also evaded prosecution. In 1946, Verschuer claimed that he had not known about the true nature of Auschwitz, or about the illegitimacy of the body parts he used, i.e., that he prompted the killing of people for extraneous reasons. Neuroscientist Julius Hallervorden, who possibly collected the brains of over 1,500 euthanasia victims for research, similarly defended his actions. In Vienna, there were also large collections of victims' brains, the last buried only in 2014. The legacy of Nazism was immense, and it tainted medical and scientific elites in the Federal Republic of Germany. Few were informed about the chance of reversing the sterilisation operation with re-fertilisation. The victims' stigma held fast, and eugenicists still argued that the victims had been justifiably sterilised. Eugenics was a prominent topic at the Nuremberg trials, as well as at the trials of Nazi physicians and of the SS Race and Settlement Office. Physician Hermann Poppendieck had trained at the Kaiser Wilhelm Institute for Anthropology, and was involved in SS-administered racial policy.[27] Although Rüdin was deprived of his Swiss nationality for his deeds, this did not bring sterilisation on the grounds of schizophrenia or 'moral idiocy' to an end in Zurich; indeed, it continued until 1970. Despite limited compensation for German victims, full acknowledgement of the injustices of sterilisation and racial research victims has not been made.

Racial hygiene and eugenics were rebranded as human genetics. This allowed for continuity of former racial experts in the Federal Republic. Many eugenicists like Lenz, Nachtsheim, Harmsen (of the Pro Familia birth control organisation) and Verschuer had influential careers in birth control provision, radiation monitoring and forensic psychiatry. That many former eugenics experts retained their positions in such fields is indicative of continuities from the Third Reich to the Federal Republic and post-Second World War Austria. The Viennese brain pathologist Hans Gross continued research on the brains of euthanasia victims. The student protests of 1968 initiated a break with the old elites, leading to critical publications by such figures as the geneticist Benno Müller-Hill. A new phase of concern began with birth control and the liberalising of restrictions on abortion, and latterly over whether human genome research and pre-embryonic implantation constituted new forms of eugenics. The German case cautions against any monolithic interpretation of eugenics, as eugenics sustained itself under both democratic and authoritarian regimes.

A new historical pitfall arose – that all state welfare could be seen in the light of abusive powers and Nazi atrocities. Problematic new interpretations of eugenics that made too much of contrasting stereotypes arose as well.[28] Here, loosely conceptualised interpretations of Nordic and Latin eugenics require critical reappraisal. 'Nordic eugenics' is taken as representing selection and sterilisation, whereas 'Latin eugenics' is seen in such contrasting terms as pronatalist and promoting reproductive health. In the middle sits Nazi eugenics, seen as driven by exterminatory impulses against Jews, the Roma and the mentally ill – both extremes lacking in the Nordic and Latin variants with intersections with German eugenics and racial hygiene.

Switzerland is an indicative case study. In analysing Swiss eugenics as putatively 'Latin', there is a need to acknowledge a structural point – Swiss policies were cantonal. The result is more of a patchwork and clusters rather than a country heading towards the Latin camp. In fact, the francophone canton of Vaud introduced sterilisation legislation in 1928. Swiss psychiatrists had taken a lead in advancing sterilisation. Rüdin, as a Swiss national, retained influence in the German-speaking cantons. Turda and Gillette cite the Swiss anthropologist Georges Montandon, as a prominent advocate of Latin eugenics. Montandon had a key role in shifting French anthropology, politically left-wing and anti-racist (as represented by the grouping *Races et Racisme*), towards the fascist and racially genocidal right. Montandon moved to German-occupied France and drove forward the roundups and deportations of French Jews. Extolling Latin virtues should not obscure activism in the unleashing of negative policies. If Montandon is an archetypal Latin eugenicist, we see the Latins in ultra-racist exterminatory mode.

Nordic eugenics presents a similarly problematic situation. Here, the issue has been that Nordic eugenics should be seen in the context of a welfare state concerned with 'unfit' mothers.[29] The Scandinavian accounts underestimate policies against the nomadic Sami (sometimes referred to as Laps). The other dimension is that of the wider international framework. In this framework the deep gulf between Nazi racial sympathisers like Norwegian Jon Alfred Mjøen (albeit limited to before he died in 1939) and pro-Allied groupings, argues Gunnar Dahlberg at Uppsala University, should be read as a swing towards anti-racist politics.[30] In Finland, General Mannerheim vacillated over what to do about foreign and Finnish Jews. While the number of deportations from the precariously independent Finland was, in the end, relatively low, for a period Finland was also firmly in the German cultural sphere. The Nordic stereotype obscures deep divisions.

What needs to be taken into account is that Nazi race theory was itself contested and polarised. Far from being monolithically uniform, publications on racial hygiene show a pluralist approach, be it on heredity, cultural or psychological issues. Even among the SS there were deep divisions between geopolitical factions of SS hygienists and those who were genetically and genealogically oriented. Multiple types of eugenic racial theory were operationalised as genocide. Such pluralism also operated in the 'Latin' and 'Nordic' contexts.

Sociobiological approaches continued to be developed. Biotypology is questionably hailed as a wholly 'Latin eugenic' characteristic. Certainly, France was a major centre of bio-typological research. But root ideas drew heavily on the German eugenicist Ernst Kretschmer's *biotypes* oriented to body and character (as outlined in *Körperbau und Charakter/*Physique and character of 1921). Another centre was Czechoslovakia. The Bata shoe factory at Zlin in southern Moravia was a modernist vortex of bio-typological research and practice in industry and administration. The Czechoslovak Eugenic Society was affiliated to the French in 1937. What this signified was that bio-typology was not 'Latin' but internationalist, modernist and progressive, and eschewed racial concepts. Clearly bio-typological clusters arose in contexts from Mexico to Zlin, but the contexts were not uniformly 'Latin'. Seen in the above perspectives, reviewing the different components of Nordic eugenics and welfare is therefore timely.

Conclusions

Eugenics has been a powerful influence in shaping diverse aspects of health care. Historiographically, eugenics has shifted from the marginal ultra-right to entering the mainstream of welfare policies and practices. On the one hand, we find practitioners; but the victims are sadly lacking a voice and identity. On the other hand, the extent of eugenics needs to be circumscribed and specified. From the start there were opponents as well as diverse opinions. Eugenics – as argued here – has its innovative side, in terms of the problems identified in epidemiological and demographic shifts. In terms of ideology and social forms, these were normally driven by expert elites. Eugenics organisations allowed for multiple disciplines to address problems regarding mental health, chronic disease and disability. The diversity of eugenic opinions allowed for the survival of programmatic ideas in times of transition. The past certainly casts a darker shadow over Germany than Britain, which has shaped medical and biologistic discourses. Looking forward, Germany has seen a problematic transition to human genetics, molecular medicine and in vitro fertilisation (IVF). Whereas in the UK, pre-embryonic selection prior to in vitro fertilisation is accepted, in Germany there are deep reservations. The dreams of the early eugenicists are now – in part – realisable. This adds to the importance of critically reappraising the different strands of eugenic histories.

Notes

1   C.P. Blacker, *Eugenics: Galton and After* (London: Duckworth, 1952).
2   Michel Foucault, *Histoire de la sexualité* (Paris: Gallimard, 1976, 1984); Donald MacKenzie, *Statistics in Britain 1865–1910: The Social Construction of Scientific Knowledge* (Edinburgh: Edinburgh University Press, 1981).
3   Alfred Ploetz, *Die Tüchtigkeit unserer Rasse und der Schutz der Schwachen: Ein Versuch über Rassenhygiene und ihr Verhältnis zu den humanen Idealen, besonders zum Socialismus. Grundlinien einer Rassen-Hygiene, 1. Theil* (Berlin: Fischer, 1895).
4   Paul Weindling, *Health, Race and German Politics between National Unification and Nazism* (Cambridge: Cambridge University Press, 1989).
5   Alfons Labisch, 'Experimentelle Hygiene, Bakteriologie, Soziale Hygiene: Konzeptionen, Interventionen, soziale Träger – eine idealtypische Übersicht', in *Stadt und Gesundheit*, ed. J. Reulecke and A. zu Castell Rüdenhausen (Stuttgart: Steiner, 1991), 37–47.
6   Pauline Mazumdar, *Eugenics, Human Genetics and Human Failings: The Eugenics Society, its Sources and its Critics in Britain* (London: Routledge, 1992); Weindling, *Health, Race*.
7   Ernst Rüdin, *Zur Vererbung und Neuentstehung der Daementia Praecox* (Berlin: Springer, 1916).
8   Jana Grimm, *Zwangssterilisationen von Mädchen und Frauen während des Nationalsozialismus: Eine Analyse der Krankenakten der Universitäts-Frauenklinik Halle von 1934 bis 1945* (doctoral dissertation, Halle: Martin-Luther-Universität Halle-Wittenberg, 2004), 65.
9   Sheila Weiss, *Race Hygiene and National Efficiency: The Eugenics of Wilhelm Schallmayer* (Berkeley and New York: University of California Press, 1987).
10   Nicholas Wright Gilham, *A Life of Sir Francis Galton: From African Exploration to the Birth of Eugenics* (Oxford: Oxford University Press, 2001).
11   Francis Galton, 'Kantsaywhere', in *Life, Letters and Labours of Francis Galton*, vol. 3, ed. Karl Pearson (Cambridge: Cambridge University Press, 1930), 414–24.
12   John Welshman, 'Eugenics and public health in Britain, 1900–40: Scenes from provincial life', *Urban History* 24, no. 1 (1997): 56–75; Mathew Thomson and Paul Weindling, 'Sterilisationpolitik in Grossbritannien und Deutschland', in *Nach Hadamar: Zum Verhältnis von Psychiatrie und Gesellschaft im 20. Jahrhundert*, ed. F.W. Kersting, K. Teppe and B. Walter (Paderborn: Ferdinand Schöningh, 1993), 137–49.

13 Karl Pearson, *Eugenics and Public Health: A Lecture Delivered at the York Congress of the Royal Sanitary Institute, July 30th, 1912* (London: Dulau, 1912).
14 F.G. Bushnell 'The present position of eugenics' *Public Health* 25 (1911–12): 384–87.
15 Paul Weindling, 'The politics of international co-ordination to combat sexually transmitted diseases, 1900–1980s', in *AIDS and Contemporary History*, ed. Virginia Berridge and Philip Strong (Cambridge: Cambridge University Press, 1993), 93–107.
16 Atina Grossmann, *Reforming Sex: The German Movement for Birth Control & Abortion Reform 1920–1950* (Oxford: Oxford University Press, 1995).
17 Weindling, *Health, Race*, 150.
18 Barbara Nemec, 'Anatomical modernity in Red Vienna: Julius Tandler's textbook for systematic anatomy and the politics of visual milieus', *Sudhoffs Archiv* 99, no. 1 (2014): 44–71.
19 Paul Weindling, 'Die Preussische Medizinalverwaltung und die "Rassenhygiene"', in *Medizin und Faschismus,* ed. A. Thom and H. Spaar (Berlin: Akademie für ärztliche Fortbildung, 1983), 23–35; Weindling, *Health, Race*.
20 Paul Weindling, 'The medical publisher J.F. Lehmann and racial hygiene', in *Die 'rechte Nation' und ihr Verleger: Politik und Popularisierung im J.F. Lehmanns Verlag 1890–1979,* ed. Sigrid Stöckel (Berlin: Lehmanns Media, 2002), 159–70.
21 Hans-Walter Schmuhl and Paul Weindling, 'Weimar eugenics in social context: The founding of the Kaiser Wilhelm Institute for Anthropology, Human Heredity and Eugenics', *Annals of Science* 42 (1985): 303–18.
22 Richard Soloway, *Demography and Degeneration: Eugenics and the Declining Birthrate in Twentieth-Century Britain* (Chapel Hill: University of North Carolina Press, 1990), 222–4.
23 C.P. Blacker, *Eugenics: Galton and After* (London: Duckworth, 1952), 305.
24 John Macnicol, 'Eugenics and the campaign for voluntary sterilization in Britain between the wars', *Social History of Medicine* 2, no. 2 (1989): 147–69.
25 Guenter Lewy, *Nazi Persecution of the Gypsies* (Oxford and New York: Oxford University Press, 2000); Joachim Stephan Hohmann, *Robert Ritter und die Erben der Kriminalbiologie: 'Zigeunerforschung' im Nationalsozialismus und in Westdeutschland im Zeichen des Rassismus* (Frankfurt am Main: Lang, 1991); Tobias Schmidt-Degenhard, *Vermessen und Vernichten: Der NS-'Zigeunerforscher' Robert Ritter* (Stuttgart: Steiner, 2012).
26 Paul Weindling, *Victims and Survivors of Nazi Human Experiments: Science and Suffering in the Holocaust* (London: Bloomsbury, 2014).
27 Paul Weindling, *Nazi Medicine and the Nuremberg Trials: From Medical War Crimes to Informed Consent* (Basingstoke: Palgrave Macmillan, 2004).
28 Marius Turda and Aaron Gillette, *Latin Eugenics in Comparative Perspective* (London and New York: Bloomsbury Academic, 2014).
29 Paul Weindling, 'International eugenics: Swedish sterilisation in context', *Scandinavian Journal of History* 24, no. 2 (1999): 179–97.
30 Gunnar Dahlberg, *Race, Reason and Rubbish* (London: Allen & Unwin, 1942).

3 Female doctors, prophylactic health care and public health

Merle Wessel

Introduction

In Sweden and Finland, medicine was the first university subject opened up to women. In 1870, women could take medical exams in Sweden for the first time. All other subjects were open to female students in 1873.[1] The first female physician with a university degree in Sweden was Karolina Widerström (1856–1949). Graduating in 1895 from the University of Helsinki, the first Finnish female doctor was Karolina Eskelin (1867–1936). The first female medical students in Sweden as well as in Finland took a special interest in fields that could be understood as feminine: paediatrics and gynaecology.[2]

In this chapter, I discuss three female doctors from Sweden and Finland – Karolina Widerström, Karolina Eskelin and Ada Nilsson (a doctor of the second generation) – and their engagement in prophylactic care in order to improve public health. The main questions I answer concern the role these three female doctors took in their national public health discourses in the early twentieth century. How did they understand the concept of public health? What was the focus of their work to improve public health? Further, I discuss the extent to which eugenic ideology played a role in their understanding of prophylactic care and public health.

I answer these questions by analysing health advice books published by Karolina Widerström and Karolina Eskelin. Widerström published two ground-breaking books – *Kvinnohygien I* (Women's Hygiene) and *Kvinnohygien II*, in 1899 and 1905 – in which she gave detailed advice on sexual hygiene, clothing, female health and the upbringing of children. The first book was reprinted seven times. Karolina Eskelin published several books and articles in Swedish and Finnish on how housewives and mothers should keep the family healthy, the house clean and their sexuality pure.[3] The Swedish doctor Ada Nilsson, together with colleagues from the liberal women's movement *Frisinnade Kvinnors Riksförbund* (FKR), established a hygiene advice office in Stockholm in 1925, following the models of Margaret Sanger and Marie Stopes, who had been active promoters and reformers of birth control in the USA and Great Britain, respectively. Nilsson wanted to provide sexual and hygiene advice to women in a relaxed and non-threatening environment.

As Finnish sociologist Sirpa Wrede argues, the role of women in the medical sphere changed during modernity. In the nineteenth century, they were active subjects in health care. During the early twentieth century, they became passive recipients, and after the Second World War women could become experts.[4] However, I argue that at least some women became leaders in providing prophylactic health care already before the Second World War, which had an impact on the conceptualisation of public health in Sweden and Finland in the interwar period and afterwards.

The chapter is divided into three parts. In the first part, I show why I see Widerström, Eskelin and Nilsson as representative of their generation as female physicians as well as first-wave feminists. The second part focuses on the content of their health advice books and a description of their practical work. I analyse the rhetoric they used to describe their patients, their work environment and the advice they provided. The last part situates their advice within the public discourse about public health before the Second World War. I show that their work influenced the conceptualisation of public health in their countries. Furthermore, I discuss how eugenic ideology was introduced into the public health discourse and how this influenced female doctors.

Female doctors in Sweden and Finland

Karolina Eskelin, Ada Nilsson and Karolina Widerström belonged to the first generation of female doctors in their countries. Comparing their biographies, various similarities can be detected. The oldest of the three, Widerström, was born in 1856 in Helsingborg. Her father was a gymnastics teacher, and her interest in the human body was stimulated from early on. Widerström passed her exams at the Wallinska Skola in Stockholm in 1879, the first Swedish school to provide girls the opportunity to receive the qualifications required for a university education. From 1880 onwards, Widerström studied medicine, first in Uppsala and later at the Karolinska Institute in Stockholm. She financed her studies by working as a gymnastics teacher and physiotherapist.[5]

Karolina Eskelin was born eleven years after Widerström, in 1867. Due to her father's profession as a sea captain, she grew up in England and Belgium. After her father's death, she moved back to Helsinki to attend the Swedish Girls' School. Her mother died soon after their return, leaving Karolina orphaned at a young age.[6] However, that did not hold Eskelin back. Although there were no formal possibilities for women to study in Finland at the time, she continued her education after graduating from a girls' upper secondary school, enabling her to enter university. To finance her education, Eskelin worked as a shop assistant. Finally, in 1885, Eskelin and her friend, Ina Rosqvist, entered the University of Helsinki as the first female students.[7]

Ada Nilsson, born 1872 in West Gothland, had a similar biography to Eskelin, having also lost her parents at a young age. Her guardian, a member of the Swedish parliament, stimulated her social interests at an early age and provided her with an extensive education. She studied at the Karolinska Institute from 1891 onwards to become a physician, like her role model Karolina Widerström.[8]

The biographies of these three women show clear similarities: they were born into middle-class families; two of them were orphaned at a young age; and the path to education was not straightforward for any of them. Eskelin and Widerström, in particular, were among the first women in their countries to pave the way for academic education for women, which made the journey easier (albeit not self-evident) for women like Nilsson. Besides being among the first female students in their countries, all three showed also great interest in political and social issues. The Swedish journalist Ulrika Knutson has described Ada Nilsson as a typical feminist of the turn of the century.[9] Nilsson showed great interest in the social conflicts of her time. She provided shelter for homeless girls and elderly women in her home; and, besides her work as physician, she was engaged in school teaching, sex education and popular education on hygiene and health matters.[10] Together with other prominent Swedish feminists like Julia Kinberg, Alma Sundquist and Elin Wägner, Nilsson founded FKR, the liberal women's organisation, which came up with pioneering proposals on several social policy issues.[11] Between 1923 and 1936, the organisation published the magazine *Tidevarvet*, to which Nilsson frequently contributed articles on various social topics such as women's rights, prostitution, abortion and birth control.

Widerström, too, was active in politics. She was member of the Stockholm city council for the Liberal Party between 1912 and 1915, and, from 1918 onwards, chairwoman of the Swedish suffragette organisation. Furthermore, she participated actively in debates about the regulation of prostitution before the First World War, and was one of the Swedish doctors who signed a petition against *lex hinke*[12] in 1911.[13] Eskelin taught gynaecology to students at the nurses' school and gave lectures on, e.g., the proper nutrition of infants, in addition to talking in schools about hygiene and physiology.[14]

All three women practised as medical doctors after finishing their studies, in addition to doing political and social work. Yet, being able to study medicine did not imply that working as a doctor was self-evident. The National Medical Board in Sweden took a critical stance against female doctors. Its members were concerned that female doctors would embark on inappropriate relationships with male doctors, or that the sex drive of male patients would be stimulated by a female physician. In addition, it was unimaginable that a female doctor could lead an institution, making men her subordinates.[15] Ada Nilsson was primarily interested in psychiatry, but, as reported in her autobiography, she could not find a mental hospital willing to employ her.[16] Therefore, she redirected her interest towards gynaecology. She began working in a hospital in Stockholm's working-class district of Södermalm, and later started her own practice there.[17]

In 1899, Widerström started her gynaecology practice in Stockholm and kept its doors open for over thirty years. Her former professor from Uppsala University, who had claimed nobody would hire a female doctor, was thereby proven wrong.[18] After her studies, Eskelin worked in several hospitals, first in Tampere, and later as a surgeon in the policlinic in Helsinki's working-class district of Kallio. In 1903–1905 and 1912, she also worked in the United States.[19]

Widerström, Eskelin and Nilsson had to overcome various gendered obstacles in order to achieve their goals. They were pioneers of their own generation and role models for the following ones. They embraced a new type of woman: independent, professional, engaged in public affairs and with an interest in social and political matters. They were among the first women to combine professional life with political careers by serving the social and political sphere not as philanthropists, but as professionals.

Health books and advice offices: Information by women for women

Female medical experts sought to disseminate health knowledge primarily through two channels: firstly, through written publications – primarily books but also articles; and, secondly, directly in health advice offices. The two channels had different, class-based target audiences. Written publications were mainly directed at the middle class, while the offices (although open to everyone) served mainly the lower classes, the working class in particular. However, both forms of advice were highly gendered; they were exclusively directed at women or, more precisely, at mothers.

As noted before, the first generation of female physicians was interested in feminine medical disciplines such as gynaecology and paediatrics. Furthermore, they were interested not only in treating sick women but also in preventing women's and family illness in general. Both Widerström and Eskelin published several comprehensive books with health and hygiene advice for women and their families. Nilsson, for her part, was more active in providing health education to the working class.

Widerström was a pioneer in providing publicly available advice related to women's health and hygiene. Her first book, *Kvinnohygien I*, was published in 1899 and reprinted regularly until the 1930s. In the preface of the first edition, she stated:

> The woman has been endowed by Mother Nature the greatest and most important parts of the life process, which result in the reproduction of the race. But long has she cared little about seeking to know these most wonderful and admirable of all life processes, or to acquire knowledge of the body and organs in which they take place.[20]

Widerström explains that women, due to their special reproductive ability, need to show a greater interest in the bodily aspects of human nature. She elevates women to a position as guardians not only of their own bodies but also of the bodies of the race (*släkte*).[21] In doing so, she justified providing health advice exclusively for women. Preserving the race (or lineage) was the responsibility of women, not only by curing illnesses but also by preventing illness.

Sirpa Wrede argues that the rising interest in prophylactic health from the late nineteenth century onwards in Finland and Sweden implied a central role for women. The woman became interesting from the point of view of society, as she was thought to be responsible for health care at home.[22] Care of the family was transformed from a private issue into a public and societal matter. Health and its conservation were becoming concerns of the nation as a whole, and women hence became public figures in the newly formulated mission.[23]

Eskelin published several health advisory and educational books, and numerous articles. One of her most prominent was *Personlig hälsovård med särskild hänsyn till bostad* (1925)/*Henkilökohtaisesta terveydenhoidosta* (1927) (Personal Health Care with Special Attention to Housing), first published in Swedish and later in Finnish. While the target audience of Widerström's book was clearly indicated in the title and preface, Eskelin did not define her audience as clearly. However, the topics she discussed – such as housing, clothing, nutrition and physical care – were probably self-evidently understood as feminine. Eskelin's health advice focused on the human body. In her introduction, she argues that a healthy body is the key to luck and happiness in life. However, the body is not healthy by itself, but needs care. Furthermore, a sick body always needs professional medical care.[24]

Eskelin hence contributed to the societal discourse about normality and pathology in Finland. As sociologist Elianne Riska argues, health and illness relate to the relationship between society and individual and the individual's societal responsibility. From a medical approach, being healthy and having a healthy body was understood as normal. The sick body had to be normalised. The doctor was responsible for observing the sick until they were healthy, i.e., normal again.[25]

Yet, the aim of these books was not to give advice on how to cure diseases (at least not in the first place); instead, they sought to give advice on how to prevent disease altogether. The mother of the family was the focus of this advice. It was the mother's responsibility to keep the family healthy, which would also help maintain national and public health. In one of her early health and hygiene books (published in 1914), Eskelin argued that Finnish experts ought to target their practical advice at housewives, as she claimed that the majority of Finnish housewives lacked fundamental knowledge about basic hygiene. She blamed the traditional orienta-tion and the underdeveloped status of the Finnish population, which made the implementation of new hygiene practices very difficult.[26] Furthermore, Eskelin demanded that mothers and housewives should be the primary recipients of health education, since they carried the responsibility for the care of children, the home and the health of the family.[27]

Eskelin wanted to achieve on a micro level the same things that were discussed by politicians and social reformers at the macro level – the national context of public health. One aspect of the public health discourse in Sweden and Finland in the early twentieth century was that health had transformed from a private issue into a public matter. The health of the individual had a direct impact on the health of the nation. Swedish social scientist Eva Palmblad argues that the education on hygiene was designed both from the point of view of the individual as well as society. The life of the individual had to be reorganised to meet the newest scientific ideas about hygiene.[28] Palmblad further argues that hygiene must be seen in a wider context than just physical hygiene. The term 'hygiene' was central in the political and scientific discourse, and referred to topics such as racial hygiene, societal hygiene, sexual hygiene and family hygiene.[29]

Eskelin's health advice, as well as Widerström's books, was connected to a general shift in the way social and health-related problems were dealt with, not only in Sweden and Finland but also in the entire Western world. In the nineteenth century, social problems were mainly addressed through philanthropic work. While most countries had some kind of state-based poor relief, upper- and middle-class women provided the majority of help for the poor. However, according to Norwegian historian Elisabeth Haavet, the development of welfare state ideas in the interwar period was associated with bringing social problems onto the political agenda.[30] Expert knowledge was now considered a requirement for solving social issues.

However, experts could not monitor all members of the population, so the smallest entity of society needed to be educated in order to preserve and promote public health. The advice Widerström and Eskelin provided in their books was very detailed but also manifold. The focus in Widerström's *Kvinnohygien I* was predominately on the sexual body and how a mother should educate her children so they develop a healthy sexuality.[31] Following Palmblad, sexual hygiene was considered an important aspect of hygiene and public health discourse.[32]

Eskelin provided a much wider focus in her books. She did discuss care of the sexual female body, but this was only one aspect of her wider understanding of hygiene and health. She also discussed the general housing situation in cities, and what the appropriate living environment for a healthy family was.[33] Furthermore, she explained what healthy clothing for men and women was about: for example, women should not wear constricting corsets; the entire family should enjoy a well-balanced diet; and the husband should rest after work.[34]

Widerström's stronger concern with sexual hygiene might be understood against the background of sexually transmitted infections (STIs) such as syphilis and gonorrhoea, which were considered leading dangers to public health in Sweden and Finland.[35] Urbanisation and industrialisation, as well as the development of the working class, not only led to a new social order but also appeared to embrace a new, looser understanding of morality.[36] The seemingly uncontrolled sexuality of the lower classes, as well as the rise of prostitution in addition to the spread of STIs and increasing numbers of illegitimate children, endangered the health of the whole nation. STIs were not only an issue concerning the lower classes. Female doctors condemned middle-class men, in particular, for carrying the diseases into their homes and to their innocent families.[37]

Eskelin's later publications focused on the overall health of the family rather than on the sexual, mainly female, body. However, she focused predominately on middle and upper working class households. She did not provide any advice directed at poor families. Female doctors such as Eskelin considered educated housewives responsible enough to be able to read books. However, lower-class women had to be educated in a more direct way on proper hygienic behaviour. For this purpose, female doctors established health and hygiene advice offices in several Nordic cities.[38]

There were two leading health advice offices in the Nordic countries at the time: the office in Stockholm, led by Ada Nilsson and her colleagues from FKR; and the office run by the Norwegian sex educator Katti Anker Møller and her daughter, Tove Mohr.[39] My focus here is mainly on Nilsson's office in Stockholm, since Møller herself was not a physician, but her daughter was. However since Møller's office was to a certain extent a model for Nilsson, it will not go unmentioned here. Nilsson's office was discussed in a contemporary article in the magazine *Tidevarvet*. Her office had opened in 1925 and was designed in accordance with the example provided by Anker Møller. Male and female physicians worked alongside each other in Nilsson's office, the article explained.[40] The article argued that modern times had "a high impact on men's and women's relationships, as well as their entire sexual life".[41] This would require a new kind of guidance and a new understanding of sexuality in addition to education.[42] The article focused on both men and women, and not primarily on the housewife, as the earlier books by Eskelin and Widerström had. The author of the article argued that men and women needed education on sexuality and sex life. Nevertheless, the article further argued that the advice office ought to provide guidance for all men and women in economically and ethically difficult times. The office was not only intended for the poor or the sick, but for all women. It should provide care and help for exhausted mothers who, for economic or health reasons, did not wish to have more children.[43]

While the health advice office was described as being open to everyone, in practice its activities appeared to be targeted at poor and sick women. Middle class women had better access to birth control, and endless broods of children were primarily a characteristic of lower and working class families.[44] In addition, working and lower class women needed child care services because they often worked outside the home in addition to carrying out their family duties.

Nilsson did not only provide advice in her office but was also active in discussing public health in numerous articles in *Tidevarvet*. She discussed the reorganisation of the Medical Board in Sweden in an article series in 1926. Nilsson argued that it was crucial to solve contemporary social and medical issues, particularly issues related to compulsory maternal health care and help for mothers. Furthermore, she argued that hospital and epidemic care should become more effective, and that the positive effects of sport and gymnastics should be acknowledged. Ada Nilsson thus concluded that good health care, accessible to everyone, is of benefit for the whole population.[45]

Nilsson argued that female doctors were not only concerned with women's health, but with the overall health of the population as well. Mental and social health was also important to female doctors, and they associated these issues with public health. Their focus on women and mothers, as well as on childrearing, indicates that they operated with a wide conceptualisation of public health. The physical healthy body had to live in a healthy and hygienic environment to stay healthy and to provide a perfect breeding place for the next generation. Hence, there was a eugenic aspect in their understanding of public health. Not only was the health of the current generation of concern but also, in particular, the health of future generations.

Eugenics and prophylactic health care: The advance of public health

The idea of improving the quality of the population through positive and negative eugenics influenced policy making, science, medicine, social reforms and economics in the early twentieth century.[46] It would be an exaggeration to consider public health before the Second World War as primarily based on eugenic ideas, let alone to consider the ideologies the same. Nevertheless, in adopting and promoting prophylactic ideas of health care, the female doctors presented here were inspired by the eugenic idea of improving the quality of the population.

Eugenics was considered a part of progressive social policy. In Finland, doctor and feminist activist Rakel Jalas argued that preventive welfare work contributed to social progress.[47] Finnish feminists were interested in eugenic measures such as sterilisation in the context of a rising rate of sex crimes.[48] However, female doctors had a wider understanding of eugenics. While the term 'eugenics' was not always used, its principles are visible in several ideas expressed by female doctors.

All three female doctors discussed here were interested in eugenic ideas or used explicit eugenic rhetoric in the formulation of their understanding of public health. However, the use of eugenic rhetoric and ideas was not limited to women in the medical profession. Eva Palmblad argues that the topic of degeneration was of interest not only to the medical profession but also to people involved in politics, sociology, psychology and anthropology. Palmblad further argues that degeneration was a socio-biological concept useful for classifying people.[49] This social-hygienic perspective on the population enriched medicine as a discipline with a new dimension. According to Palmblad, the connection of medicine and social science resulted in a stronger link between public health and the social economy, while simultaneously increasing the political and social authority of medical experts.[50] On the one hand, the fear of degeneration and the notion of eugenic measures as a possible solution to this threat emphasised the national importance of the health of future generations. On the other, the association of social and medical problems with physical and moral degeneration provided doctors with a new role in society: the doctor was transformed from an expert on the body to an expert on the mind, the body and society.

Nilsson took a very positive stand on the new Swedish population policy in the 1920s and 1930s. In an article published in *Tidevarvet* in 1932, she claimed that the policy to increase the quality of the population was a most successful social initiative, more successful than any previous maternal and child care programme.[51] Nilsson looked at the population question from the perspective of economics. She considered birth control the most promising method for preventing degeneration among the population. She argued that it was the responsibility of the medical profession and the policy makers to provide society with birth control, and hence contribute positively to the development of population quality and public health.[52]

Nilsson, as a female physician and gynaecologist, argued for a stronger interaction between policy makers and medical professionals. From her point of view, the diffusion, or degeneration, of the nation's health was mainly happening because of disturbed sexuality. Sexuality and reproduction should be regulated through public health measures to improve the health of the people and the quality of the population. According to Nilsson, this was important not only for social reasons, but also for economic reasons.

More generally, eugenicists at the time focused on women and female sexuality.[53] Female reproduction was of special interest to the modern state because reproduction was both a private and a public matter.[54] However, in Finland, the concern over female sexuality was based not only on gender, but also on class. The class-based population policy in Finland was mainly concerned with women and their reproduction of the lower classes. Mothers constituted the main target group for family and housing policy. Hence, health experts and policy makers were particularly interested in issues concerning mothers and female sexuality.[55]

The class aspect was influential in Sweden as well. Karolina Widerström argued that uneducated women, in particular, had a tendency to organise their lives in inefficient ways. According to her, they wasted more time and energy in performing everyday tasks compared to educated women.[56] Widerström considered the body to be a resource that needed to be healthy and productive in daily household work and in the greater context of the reproduction of society. Moreover, she argued that women should care for their bodily hygiene from an early age. Every woman who wanted to be a mother should constantly care for her body, for example by maintaining good hygiene and by strengthening her bones, organs and nervous system. Widerström was concerned about the fact that only a few women were well suited to or equipped for motherhood; she was also concerned that women who were poorly equipped for motherhood became pregnant and bore children.[57]

The paragraph above illustrates Widerström's eugenic notions in several respects. For one, she considered a hygienic and healthy body as a source of success in life. This healthy body did not develop by itself but needed active care to prevent harms. Furthermore, Widerström divided mothers into the 'fit' and the 'unfit'.[58] This division relates to two ideas proclaimed by other eugenicists: firstly, the fear of a shortage of women capable of producing the next generation.[59] This was the leading idea of most eugenicists. Although the size of the population increased, its quality was constantly decreasing due to a lack of good population material. Secondly, there were women who, despite having the ability to reproduce, should be prevented from doing so as their offspring might cause societal harm. Widerström's argumentation can be related to Nilsson's claim that a beneficial population policy must be accompanied by preventing, through contraception, the birth of too many children or of defective children.

Karolina Eskelin was also concerned about the female body and sexual organs in the context of prophylactic health care and hygiene. In her book *Gynekologisk sjukvård* (Gynaecological Health Care), she argued that women of childbearing age, in particular married women, ought to take special care of their sexual organs. Eskelin advised regular consultations with a doctor and daily washing of the vulva.[60] However she recommended this special attention to the female sexual organs only for married women and women of reproductive age. She did not see any need for special care before menarche (the onset of menstruation) or after the menopause.[61] Prophylactic care and hygiene should focus on the female reproductive body, i.e., the body which produces the next generation. Eskelin's aim was not only to keep women healthy for their own sake, but also so that they were able to produce healthy and hygienic offspring. By advocating prophylactic care for the female body she had not only the private, female body and women's individual well-being in mind, but also that of the public, reproductive body, whose uncleanliness and illness might harm societal well-being.

To sum up, prophylactic health care advocated by the female doctors discussed here showed specific links to the eugenic ideas of the early twentieth century. Prophylactic health care advice focused on the female reproductive body. Women were advised on how to keep their sexual organs clean and their bodies healthy in order to be able to reproduce healthy offspring. Unclean or unhealthy women were advised to prevent pregnancy through birth control, as Ada Nilsson suggested. The individual female body was not the only concern of prophylactic health care; the public, national woman's body was also to be cared for. The concern that an unhealthy female body would produce defective offspring and affect the present and future health of the nation was great. Prophylactic health care for women was about overall societal well-being, and not just about the health of the individual. Eugenic and public health ideas intersected in the aim to create a better future society and end the degeneration of the population.

Conclusions

The first generation of female doctors in Sweden and Finland in the early twentieth century took a special interest in women's health and the female body, and promoted the well-being of women. Karolina Widerström, Karolina Eskelin and Ada Nilsson were among the first professional women to draw special attention to the health and hygienic needs of women in the public sphere and in policy making. They were also the first to provide other women with extensive and open information about the female body and sexuality – through books, lectures and in health advice offices.

Female medical experts followed a trend that combined concern for the individual health of the citizen with social policy making.[62] Health and hygiene became political issues. The physician became a central figure not only in curing diseases, but also in preventing illness in the first place. This made them crucial actors in societal life.[63] Health was no longer a private concern but a societal, national and political matter.

The new female doctors acquired a special place in establishing the new role of medical experts in the public health discourse of the early twentieth century. Their focus was on providing various forms of health education to women (particularly housewives) in order to prevent the spread of diseases within the home and the family, and to keep the reproductive female body healthy and clean, in addition to guaranteeing the health of future generations. The female doctors wanted to educate ordinary housewives. This was a new aspect in medical care: women were both providers and recipients of care. The former private role of women as carers for the home was now transformed into a public role.[64] Women doctors continued their female duties of caring at a societal level, legitimated by their new expert status and monitored by (male) policy makers.

However, the prophylactic health advice from female doctors drew on the discourse about the degeneration of the population, and they regarded eugenic ideas as possible solutions for the challenge ahead. Female doctors were mainly concerned with providing information for women of reproductive age in order to ensure a healthy future generation.[65] They also provided extensive advice on childrearing, as well as on housing, nutrition and clothing, in order to promote public health.

The first generation of female doctors had a significant impact on the development of prophylactic health care measures in Sweden and Finland and the centralisation of the female body in the public health discourse. On the one hand, this resulted in extensive welfare benefits for and improvement in the individual health of both mothers and children. On the other hand, the attention was partly drawn so heavily to the female body and sexuality that the public health discourse became a restrictive organ to control and shape the female body as public concern for the nation's well-being, and disregarded the individual well-being and rights of the woman, for example, through the restriction of reproduction by eugenic sterilisation.

Notes

1 Ulrika Nilsson, 'Kön, klass och vetenskaplig auktoritet: Om kvinnliger läkarpionjärer', in *Vetenskapsbärarna*, ed. Sven Widmalm (Hedemora: Gidlung, 1999), 144.
2 Ulrika Nilsson, *Det heta könet: Gynekologin i Sverige kring förra sekelskiftet* (Stockholm: Wahlström & Widstrand, 2005), 63–4.
3 See, e.g., Karolina Eskelin, *Gynekologisk sjukvård* (Porvoo: WSOY, 1924); Karolina Eskelin, *Personlig hälsövård med särskild hänsyn till bostad* (Helsinki: Föreningen för bekämpandet af tuberkulosen, 1925), first published in Swedish and later in Finnish as *Henkilökohtaisesta terveydenhoidosta* (Porvoo: WSOY, 1927).
4 Sirpa Wrede, 'Befolkningspolitik och kvinnokontroll: Mödrarådgivningens dolda ideologi i Finland från sekelskiftet till Efterkrigstiden', in *Kvinnors hälsa och ohälsa. Social kontroll av kvinnor*, ed. Ulrica Hägglund and Elianne Riska (Åbo: Åbo Akademi, 1991), 54.
5 Nilsson, *Det heta könet*, 65.
6 Tuomo Olkkonen, 'Suomen ensimmäinen naistohtori', *Opusculum* 5, no.3 (1985): 122–8, 122.
7 '100 vuotta naisten tieteellistä työtä: Karolina Eskelin ja Tekla Hultin – ensimmäiset naistohtorimme', *Naistutkimustiedote* 16, no. 4 (1996): 13–16, 13.
8 Ulrik Knutson, *Kvinnor på gränsen till genombrott. Grupporträtt av Tidevarvets kvinnor* (Stockholm: Bonnier, 2004), 31.
9 Ibid., 29.
10 Ibid., 30.
11 Hjördis Levin, *Kvinnorna på barrikaden. Sexualpolitik och sociala frågor 1923–1936* (Stockholm: Carlsson, 1997), 15.
12 Prohibiting public advertisements for contraception, *lex hinke* was a law implemented in Sweden between 1911 and 1938.
13 Nilsson, *Det heta könet*, 256.

14   Olkkonen, 'Suomen ensimmäinen naistohtori', 124–5.
15   Nilsson, 'Kön, klass och vetenskaplig auktoritet', 156–7.
16   Ada Nilsson, *Glimtar ur mitt liv som läkare* (Stockholm: Natur och Kultur, 1963), 37.
17   Ibid., 59.
18   Nilsson, 'Kön, klass och vetenskaplig auktoritet', 164.
19   '100 vuotta', 14.
20   "Kvinnan har åt sig av vår moder naturen fått överlämnad den väsentliga och större parten av de livsprocesser, hvilka åstadkomma släktets fortplantning. Men hon har länge föga vårdat sig om att söka närmare lära känna dessa de underbaraste och beundransvärdaste av alla livsprocesser eller att taga kännedom om de organ, inom hvilka de försiggå." Karolina Widerström, *Kvinnohygien I: De kvinnliga underlifsorganen, ders förrättningar och yård* (Stockholm: Norstedt & Söner, 1903), 3.
21   See Chapter 6 by Annika Berg and Teemu Ryymin for a discussion on translating the Swedish word *släkte*.
22   Wrede, 'Befolkningspolitik och kvinnokontroll', 58.
23   Eva Palmblad and Bengt Erik Eriksson, *Kropp och politik: Hälsoupplysning som samhällsspegel från 30- till 90-tal* (Stockholm: Carlsson, 1995), 23.
24   Eskelin, *Personlig hälsövård*, 5–7.
25   Elianne Riska, 'Kvinnors sjuklighet: Den bortglömda siffran i hälsoforskningen', in *Kvinnors hälsa och ohälsa: Social kontroll av kvinnor*, ed. Ulrica Hägglund and Elianne Riska (Åbo: Åbo Akademi, 1991), 21.
26   Karolina Eskelin, *Om hygienin i allmogehemmen och späda barns vård* (Helsingfors: Föreningen Martha, 1914), 3–4.
27   Ibid., 5.
28   Eva Palmblad, *Medicinen som samhällslära* (Daidalos: Gothenburg, 1990), 12.
29   Ibid., 15.
30   Inger Elisabeth Haavet, 'Milk, mothers and marriage: Family policy formation in Norway and its neighbouring countries in the twentieth century', in *The Nordic Model of Welfare: A Historical Reappraisal*, ed. Niels Finn Christiansen et al. (Copenhagen: Museum Tusculanum Press, 2006), 189–214, 191–2.
31   Widerström, *Kvinnohygien I*, 30.
32   Palmblad, *Medicinen som samhällslara*, 15.
33   Eskelin, *Personlig hälsovård*, 8ff.
34   Ibid., 43ff.
35   Levin, *Kvinnor på barrikaden*, 45.
36   Ibid., 18.
37   Karolina Widerström, *Kvinnohygien II: Om den veneriska sjukdomarna och deras bekämpanda* (Stockholm: Norstedt & Söner, 1905), 28.
38   Levin, *Kvinnor på barrikaden*, 216.
39   Nils Roll-Hansen, 'Norwegian eugenics: Sterilization as social reform', in *Eugenics and the Welfare State: Sterilization Policy in Denmark, Sweden, Norway and Finland*, ed. Gunnar Broberg and Nils Roll-Hansen (East Lansing: Michigan State University Press, 2005), 151–94, 161.
40   I.B. 'Efter sex veckor: Erfahrenheter från Tidevarvet's rådgivningsbyrå', *Tidevarvet* 31 (1925): 1.
41   "Detta inverkar i oerhörd grad på mäns och kvinnors inbördes förhållanden, på hela det sexuella livsområdet." Ibid.
42   Ibid.
43   Ibid., 4.
44   See for more on this, for example Levin, *Kvinnor på barrikaden*; Hera Cook, *The Long Sexual Revolution: English Women, Sex and Contraception, 1800–1975* (Oxford: Oxford University Press, 2004).
45   Ada Nilsson, 'Folkhälsan och Medicinalväsendet', *Tidevarvet* 46 (1926): 2.

46 Positive eugenics describes inducements for reproduction, for example, money endowments, medical care or maternity leave. Negative eugenics refers to the restriction of reproduction through, for instance, contraception, marriage restrictions or sterilisation. See also Chapter 2 by Paul Weindling in this volume.

47 Marjatta Hietala, 'From race hygiene to sterilization: The eugenics movement in Finland', in *Eugenics and the Welfare State. Sterilization Policy in Denmark, Sweden, Norway and Finland*, ed. Gunnar Broberg and Nils Roll-Hansen (East Lansing: Michigan State University Press, 2005), 195–258, 229.

48 Ibid.

49 Palmblad, *Medicinen som samhällslara*, 19.

50 Ibid., 31.

51 Ada Nilsson, 'Kommentarer till befolkningspolitiken', *Tidevarvet* 34 (1932): 3.

52 Ibid.

53 For a more extensive discussion of this phenomenon, see Maija Runcis, *Steriliseringar i folkhemmet* (Stockholm: Ordfront, 1998).

54 Wrede, 'Befolkningspolitik och kvinnokontroll', 93.

55 Ibid., 86.

56 Widerström, *Kvinnohygien I*, 39.

57 Ibid., 58.

58 See also Chapter 1 in this volume for Francis Galton's ideas on eugenics.

59 Mariana Valverde, 'When the mother of the race is free: Race, reproduction, and sexuality in first-wave feminism', in *Gender Conflicts: New Essays in Women's History*, ed. Franca Iacovetta and Mariana Valverde (Toronto: University of Toronto Press, 2002), 3–26, 7–8; Hietala, 'From race hygiene to sterilisation', 209.

60 Eskelin, *Gynekologisk sjukvård*, 148.

61 Ibid., 144, 150.

62 Palmblad, *Medicinen som samhällslara*, 15.

63 Ibid., 11.

64 Haavet, 'Milk, mothers and marriages', 191.

65 Ibid.,192.

4   The Nazis' cloven hoof:

Finnish critiques of legal sterilisation

Ainur Elmgren

Health care and civil rights

The critics of invasive eugenic measures in Finland have been described as "marginal figures".[1] Professionals in health care and education preferred to publish their criticism of eugenics and sterilisation under pseudonyms. In contrast, cultural journalists and writers felt freer to come forth under their own names, or under well-known pseudonyms. However, in some cases they came to regret this, as in the case of the Finnish poet and political columnist Katri Vala, who lamented in a letter to her husband in 1936: "I am a lightning conductor for the wrath of the reactionaries . . . Few have sacrificed as much as I have."[2]

Although Katri Vala (1901–1944) and her brother Erkki (1902–1991) wrote editorials under pen names, their identities were well known. In the late 1920s and the 1930s, their public personas were strongly connected to the literary journal *Tulenkantajat* and other left-liberal publications. Editor-in-chief Erkki Vala – a vocal proponent of freedom of speech and opponent of fascism – was no stranger to public controversy, and used his journal to champion unpopular causes.

The Swedish Sterilisation Act proposal coincided with a general tightening of political rights in Finland. Hence, the sterilisation debate needs to be seen in the context of this atmosphere of repression and obstruction. In 1930, anti-communist laws limiting freedom of speech and association had been introduced under pressure of the extra-parliamentary Lapua Movement. Favourable to the Lapua movement, the nationalist student organisation Akateeminen Karjala-Seura (Academic Karelia Society, AKS) was influential in the ousting of Vala from the editorial board of the first edition of *Tulenkantajat* before the magazine folded for financial reasons in 1930. In 1932, Lapua's most militant wing attempted a coup, and a new amendment to limit press freedom was introduced in response. The scattered movement reorganised as a fascist-inspired party, the Patriotic People's Movement, which demanded the prohibition of the Social Democratic Party. Erkki Vala had joined the latter in solidarity, and was inspired to relaunch *Tulenkantajat* in 1932.

The Vala siblings' civil rights activism took place in a wider European context of a generation of intellectuals and artists, coming of age after the First World War and the Bolshevik Revolution, and confronting the ready-made frontlines of their precedents – in the Finnish case, those of the Civil War in 1918. They could choose conformity in the safe haven of 'non-political' expertise – the equivalent of the *chiens de garde* decried by French Marxist Paul Nizan in 1932.[3] For Nizan, this detachment from politics, this supposed neutrality and objectivity, was a smokescreen to hide the intellectuals' subservience to the state and support of the dominant classes. The other choice, which attracted both left- and right-wing youth, was to devote themselves to a struggle for society's renewal – either by overthrowing the capitalist system of exploitation or through a 'national rebirth' or 'awakening'. The Vala siblings did not so much seek out any of these missions as end up being pushed towards a Marxist analysis of society while trying to maintain their liberal patriotism. When the Valas protested against the Sterilisation Act, they attacked those ostensibly neutral experts who, in their opinion, ignored progressive opinions and participated in an ideological struggle to limit human rights and steer the entire Finnish society closer to Nazism.[4]

The question of the people's health and the question of civil rights had been connected at least since the election reform of 1906, when nine criteria were introduced to limit a citizen's right to vote and right to be elected. It has been estimated that up to 15 per cent of the population, meaning about 200,000 Finns, were not eligible to vote in the early twentieth century.[5] Besides the thousands of Finns who had lost their civil rights for siding with the Reds in the Civil War of 1918, there were also numerous persons who were categorised in accordance with the law as destitute, sick and feeble-minded – and consequently ineligible to vote.

Constitutional authority Rafael Erich explained in 1908 that the individual did not exercise their political rights for their own personal benefit, but for the general good and the public interest.[6] The prerequisite for the use of political rights was the individual's moral, free, self-aware and personal activity on behalf of the state – that is, for a higher goal than the individual's personal benefit. Nature herself had put limitations on these abilities: part of the population would always be careless, unworthy and irresponsible – and thus incapable of acting as citizens. The sterilisation committee echoed this view in its 1929 memorandum: "A commonly accepted principle of justice is that the individual's right has to cede, when his and the society's interests are in conflict with each other."[7]

Those who were left without political rights were largely the same groups whose procreation concerned the eugenicists.[8] A healthy national body consisted of healthy citizens – health became a prerequisite for good citizenship.[9] The politically restless years of the early twentieth century convinced many conservative authorities of the wisdom of such caution. The political anxieties of both Finnish- and Swedish-speaking conservatives found their expression in biologist and medical metaphors of 'disease', 'infection', 'chirurgical operation' and 'the chancre of anarchy' after the Civil War of 1918.[10] Although social reforms were deemed necessary to 'cure' the working class, they were embedded in patriotic ideology that emphasised obedience, unity and moral as well as physiological purity. Eugenic legislation was an additional tool to mould the Finnish people into a single healthy national body, and to restrict the possible political influence of the 'unfit' – who, as Finnish eugenicist Harry Federley claimed, had taken over Bolshevist Russia.[11]

In 1925, a committee for the preparation of a law on eugenic sterilisation was founded in Finland, and its work continued to the following decade.[12] The journal for professionals in jurisprudence, *Lakimies*, simultaneously discussed eugenic motives for a reform of the marriage law.[13] The marriage law of 1929 limited the right of epileptics and deaf-mutes to marry to apply only under condition of sterilisation: the mentally ill, imbeciles and close blood relatives were not permitted to marry at all.[14] This did not stop illicit unions from producing offspring, but sterilisation provided a solution. The reports of the parliamentary committee in preparation for the 1935 Sterilisation Act reveal that the committee left for future consideration the possibility of expanding compulsory sterilisation from "the idiot, the imbecile, and the mentally ill" to epileptics, alcoholics and criminals.[15] Crimes that could prove an individual's "unnatural sexual drive" – either in intensity or orientation, and potential "danger to another person" – were already included in the act as valid reasons for sterilisation.[16] The second paragraph of the Sterilisation Act permitted voluntary sterilisation if there was reason to believe that the individual would sire 'deficient' offspring, or if their sexual drive or orientation would compel them to commit crimes. During the committee's final year of preparatory work, sterilisation proponents frequented conferences on crime prevention to publicise the proposals.[17]

Previous research has revealed the extent to which the sterilisation law was supported by contemporaries.[18] However, criticism was voiced already in the 1920s. In 1928, a columnist in *Kurikka*, the satirical journal of the Social Democratic Party, commented on the sterilisation committee's work: "The purpose is good, but it's a different story how such a law will work out in practice." With a touch of crude humour, he noted that governments had "on occasion cut the heads off their political opponents, why would they shy away from another kind of operation". How could anyone, potentially 'unfit', be trusted with the power to decide another's 'fitness'? "Thank God that we did not have such a law during those years of 'weeding'; in what shape would the survivors have returned from the prison camps!"[19] The euphemism 'weeding' referred to the bloody aftermath of the Finnish Civil War, when thousands of Red prisoners-of-war were put before summary military courts or languished in prison camps around the country. In 1931, a satirical verse in *Kurikka* compared anti-socialist purges to the eugenic sterilisation of farm animals in order to produce 'good bourgeois pigs'.[20]

The struggle for civil rights

In 1934, the same year the Sterilisation Act was proposed, a law to prevent agitation harmful to society and legal order was passed (popularly known as *kiihotuslaki*, 'agitation law') that limited the freedom of the press. *Tulenkantajat* opposed both laws openly. After the law on the protection of the republic was abolished in 1935, the 1934 'agitation law' continued to be enforced against the press, sometimes rather arbitrarily. Erkki Vala was fined in 1935 and briefly imprisoned in 1936 for crimes against this 'agitation law'.[21] A sarcastic comment illustrates his experiences as a well-known journalist during these years:

the only way to avoid press trials in our clerical state is to begin a campaign for general dismemberment of human beings through capital punishment, castration and caning. This is not [seen as] agitation, but true patriotism.[22]

Both Katri Vala and her brother were personally touched by the issue in more ways than one. Both were suffering from tuberculosis (TB), considered a *kansantauti* ('people's disease') because of its prevalence.[23] In combination with wartime deprivation, its consequences were often lethal. Tuberculosis brought Katri Vala's life to a premature end in 1944. Their younger brother, the translator Niilo Wadenström, and their mother, Alexandra Wadenström, died of the same disease in 1945.[24] Erkki's son, Klaus Vala, spent some time at a TB sanatorium as a teenager in the late 1940s.[25]

Health and sexuality questions intimately shaped the lives of many of the young intellectuals' friends and acquaintances. The first literary treatment of the sterilisation question, the novel *Hedelmätön puu* (The Fruitless Tree, 1932), was written by Unto Koskela, who belonged to the wider circle of young writers and poets around the first *Tulenkantajat*.[26] The novel's account of sterilisation as a prerequisite for marriage, and its traumatic consequences, was partly based on Koskela's own experience of epilepsy.[27] The heredity of epilepsy was poorly understood at the time, and the legal restrictions were based on accumulated custom and prejudice rather than scientific study. In Sweden and Finland, congenital epilepsy had been considered a legal impediment to marriage since the eighteenth century.[28] It is not clear if contemporaries were aware of the novel's autobiographical character. Critics praised it as the first Finnish psychological novel.[29] Katri Vala's lukewarm review in *Tulenkantajat* lauded the protagonist's "responsible" decision to request sterilisation, but called for a novel on a different topic: the suffering of those who were forced into childlessness by poverty.[30] Vala's own concerns may have coloured her review. In 1931 she had given birth to a girl who lived for only a few hours. After this tragedy, Vala's poetry increasingly dwelt on topics such as suffering, motherhood and the protection of children.[31]

There were other entry points to the broader topic of health care and coercion. As TB patients, the Wadenström-Vala family had experiences of different health care strategies, some more coercive than others, including institutionalisation and hygiene education.[32] *Tulenkantajat* addressed this topic in the 1930s, alerting its readers to perceived abuses in the institutionalisation of TB patients and connecting the abuses to the questionable state of democracy and civil rights in Finland.[33]

Another less openly discussed affliction was mental illness. Erkki and Katri's father, Robert Wadenström, had spent his final years in a mental hospital, and their youngest sibling, Niilo, was considered mentally troubled.[34] In *Tulenkantajat*, problems in the treatment of institutionalised mental patients were also connected to democracy issues.[35] This may have contributed to the siblings' strong opinions against enforced sterilisation of those considered 'unfit', turning with passion against the "dangerous proposal" in 1934, which would enable "arbitrary abuse of power", and which represented "downright barbarism" to them.[36]

Tulenkantajat provided a platform for some of the most publicly visible scientists opposing sterilisation. Väinö Lassila, Professor of Anatomy at the University of

Helsinki and champion of pacifism and civil rights, provided the voice of the rational and socially responsible scientist. In *Tulenkantajat*, Lassila referred to the holistic concept of 'people's health', written as two words – *kansan terveys*.[37] He emphasised the importance of prophylactic care, arguing for the economic advantages of rehabilitation versus institutionalisation of supposedly incurable cases. In his critiques of sterilisation, Lassila noted the lack of scientific evidence of its efficiency, cast doubt on its economic benefits and debunked racial theories imported from Germany.[38]

Tulenkantajat also gleaned arguments from the paediatrician Torild Brander, who criticised the Sterilisation Act's definition of intelligence and imbecility for being too vague and likely to cause arbitrary selection.[39] Not only experts were cited. An anonymous 'man of the people' turned both scientific and socioeconomic concerns against the proposal: "When science as yet cannot give an undisputed answer on the effects of sterilisation, who will take care of those idiots that sterilisation will possibly bring into existence?"[40] Even among the enlightened bourgeoisie, critics were to be found, such as the governor of Åland, a medical doctor by profession, who had requested that the act would not be passed before other countries had tested the procedure.[41] Consequently, no sterilisations were carried out in Åland.[42]

Besides doctors and experts of the natural sciences, *Tulenkantajat* interviewed scholars of the humanities, who presented historical arguments against the supposed benefits of sterilisation. Oskar von Schoultz, Senior Lecturer in Russian Literature at the University of Helsinki, listed famous personalities who, despite suffering from epilepsy, had contributed to the accomplishments of humanity.[43] The result of an implementation of the Sterilisation Act would be nothing less than a barbaric people "without Porthans or 'Dostoyevskys'". Both the trailblazing Finnish eighteenth-century historian Henrik Gabriel Porthan and the revered Russian author Feodor Dostoyevsky were descended from ancestors who had suffered from various congenital diseases or mental illness.[44]

In *Tulenkantajat*, the most important argument against the Sterilisation Act was that it would place power over the individual in the hands of officials and professionals, who would be able to exercise inordinate power arbitrarily and obliquely: "The most dangerous [end] is giving the authorities rights and freedoms over the treatment of citizens that no organ of elected representatives can control." *Tulenkantajat* did not oppose sterilisation of the truly sick, Erkki Vala admitted in one instance, but could not "accept that another new and terrifying weapon without effective control is put in the hands of the authorities that evidently function in a class society and whose frontline is drawn against the lowest and poorest layers of the people".[45]

Foreign experts with antifascist credentials supplied proof of the dangers of such a 'weapon'. German sexologist Magnus Hirschfeld had personally experienced persecution in Nazi Germany. Hirschfeld's most important argument against eugenic sterilisation was based on scientific scepticism. He noted that most of the afflictions that sterilisation targeted were not conclusively proven to be hereditary, and that many highly talented individuals had been proven as descended from 'unfit' ones, and vice versa.[46] Norwegian doctor Karl Evang also criticised Nazi racial hygiene policies.[47] Both Hirschfeld and Evang were socialists, and identified a serious danger in political abuse of eugenic laws. However, in his contemporary book *Rasepolitikk og reaksjon* Evang stated that the 'socialist planned society' would include 'the rational idea' of limiting harmful hereditary traits.[48]

Evang's arguments were selectively picked to support the editorial line against sterilisation. Occasionally, other opinions slipped through. For *Tulenkantajat*, Kaisu Snellman, a lecturer on sexual hygiene, interviewed American birth control activist Margaret Sanger, whose opinions on sterilisation differed radically from the journal's position. Sanger endorsed compulsory sterilisation of certain groups with hereditary disabilities.[49] In the interview, she maintained that sterilisation was needed in cases where other birth control methods would fail, and that sterilisation was not harmful to the individual – contrary to abortion, which she vehemently opposed.[50]

Tulenkantajat attempted to deter support by collecting examples of coercive sterilisation from many different sources and presenting them as Nazi atrocities.[51] According to a dramatic account from Halle, Germany, thousands of children and adults had been coercively sterilised – some of whom were merely malnourished, not congenitally 'unfit'.[52] When a German gynaecologist lectured about eugenics in Helsinki, *Tulenkantajat* summarised his policy as "kill the weak!"[53] Threats by individual MPs to tighten the Sterilisation Act, according to *Tulenkantajat*, revealed the "Nazis' cloven hoof", the actual ideology behind the eugenics programme.[54] However, as studies on the British eugenics debate also have shown, the Nazi scare had little effect on leading representatives of a society that identified itself as democratic and rational.[55]

After the passing of the Sterilisation Act, Erkki Vala linked it to other attacks on civil rights, such as the proposal to widen the scope of capital punishment in 1935, and defined the "greatest danger to democracy" as "the continuous limitation of human rights".[56] He came to see the Sterilisation Act as part of a greater programme to exercise arbitrary power over the people. Using Orientalist stereotypes to satirise the nationalist image of Finland as a bulwark against the barbaric East, Vala decried the "attempt to turn Finland into a kind of mandarin state, where an ordinary citizen may be gagged, thrown into prison, sterilised and executed just as in some sort of ancient Oriental satrapy".[57] As a countermeasure to the sanitising euphemisms in the pro-sterilisation discourse, Vala used the term *kuohitseminen* (castration, primarily of animals).[58]

Tulenkantajat quoted some of the Finnish proponents of sterilisation, such as Harry Federley and Karin Neuman-Rahn (nurse and mental health expert), to reveal their ideological connections. According to Federley, the time "when it was generally believed that human beings were all alike at birth" was finally past.[59] Neuman-Rahn praised the German people who reputedly saw "in this [eugenic] law a religious necessity".[60] The economic arguments for sterilisation were linked to the threat of militarisation at the expense of social policy. Vala commented that Germany had been able to finance its new and enormous armament programme "by declaring social care work semi-criminal".[61] The connection between coercive sterilisation and a feared rise of fascism in Finland, through legal or illegal means, was most explicitly made by an anonymous letter to the editor which supported the idea of a 'popular front' between liberals and leftists:

> [C]apital punishment, the sterilisation act [and] the national question in the service of Fascism . . . are serving the same cause: the rise of Fascism to power and preparations for a coming war. And if we intend to stop the rise of Fascism, its opponents also have to submit thousands of minor issues to serve the greater whole: resistance to Fascism. And this can be done through the united mass struggle of the intellectuals, the workers and the farmers against each and every appearance of Fascism and its attempts to take control.[62]

The idea of a 'popular front' worried the authorities to such an extent that even Professor Lassila became the target of police surveillance. According to *Etsivä keskuspoliisi*, the secret police, the illegal Finnish Communist Party had agreed to support Lassila's candidacy during the parliamentary elections of 1936 on the list of the liberal National Progressive Party.[63] In 1936, a leak revealed that the secret police had compiled 'popular front memorandums' listing individuals and organisations susceptible to communist infiltration. These documents had been supplied secretly and illegally to prosecutors and judges to influence their decisions. The memorandums included Väinö Lassila and Erkki Vala, and cast doubt on anyone involved with 'anti-fascist' or 'human rights' activities. In the far-right press, Lassila was subsequently nicknamed *ihmisoikeus-Lassila* ('human rights Lassila').[64]

Erkki Vala himself did not shy away from politically tainted terminology. He called for a "united front of sensible people" against sterilisation, using another term with a political connotation of communist collaboration.[65] Ironically, Vala also called for the co-operation of all 'healthy' elements of the Finnish people to fight against the 'sick brains' that had conceived the 'unnatural' idea of negative eugenics.[66]

Eugenic class war

The greatest threat of the Sterilisation Act identified by Erkki Vala was that it appealed to authorities who wanted to reduce spending on the poor. Indeed, the motivation for the adoption of negative racial hygiene was "a bundle of reasons, encompassing the sexuality and fecundity of degenerates, the laws of heredity, and economic factors".[67] Already in 1926, the sterilisation committee had been approached by municipal authorities complaining about the financial burden of poor relief.[68] Critics of the law warned of the likelihood that social arguments for sterilisation – for example when an individual was deemed to be unable to support offspring – would favour the wealthier classes. The law would thus turn into a 'class law'.[69] However, the Social Democrat newspaper also published opinion pieces that advocated a 'moderate' version of the act, arguing that it only targeted a minority.[70]

In the general Finnish discussion on sterilisation, eugenic arguments were intermingled with social, medical and economic concerns. It was this tangled mass of arguments that led to the broad acceptance of the law, even though critics, such as Vala, tried to expose the weaknesses that they perceived in every individual argument. The situation might be compared to the debate in Great Britain, where a sterilisation law was not passed despite an ongoing public debate in the late 1920s and 1930s. Apparently, the eugenics society of Britain insufficiently utilised such a broad arsenal of arguments in favour of sterilisation, focusing on racial eugenics and therefore failing to build broad networks of support.[71] In the Finnish case, economic arguments seemed to have a stronger persuasive power over politicians than other types of argument.

Tulenkantajat argued that a ratification of the Sterilisation Act would deny that humanity could be elevated through education and the bettering of societal conditions: "For us, it is incomprehensible that, for example, any socialist could accept this."[72] Vala criticised the economic arguments as inhuman, and posed the rhetorical question: "Was the law proposal sent to the parliamentary committee on economic affairs and not the constitutional committee because the question is viewed solely as a matter of poor relief?"[73] On the pages of *Tulenkantajat*, the parliamentary debates revealed the true intentions of some politicians, who "seemed to understand well that it was [a class law]", because they proposed that "sterilisation should be commissioned for free in state hospitals" – obviously assuming that the sterilised would be chosen from among the proletariat.[74] Lassila expressed concern over the "social reasons" glossed over in the law proposal, which referred to the opinion of an anonymous "respected source" that the parents' economic misery and other social circumstances would be reason enough for sterilisation.[75]

Finally, the Sterilisation Act was passed by a clear majority in parliament, with 144 MPs in favour and 14 against. The opponents did not constitute a single coherent political grouping, comprising Social Democrats, Swedish-speaking liberals, conservative Christians and centrist members of the Agrarian Union. A vicar and member of the Patriotic People's Movement condemned the law as "immoral" and "unnecessary", but stated that opposing such a popular law was bound to fail.[76] With headlines such as "Sterilisation Humbug Arouses General Resistance", *Tulenkantajat* tried disprove that the law was widely supported. It declared that people in all parties were resisting the "madness" and voicing their disgust towards this law "that deeply offends the individual's rights and the notion of humanity".[77] However, few examples were to be found in the press.[78] Even according to its own words, *Tulenkantajat* appeared as the only newspaper in Finland that had opposed the act.[79] In his editorials, Erkki Vala persistently claimed that 'the people' remained suspicious of the act, even though they could not get their voices heard.[80] In other words, *Tulenkantajat* tried to present the will of the people so it appeared consistent with its own position.

A year after the act was passed, *Tulenkantajat* confirmed that the municipalities that applied for permission to sterilise individuals were disproportionately targeting the poorer classes.[81] Other contemporaries, such as an anonymous author in the social workers' trade paper *Huoltaja*, likewise expressed concern, noting that women were also disproportionately targeted by the law.[82] Indeed, promoters of the Sterilisation Act like Harry Federley had stated openly that its most important effect would be economic.[83] The suspicion that sterilisation was being used as a political weapon also seemed to find some confirmation. Under an alarming headline, "Sterilisation of Society's Oppositional Elements Starts Now", Erkki Vala noted that the proposed form for a doctor's statement on sterilisation of a patient required information on "opposition towards society [*yhteiskuntavastaisuus*]" in the patient's family tree.[84] Erkki Vala's *Tulenkantajat* collaborator, Marxist literary critic Raoul Palmgren, stated that the sterilisation law belonged to the numerous "grotesque" forms of the latter stage of capitalism, when human rights were declared treasonous.[85]

Vala's strategy resembled Catholic criticism of eugenic sterilisation in the United States in the 1930s. Instead of resorting to arguments founded on religious dogma, Catholic critics utilised the moral argument of universal natural rights along with scientific arguments, casting doubt on the efficacy of the methods that the sterilisation advocates promoted.[86] Vala, too, quoted scientists and experts, sometimes selectively. These arguments were intermingled with the social question and criticism of the capitalist class society. Vala, undoubtedly supported by Marxist colleagues, considered a critical analysis of capitalism and the class society to be scientifically founded. At the same time, he did not hesitate to refer to the authority of principled opponents of sterilisation that were not Marxist, such as the Catholic Church.[87] Simultaneously, the fact that sterilisation laws were about to be passed in Scandinavian countries was vehemently denied or simply kept quiet about in the otherwise pro-Scandinavian *Tulenkantajat*.[88]

Although repression and coercive means coloured the image of public health initiatives during the sterilisation debate, this was also the time of a slow but steady breakthrough of the idea that the citizen had a *right* to health care.[89] There was a growing demand for sexual health education and information about contraception. In 1934, as the plan for a public sexual advice station was presented to the City of Helsinki, Katri Vala defended it against moralist attacks.[90] She dismissed worries about "illegal marital life" and "diminishing birth-rates", stating that a law limiting the natural and healthy impulses of free individuals was obsolete. Immigration from overpopulated countries could easily compensate for the lack of new births. She shared some concerns with her contemporary progressive eugenicists; but, instead of blaming the lower classes for producing deficient offspring, she condemned the ideal bourgeois marriage as a breeding-ground of "spiritual suffering, disease, poisoned life and unhappy children".[91] The precondition for healthy life was societal change and the end of a system based on the exploitation of large parts of the population, which was also the cause of degeneration among the middle and upper classes.

Understanding the priority of economic arguments in the public discourse, Professor Lassila argued after the passing of the Sterilisation Act that the capital invested in prophylactic social and health care would be repaid a hundredfold. Children were "the true Greater Finland", and the children of the poor deserved generous support. These were the foundations of a health care for a society built on democracy. When democratic rights were threatened, all its gains were put at risk. Institutionalisation and enforced labour under denigrating circumstances were made possible by legislation, but threatened the well-being of the whole nation by attacking the poor and the feeble-minded and increasing suffering and disease.[92]

"In a classless society, the situation would be different"

The resistance to the sterilisation law was not free of instrumental thinking. While the pro-sterilisation activists saw the individual as subjected to a greater good, the health of the nation, the anti-sterilisation activists of *Tulenkantajat* claimed that it was the capitalist class society that provided an obstacle to a rational application of such a law – which opened up the possibility that in a socialist, classless society, the situation might be different. Most of the opinions expressed in *Tulenkantajat*, especially by the Vala siblings, did not draw such a conclusion, but remained adamant in the defence of individual rights. As a voluntary choice by the individual, sterilisation was an acceptable measure that ought to be legal. However, as the case of Unto Koskela showed, the reasons for this voluntary decision often stemmed from societal pressure: a belief in the heredity of diseases and the responsibility of the individual to submit their personal desires to the needs of the greater whole. Perhaps with this in mind, Lassila opposed the legalisation of voluntary sterilisation with the argument that current contraceptive methods were adequate for the person potentially able to make a voluntary decision.[93]

What circumstances would make sterilisation an actual free choice by the individual, and not an imposition by society under external pressure? Some Social Democrats, such as Karl Evang or Karl Harald (K.H.) Wiik expressed the belief that a classless society would provide a neutral basis for sterilisation decisions.[94] They did not explain how such a society would make the individual's unalienable rights obsolete. Facing the fact that the law was about to be passed with a clear majority in parliament, Erkki Vala proposed a compromise specifying that the Sterilisation Act would only concern "voluntary sterilisation" and that all references to coercion would be removed. Anything else would mean the loss of ideas about justice and humanism that were the fruit of "centuries of struggle".[95] Vala's position on the question of voluntary versus coercive sterilisation vacillated between pragmatic acceptance and principled opposition until the law was passed, after which the sterilisation question was easier to integrate in a broader struggle against fascism.

Katri Vala was the only author who consequently addressed sterilisation and contraception as something that should be a personal choice, despite her conviction of the sanctity of motherhood. She defended the choice against reproduction as 'natural' at a time when freedom and humanity were increasingly under attack: "The world is now a powder keg, or a barrel of poison gas. That is not a suitable place for a new human life."[96] She also defended unmarried couples against accusations of immorality, reminding them of their often harsh economic circumstances.[97] She avoided judgement of any individual as less deserving of rights on hereditary grounds.

Tulenkantajat presented other answers to the social ills that Finland's leading eugenicists tried to treat with enforced sterilisation. Instead of coercive negative eugenics, the journal focused on positive measures that also belonged to the arsenal of eugenicists. Sexual education and health policies required more far-reaching planning and investment, anathema to conservatives who argued that a person with a 'healthy' moral sense would only approach sexuality on an instinctive, subconscious level.[98] Lassila emphasised the importance of pre-emptive health work, based on encouragement instead of coercion.[99] Kaisu Snellman found that women's changed position in society connected the issues of citizenship and health care. A re-evaluation of women's "most important functions", reproduction and child care, was needed to reconcile them with her political emancipation:

> Where woman is not liberated, this is a way to liberate her, and where she has truly achieved equality with man, voluntary motherhood is one of the most important preconditions for its preservation.[100]

Like Scandinavian progressive female doctors in the 1920s, she connected women's liberation with a general change for the better in society.[101] Her activism contributed to the founding of the first sexual advice station in Helsinki.[102]

In sum

Erkki Vala had no articulated stance on eugenics, but reacted to threats against individual liberties. He differentiated very clearly between methods for the advancement of social welfare on the basis of whether they endangered his idea of civil rights and social justice. His emphasis on individual rights as a cornerstone of social justice set him apart from many leftist and liberal supporters of eugenics. However, he was prepared to at least rhetorically accept compromises, as long as they allowed the individual to make a free and informed choice. Vala used other people's arguments instrumentally, when they bolstered his own argument. He quite clearly avoided disclosing playwright George Bernard Shaw's full opinion on eugenics. *Tulenkantajat* did not deal with eugenics explicitly, but did discuss methods of health policies that others would classify as 'positive eugenics'.

Erkki Vala, Katri Vala, Väinö Lassila and their allies are examples of public intellectuals using their visibility to give voice to unpopular causes. The arguments and examples they used to sway public opinion may not have had the desired effect, but they reveal the ideological limits of the public health debate in twentieth-century Finland which were to have effects until the legal requirements for sterilisation were reformed in 1970. *Tulenkantajat* was fighting windmills in the 1930s. Its ideas of the right of the individual to education and personal liberty would be resurrected after the war, but not until the late 1960s would they acquire wide support. The Sterilisation Act of 1950 was even stricter and applied even more diligently than the act of 1935.[103] From the perspective of civil rights, the restrictions on the right to vote for citizens receiving poor relief or under guardianship were not removed until 1948 and 1972, respectively.[104]

Notes

1 Minna Harjula, *Vaillinaisuudella vaivatut: Vammaisuuden tulkinnat suomalaisessa huoltokeskustelussa 1800-luvun lopulta 1930-luvun lopulle* (Helsinki: SKS, 1996), 166.
2 Kerttu Saarenheimo, ed., *Katri Vala: Eikä minussa ollut pelkoa: Runoilijan omakuva kirjeiden, päiväkirjojen ja kirjoitusten valossa* (Juva: WSOY, 1991), 158–9.
3 Paul Nizan, *Les chiens de garde* (Marseille: Agone, 2012), 24, 73–4, 86–9.
4 'Yksipuolista asiantuntemusta', *Tulenkantajat*, no. 40 (1934): 5.
5 Minna Harjula, 'Köyhä, kelvoton, kansalainen? Köyhäinapu yleisen äänioikeuden esteenä Suomessa', *Janus* 18, no. 1 (2010): 4–19.
6 R[afael] Erich, 'Yleisen äänioikeuden rajoituksista', *Lakimies* 3, no. 6 (1908): 111–37.
7 Quoted in Markku Mattila, 'Rotuhygienia ja kansalaisuus', in *Kansalaisuus ja kansanterveys*, ed. Ilpo Helén and Mikko Jauho (Helsinki: Gaudeamus, 2003), 122.
8 Ibid., 110, 112–13.
9 Ilpo Helén and Mikko Jauho, eds, *Kansalaisuus ja kansanterveys* (Helsinki: Gaudeamus, 2003), 14.
10 Ainur Elmgren, *Den allrakäraste fienden: Svenska stereotyper i finländsk press 1918–1939* (Lund: Sekel, 2008), 186f.
11 Mattila, 'Rotuhygienia', 115–16.
12 Marjatta Hietala, 'Eugeniikan ja rotuhygienian tausta ja seuraukset', *Tieteessä tapahtuu*, no. 8 (2009): 14–19.
13 Kustavi Kaila, 'Aviokaariehdotuksen säännökset avioliiton päättämisestä ja purkamisesta', *Lakimies*, no. 1 (1924): 265–83.
14 Mattila, 'Rotuhygienia', 111.
15 Harjula, *Vaillinaisuudella vaivatut*, 163.
16 Eliina Kestilä, *Liian huono kansalaiseksi? Kansalaisihanne sterilisaatioasiakirjoissa v. 1935–1949* (Helsinki: University of Helsinki, 2001), 4.
17 Anonymous, 'Rikollisuuden vastustamispäivät', *Suomen Sosialidemokraatti* 8 January 1934, 2; E.J. Jatkola, 'Rikollisuuden lisääntyminen', *Länsi-Savo* 7 June 1934, 1, 4; Anonymous, 'Taistelu rikollisuutta vastaan', *Etelä-Suomen Sanomat* 8 November 1934, 1.
18 Marjatta Hietala, 'Rotuhygienia', in *Mongoleja vai germaaneja? Rotuteorioiden suomalaiset*, ed. Aira Kemiläinen, Marjatta Hietala and Pekka Suvanto (Helsinki: SHS, 1985).
19 Hiski Tuppurainen, 'Kurikoimista', *Kurikka*, no. 21 (1928): 2.
20 'Rodut vaihtuvat', *Kurikka*, no. 21 (1931): 21.
21 Erkki Sevänen, *Vapauden rajat: Kirjallisuuden tuotannon ja välityksen yhteiskunnallinen sääntely Suomessa vuosina 1918–1939* (Helsinki: SKS, 1994), 134.
22 'Merkillepantavia asioita', *Tulenkantajat*, no. 7 (1935): 2.
23 See Chapter 5 by Minna Harjula in this volume.
24 Interview by Eero Saarenheimo, tape 1, side A, transcript, SKS 25318 file 3, Erkki Vala, Archive of the Finnish Literature Society.
25 Klaus Vala, *Montparnassen juhlasekoitus* (Helsinki: Helka Vala, 2003), 61, 92–8.
26 Unto Koskela, *Hedelmätön puu* (Jyväskylä: Gummerus, 1932).
27 Tapio Niemi, *Outo mies – outo reitti: Raumalaiskirjailija Unto Koskelan lyhyt elämä* (Vammala: Vilpatek, 2004), 192.
28 Harjula, *Vaillinaisuudella vaivatut*, 151.
29 Niemi, *Outo mies*, 193.
30 K. H. [Katri Vala], 'Psykologinen romaani', *Tulenkantajat*, no. 2 (1933): 3.
31 Kerttu Saarenheimo, *Katri Vala: Aikansa kapinallinen* (Helsinki: WSOY, 1984), 204–26.
32 Hanna Kuusi, 'Tuberkuloosin torjunta ja moderni kansalainen', in *Kansalaisuus ja kansanterveys*, ed. Ilpo Helén and Mikko Jauho (Helsinki: Gaudeamus, 2003), 33–57.

33   '"Demokraattinen" Suomi v. 1936', *Tulenkantajat*, no. 42 (1936): 6; 'Meillä sitä ei voi tapahtua', *Tulenkantajat*, no. 48 (1936): 11.
34   Vala, *Montparnassen juhlasekoitus*, 40.
35   'Miten huoltolakeja pannaan käytäntöön', *Tulenkantajat*, no. 15 (1937): 2; 'Todistuskappaleita "demokraattisesta Suomesta" v. 1937', *Tulenkantajat*, no. 15 (1937): 7–8.
36   'Pakollinen sterilisatio – vaarallinen lakiehdotus', *Tulenkantajat*, no. 34 (1934): 1.
37   Väinö Lassila, 'Kansan terveys ja sosiaalinen uudistustyö', *Tulenkantajat*, no. 30–31 (1935): 6. For an extensive discussion on this concept, see Chapter 5 by Minna Harjula in this volume.
38   'Sterilisatiolain perustelut perustuvat epätieteellisiin katsomuksiin', *Tulenkantajat*, no. 41 (1934): 8; 'Sterilisatiolakiehdotuksen yksityiskohdat tarkasteltavina', *Tulenkantajat*, no. 42, (1934): 1, 6.
39   'Vähämielinen ja suvun jatkaminen', *Tulenkantajat*, no. 30–31 (1935): 5, 12.
40   'Mitä kansan keskuudessa ajatellaan sterilisatiolaista', *Tulenkantajat*, no. 43 (1934): 8.
41   'Miksi Ahvenanmaan maaherra vastusti sterilisatiolakia?' *Tulenkantajat*, no. 39 (1934): 8.
42   Marjatta Hietala, 'From race hygiene to sterilization: The eugenics movement in Finland', in *Eugenics and the Welfare State: Sterilization Policy in Denmark, Sweden, Norway, and Finland*, ed. Gunnar Broberg and Nils Roll-Hansen (East Lansing: Michigan State University Press, 2005), 195–258, 235.
43   'Kaatumatauti ja nerous', *Tulenkantajat*, no. 42 (1934): 8.
44   'Porthaneja uhataan – kansaa raaistetaan', *Tulenkantajat*, no. 42 (1934): 6.
45   'Liiallista virkavaltaa', *Tulenkantajat*, no. 33 (1934): 1.
46   'Kaksi tunnettua lääkäriä sterilisatiolainsäädännöstä', *Tulenkantajat*, no. 36 (1934): 5.
47   'Lääkäri ja yhteiskunta', *Tulenkantajat*, no. 4 (1934): 3.
48   Jon Røyne Kyllingstad, *Measuring the Master Race: Physical Anthropology in Norway, 1890–1945* (Cambridge: Open Book, 2014), 108–9. See also Chapter 6 by Annika Berg and Teemu Ryymin in this volume.
49   Nancy Ordover, *American Eugenics: Race, Queer Anatomy, and the Science of Nationalism* (Minneapolis: University of Minnesota Press, 2003), 137–58.
50   Kaisu Snellman, 'Margaret Sanger, syntyväisyyssäännöstelyn suuri esitaistelija, käynyt Helsingissä', *Tulenkantajat*, no. 25 (1934): 4.
51   'Uusimmat kauhutiedot Saksasta – sterilisatiolaki käytännössä!' *Tulenkantajat*, no. 41 (1934): 3; 'Saksan sterilisatio', *Tulenkantajat*, no. 26–7 (1935): 4, 7–8.
52   'Nälkiintyneitä lapsia sterilisoidaan Saksassa', *Tulenkantajat*, no. 42 (1934): 2.
53   'Lyhyitä tietoja', *Tulenkantajat*, no. 35 (1934): 6.
54   'Natsilainen pukinsorkka ja edustaja Paksujalka', *Tulenkantajat*, no. 44 (1934): 2.
55   G. R. Searle, 'Eugenics and politics in Britain in the 1930s', *Annals of Science* 36, no. 2 (1979): 159–69; Bradley W. Hart and Richard Carr, 'Sterilisation and the British Conservative Party: Rethinking the failure of the Eugenics Society's political strategy in the nineteen-thirties', *Historical Research*, no. 242 (2015): 716–39.
56   Erkki Vala, 'Demokratian suurin vaara: Ihmisoikeuksien jatkuva rajoittaminen', speech for Nuortasavaltalaiset (Young Republicans) 25 April 1935, manuscript, file 8, Archive of the Finnish Literature Society.
57   '"Sielun terveys", eli luonnottomuus huipussaan', *Tulenkantajat*, no. 9 (1935): 9.
58   'Kun tie kääntyy raakalaisuuteen', *Tulenkantajat* no. 8 (1935): 1.
59   From Federley's speech at 'The Week of Prevention of Crime', 7–13 January 1934, published in the journal *Sielun terveys*, no. 2 (1935); quoted in 'Sielun terveys', 1.
60   Ibid.
61   Vala, 'Demokratian suurin vaara'.
62   'Mitä olisi tehtävä?', *Tulenkantajat*, no. 8 (1935): 8.
63   Maria Wahlberg, *Syyllisiä kunnes toisin todistetaan: Etsivä keskuspoliisi ja kulttuuriliberaalit 1934–1937*, Suojelupoliisi, tutkimusraportti, no. 2 (2012), 32–3.

64 'Laukauksia', *Luo lippujen!*, no. 4 (1939): 91; see also 'Tapaus Väinö Lassila', *Ylioppilaslehti*, no. 3 (1939): 1–2.
65 'Sterilisoimishumpuuki herättää yleistä vastusta', *Tulenkantajat*, no. 9 (1935): 3.
66 'Sielun terveys', 1.
67 Markku Mattila, *Kansamme parhaaksi: Rotuhygienia Suomessa vuoden 1935 sterilointilakiin asti* (Helsinki: SHS, 1999), 292.
68 Mattila, 'Rotuhygienia', 119.
69 Harjula, *Vaillinaisuudella vaivatut*, 163.
70 Oiva Elo, 'Vain vähämielisiin olisi sterilisointi ulotettava', *Suomen Sosialidemokraatti* 27 March 1933, 1, 4.
71 Hart and Carr, 'Sterilisation and the British', 716–39.
72 'Sterilisatiolain perustelut perustuvat epätieteellisiin katsomuksiin', *Tulenkantajat*, no. 41 (1934): 8.
73 'Mitä kansan keskuudessa ajatellaan sterilisatiolaista', *Tulenkantajat*, no. 43 (1934): 8.
74 'Sielun terveys', 1.
75 'Sterilisatiolakiehdotuksen yksityiskohdat tarkasteltavina', *Tulenkantajat*, no. 42 (1934): 1.
76 Harjula, *Vaillinaisuudella vaivatut*, 163.
77 'Sterilisoimishumpuuki', 3.
78 Mattila, *Kansamme parhaaksi*, 334.
79 'On tapahtunut suuri erehdys', *Tulenkantajat*, no. 10 (1935): 1.
80 'Pakollinen sterilisatio – vaarallinen lakiehdotus', *Tulenkantajat*, no. 34 (1934): 1; 'Mitä kansan keskuudessa', 8; 'Sterilisoimishumpuuki', 3.
81 'Köyhäinhoitoviranomaiset anovat hoidokkejaan sterilisoitaviksi', *Tulenkantajat*, no. 2 (1936): 2.
82 Kestilä, *Liian huono kansalaiseksi*, 19.
83 Mattila, *Kansamme parhaaksi*, 342–3.
84 Majava, '"Yhteiskuntavastaisia" aineksia aletaan siis nyt sterilisoida', *Tulenkantajat*, no. 32 (1935): 2.
85 Raoul Palmgren, 'Kansallisen nousun legenda', *Kirjallisuuslehti*, no. 18–24 (1935): 464.
86 Sharon M. Leon, *An Image of God: The Catholic Struggle with Eugenics* (Chicago: University of Chicago Press, 2013), 132.
87 'Pakollinen sterilisatio', 1.
88 Ibid,
89 Helén and Jauho, *Kansalaisuus ja kansanterveys*, 25.
90 'Sukupuolineuvonta-asema', *Helsingin Sanomat* 9 July 1934, quoted in Saarenheimo, *Eikä minussa ollut pelkoa*, 154–6. See also Saarenheimo, *Aikansa kapinallinen*, 200–201.
91 Saarenheimo, *Eikä minussa ollut pelkoa*, 155–6.
92 Lassila, 'Kansan terveys', 6.
93 'Sterilisatiolakiehdotuksen yksityiskohdat tarkasteltavina', *Tulenkantajat*, no. 42 (1934): 6.
94 'Sielun terveys', 9.
95 'Kun tie kääntyy raakalaisuuteen', *Tulenkantajat*, no. 8 (1935): 1.
96 Pecka, 'Se syntyväisyyden väheneminen', *Tulenkantajat*, no. 38 (1934): 2; 'Äitiyshuoltolakiehdotus – farssiko?', 2.
97 Pecka, 'Uutta puritanismiako?' *Tulenkantajat*, no. 6 (1934): 2; 'Miksi isänmaallinen ylioppilasnuoriso opiskelee?' *Tulenkantajat*, no. 37 (1934): 2; cf. Saarenheimo, *Eikä minussa ollut pelkoa*, 129–30.
98 K. S. Laurila, *Taistelu taiteesta ja siveellisyydestä* (Helsinki: WSOY, 1938), 135–6; Raoul Palmgren, 'K.S. Laurilan pamfletti', *Tulenkantajat*, no. 8 (1939): 5–6.
99 Lassila, 'Kansan terveys', 6–7.

100 Kaisu Snellman, 'Syntyväisyyssäännöstely', *Tulenkantajat*, no. 22 (1934): 1–2.
101 See Chapter 3 by Merle Wessel in this volume.
102 'Sukupuolineuvontaa päätetty järjestää Helsinkiin', *Tulenkantajat*, no. 36 (1934): 1, 8.
103 Mattila, 'Rotuhygienia', 111–12. See also Chapter 5 by Minna Harjula in this volume.
104 Mattila, 'Rotuhygienia', 113.

5   Universal, but exclusive?

The shifting meanings of pre- and post-war public health in Finland

Minna Harjula

Introduction

The idea of public health was typically expressed with the concepts of *kansanterveys* and *kansantauti* in Finland in the twentieth century. *Kansanterveys* – which literally refers to the health of the nation or people – replaced hygiene as the guiding concept in health policy by the mid-1940s. At the same time, the prevention of certain widespread diseases called *kansantauti* – disease of the nation or people – was defined as one of the main tasks in promoting public health. The key role of these interconnected concepts was strengthened in 1972 when they were included in new legislation. This new legislation on public health (*kansanterveyslaki*) gave all citizens universal access to primary health care services.[1]

An essential part of the terminology in public health, the Finnish word *kansa* carried rhetorical power. Besides nation and people, *kansa* could refer to the population, the lower classes and sometimes even to the state. A special feature in the Finnish language is the close resemblance between the terms *kansa* and *kansalainen* (citizen). Due to the interconnection of these terms, the categories of formal, juridical citizenship and informal citizenship – characterised by belonging, community membership and civic virtues – are conceptually linked and vaguely separable. As a result, the key terms of public health referred to the collective, national entity in a way that remained open to overlapping and different readings.[2]

This chapter examines how the idea of public health evolved in Finnish health policy from the early twentieth century to the 1970s, by analysing the ideological premises and practical results of the various uses and changing meanings of the two interrelated key concepts. The chapter focuses on how the sphere of the concept of *kansanterveys* evolved, how the inclusion of all citizens became the aim in dominant usages of the concept, and how the development was linked to the conceptualisations of *kansantauti*. Even though the trend of development was towards universalism, the chapter shows the inclusive and exclusive tensions in the changing use of the concepts. The research material consists of legislation, committee reports, the reports of health care authorities, and medical and public health journals written in Finnish. Due to the linguistic differences, the results cannot be generalised across the discussions and practice of the Swedish-speaking minority in Finland, as their conceptualisation of the equivalent terms (*folkhälsa, folksjukdom*) were presumably more directly influenced by models from the other Nordic countries.[3]

New conceptualisations and changing interpretations of health

The terms *kansanterveys* and *kansantauti* were adopted in the Finnish language at the turn of the twentieth century. The digitised indexes of Finnish newspapers, periodicals and national bibliography indicate that the term *kansanterveys* was usually spelled as two separate words – *kansan terveys* – in the late nineteenth century. It was gradually formulated as a compound word, written without a space, in the early decades of the twentieth century. The formation of the compound *kansanterveys*, and its frequent use since the mid-1930s, clearly indicates the establishment of the Finnish variant of the concept of public health. Both the phrase *kansan terveys* and the word *kansanterveys* contained the idea of health as a special national phenomenon which was different from – but deeply related to – individual health.[4]

The previously dominant term in public health, *hygienia* (hygiene), was used in parallel with *kansanterveys*. *Hygienia* covered both *yksilökohtainen hygienia* (personal hygiene) and *yleinen hygienia* (general hygiene) in the late nineteenth century. Even though general hygiene aimed at "improving the health conditions of whole nations and society",[5] the term as such did not carry strong meanings of membership and belonging like the term *kansa*. With the word *kansa,* health promotion clearly became a collective mission.[6] Since the late nineteenth century – both spellings included – the concept *kansanterveys* was more frequent in the popular educational periodical on health care, *Terveydenhoitolehti*, than in the medical journal *Duodecim,* both of which were published by the Finnish-speaking society of physicians. This reflects the early function of the concept in propagating the imperative of health to the people.[7]

Alongside *kansanterveys*, the concept of *kansantauti* was deeply interconnected with the idea of public health in Finland. The similar German concept of *Volkskrankheit* was translated as 'disease of the people' or 'national disease' in the *British Medical Journal* (*BMJ*) at the turn of the century, but never adopted in English.[8] At the same time, the Finnish concept occurred for the first time in newspapers, periodicals and medical journals.[9] As a translation for the Swedish word *folksjukdom*, in 1909 the Finnish medical dictionary used *kansantauti* instead of the previously introduced term *väestöntauti* (disease of the population), which was never actually adopted in common usage. The neutral term *väestö*, referring to all inhabitants of a certain area, was replaced by *kansa*.[10] This opened up the concept to various new political and moral interpretations.

In the contemporary Finnish dictionary, *kansantauti* is defined as a disease with high incidence. The most recent definition by the National Institute for Health and Welfare (2015) emphasises "the significance of the disease for the health of the population, for *kansanterveys*", but admits that there is no specific definition of the significance of diseases.[11] The similar indefiniteness characterises the discussion on *kansantauti* throughout the century. Usually, the concept was used as a self-explanatory term even in academic and official contexts. A rare early definition in *Terveydenhoitolehti* (1898) described *kansantauti* as a domestic, continual, deep-rooted, destructive disease, and distinguished it from global, short-lived pandemics.[12] According to an article in 1917, even certain epidemics could be called *kansantauti*.[13] Since the 1950s, the few analytical texts emphasised the interpretative, value judgemental nature of the concept: some diseases were said to be elevated to an honorary position, or "made as a new *kansantauti* with powerful propaganda".[14] Clearly, the high incidence of a certain disease alone did not imply it was defined as *kansantauti*, since all diseases causing high mortality, morbidity or incapacity for work have not been automatically referred to by this term. Presumably, the changing definitions of *kansantauti* have reflected the prevailing notions concerning the possibilities, prerequisites, means and goals to maintain and promote health.

While a wide variety of diseases were labelled as *kansantauti* in the medical journal *Duodecim* throughout the twentieth century, the concept's usage indicates two main constructions which followed the pattern of epidemiological transition. First, the long-term dominance of tuberculosis (TB) peaked in the 1930s and slowly faded away in the 1950s. Secondly, the predominant position of chronic diseases – heart diseases, cancer, diabetes – was established from the 1970s onwards. There was, however, a notable transition period, from the 1940s to the 1960s, when various diseases of very different nature – such as goitre, anaemia, rheumatic diseases and mental problems – were equally given the epithet *kansantauti*. Such an unestablished and vacillating interpretation of the concept suggests a period during which the direction and form of health policy was reformulated.[15] This reading is supported by the fact that the concept of *kansanterveys* was officially adopted in administrative language at the same time.[16] Thus, the periodisation of the following sections is based on this turning point.

Mothers and children first: Nation and health in Finland until the 1940s

The key concepts based on the term *kansa* were gradually adopted in public health while Finland still was a part of the Russian Empire (up to 1917). Essentially, health was a part of nation-building from the late nineteenth century onwards. Alongside the early implementation of universal suffrage in 1906, active citizenship became a virtue and also a duty in Finland. Instead of governmental health reforms, the focus was on elevating the people – especially the lower classes – to the level of responsibility and awareness required by modern citizenship. The existence of different social classes was considered self-evident, and the word *kansa* was often used to signify the common people, who needed health education and guidance of the educated class. Civic organisations which were led by educated middle-class people became the main forums for civic education in health. For the working class, the promise of a better future created acceptability of health information; but, at the same time, the moralistic message which ignored the social realities of life among the poor provoked reluctance.[17]

Christine Brecht and Sybilla Nikolow have pointed out that, as a political slogan, the German concept *Volkskrankheit* – which especially referred to illness of the lower social strata – motivated social reforms of living and housing conditions in mid-nineteenth-century Germany. A new interpretation of *Volkskrankheit*, affected by new germ theory, defined everybody (regardless of social background, age or gender) under threat of infection by the turn of the century.[18] In the Finnish language, the concept of *kansantauti* allowed for both readings at the turn of the century. *Kansantauti* was often defined as a problem of the lowest classes.[19] This interpretation was supported by the ideas of social hygiene, introduced as new scholarship from civilised countries in early twentieth-century Finland.[20] While emphasising the need for social reforms, it carried the idea of social hierarchies. In contrast, the reading which perceived *kansantauti* as a problem of all the people harmonised social and political differences, and aimed at creating solidarity:

> As tuberculosis is a *kansantauti*, it must therefore be fought by united efforts . . . this opens up a field of work where all interested citizens, regardless of their class and political opinion, can work side by side. Because of the nature of the task, it is cut out for bringing the different strata of the people [*kansa*] together.[21]

As the civil war (1918) soon after independence (1917) divided the nation, questions of how to unify the nation and who belonged to the nation became crucial. Besides the political division of the ruling whites and rebellious reds, the new branch of hygiene called *rotuhygienia* (racial hygiene, eugenics) gained ground in defining the biological and moral conditions for decent citizenship in Finland.[22] In Germany, for example, ideas of social and racial hygiene expanded the concept of *Volkskrankheit* from epidemic diseases to all forms of deviant behaviour, such as prostitution and juvenile delinquency, during the inter-war years.[23] Due to the comparatively late massive epidemic which resulted in one of the highest death rates in Europe, TB was still called 'our only real *kansantauti*' in Finland in the 1920s. Thus, social or mental problems were seldom included in the concept.[24]

The concept of population policy (*väestöpolitiikka*) linked ideas of public health and racial hygiene in the 1920s and 1930s.[25] In the context of decreasing birth rate and high infant mortality, it was particularly the health of mothers and children that was defined as a matter crucial for the survival of the nation. The focus on children opened up brighter future horizons without adversarial ideological fights. With the slogan 'There are too few of us', population policy served as a national and patriotic tool even during and after the Second World War.[26]

In the first official definition of *kansanterveys,* written for the new Department for Public Health (*Kansanterveysosasto*) by the supervising governmental organisation, the National Board of Health in 1944, the department's areas of responsibility were:

- governmental and municipal doctors
- school doctors

- midwives
- public health nurses
- maternity and child health clinics
- tuberculosis, rheumatism, etc. (general *kansantauti*)
- drinking water and latrines
- population policy
- training of midwives and nurses
- popular education on *kansanterveys*
- cooperation with and supervision of civic organisations for *kansanterveys*.

Population policy was outlined as one of the sectors of *kansanterveys*. In addition, a significant number of the other sectors the new department was responsible for – school doctors, midwives, public health nurses, maternity and child health clinics – were in a joint effort to promote the quality and quantity of the population. The responsibility for drinking water and latrines indicates that even sanitary reforms were included in the concept of *kansanterveys*. However, areas such as nutrition, housing, occupational and factory hygiene, vermin and epidemics were excluded from the scope of the Department for Public Health.[27]

Along with the concept of population policy, the earlier discourse on racial hygiene with the main emphasis on negative measures to eliminate the threat posed by degenerated individuals faded away. The new, publicly expressed focus was on positive action to prevent maternal and infant mortality and to encourage 'decent' couples to start families. There were, however, obvious discrepancies between discourse and practice. Even though the practices of coercive sterilisation (1935, 1950), compulsory abortions (1950) and marriage bans for the mentally ill and mentally disabled (1929), and marriage restrictions for epileptics, deaf people and those with venereal diseases (1929) were followed until the 1960s–1970s, the topic was discussed only briefly in the first plan for public health written by the National Board of Health in the early 1940s.[28]

Essential for the politically divided nation state after the civil war was that the scope of the concept of *kansanterveys* was the whole nation, regardless of social class. As a consequence, the word *kansa* can no longer be translated as 'lower classes' or 'common people' in this context. As a result of the national, all-inclusive view, *kansanterveys* was described as the responsibility of the state in the 1940s. State-run activities were characterised as reliable, determined, uniform and being above political disputes, which reflected the new idea of the state as the supervisor of the common good. Ideologically, the change was significant, as in the early 1920s the state was still considered slow, inflexible and bureaucratic – and, as such, suitable for governing only those health sectors that involved coercion. Until then, the regional supply of health services was largely based on local initiatives and private practices. Civic organisations – the Finnish Red Cross (1876), the Associations for Prevention of Tuberculosis (1907), the Mannerheim League for Child Welfare (1920) and the Public Health Association of Swedish Finland (*Folkhälsan*, 1921) – had a pioneering role in preventative action.[29]

The emphasis on the state signified a change of focus from the local to the national. The new Department for Public Health in the National Board of Health was entrusted with the task of launching initiatives and designing and mapping future health needs for the whole country. Despite these efforts, a special governmental institution for education, research and propaganda was never established in Finland, but the National Board of Health took charge of coordinating the work of civic organisations in the early 1940s. The officials of the National Board of Health took the leading role in promoting public health. They acted as representatives of state and medicine, and were also active in non-governmental organisations (NGOs).[30]

The core of public health work – in Finnish referred to as *kansanterveystyö* (literally, 'work for the health of the people/nation') – was a new preventative attitude to health care. It was represented as the efficient opposite to expensive curative treatment in hospitals, and characterised as a good investment and the most sensible policy. Public health work was the task of local government – town or municipality – the total number of which ranged from 500 to 600 in 1940–1970. The emphasis was on rural Finland, as almost 80 per cent of the population lived in the countryside in the 1940s.[31] Essentially, a precondition for the practical work was that the local, rural officials and local politicians – who represented the established local democracy – were persuaded and educated to break from traditional, parsimonious management of municipal finances and to adopt the new thinking.[32] In addition to persuasive information, a large set of legislation on regional service provision was passed to establish the new way of thinking about public health at a local level. The municipalities were obliged to appoint midwives (1920, 1936, 1944), municipal doctors (1943), public health nurses (1944), school doctors (1952) and school dentists (1956), and to establish maternity and child health clinics (1944) and provide a certain number of hospital beds.[33]

The services of maternity and child health clinics, public health nurses, midwives and school health care were free of charge, which reflected the increased responsibility of the state in health care. The public provision and funding made it an undisputed right and obligation of a citizen to use these services. Furthermore, health services and social benefits were coupled in order to increase the usage of the services: after 1949, in order to be eligible for maternity allowance, pregnant women had to attend a maternity clinic. The uneducated public was shepherded to avail themselves of the publicly provided services in the interest of safeguarding the health of the nation. As these services and benefits were provided for every child and mother – regardless of wealth, social class or residence – every family became integrated: by the mid-1950s, the free maternity and child health clinics reached 95 per cent of pregnant women and 90 per cent of newborn babies.[34]

Curative treatment was still of limited availability, especially in rural areas: 20 per cent of rural municipalities had no practising physician in the late 1930s. Despite the new legislation on municipal doctors in the 1940s, the number of physicians per head remained the lowest in Europe in the mid-1950s. Even though municipal doctors were employed by the local government, they charged their patients as well. The municipal doctors were required to provide services free of charge to those people whom the poor law authorities deemed in need of poor relief, but the stigmatised system presumably prevented people from using the service.[35]

The prevention of widespread diseases called *kansantauti* was a central focus of public health work, but the lack of health services was a problem. Despite the coercive legislation on TB in Norway (1900) and Denmark (1905), similar measures were not considered possible in preventing the major *kansantauti* in Finland until a sufficient number of hospital beds were available. This indicates the reciprocity of health-related obligations and rights. Obligatory X-ray examinations and coercive treatment were introduced in Finland only in 1948, when the provision of a nationwide network of TB hospitals and free outpatient clinics were established by law.[36]

In addition to TB, rheumatism was singled out as a *kansantauti* in the statute of the Department of Public Health in 1944. This is the first official indication of a chronic, non-infectious disease to be included in the concept. Similarly, the medical journal *Duodecim* included rheumatism and cancer as chronic diseases among *kansantauti* in the 1930–1950s.[37] In addition to these two diseases, the Plan for Public Health *(Kansanterveysohjelma*, 1942) listed caries, trachoma and intestinal parasitic diseases as *kansantauti*. According to the plan, the fight against all these diseases was naturally considered to be the responsibility of the National Board of Health.[38] However, Severi Savonen, the plan's author and a leading official in the National Board of Health, stated that most chronic diseases were irrelevant from the point of view of the population policy because those who suffered from these diseases were usually old, unproductive people:

We all die eventually, so we cannot reduce mortality as such at all. The issue at stake is to lengthen the productive period of life; in other words, to develop measures against infant mortality, epidemics, tuberculosis, etc. This kind of action is important for population policy, whereas, for example, measures for the prevention of cancer, which is a disease of the elderly, do not carry as much significance in this sense.[39]

Basically, the strong focus on population policy meant that the need for health care for other age groups was overlooked in the practice of public health. Moreover, still in the mid-1950s, the textbooks of medicine presented chronic diseases as incurable and degenerative. For example, cardiovascular diseases were seen as the inevitable results of ageing.[40] As top priority was given to the raising of a healthy young generation, non-infectious chronic diseases were not the focus of public health until the 1960s.

Health for all with health centres in the 1970s?

The exceptionally high death rates of adults provoked a crisis in Finnish health policy which resulted in a broadened view of *kansanterveys* during the 1960s. The statistics showed that while infant mortality kept decreasing, mortality among

Finnish men was twice as high as in the other Scandinavian countries, and the figures for both men and women were generally the highest in Europe. A detailed analysis of the causes of death was possible since the reform of mortality statistics in 1936. The first introductory studies showed that – instead of epidemic diseases, TB or diseases of newborn children – it was cardiovascular diseases and cancer that took the Finns to their early graves.[41] The governmental Committee for Public Health (*Kansanterveyskomitea*, 1960–1965), appointed to find solutions, stated that the figures clearly showed the preferential status of young age groups in Finnish health care. Therefore, a systematic inclusion of older citizens in the sphere of health care was declared fundamental in promoting public health.[42]

Besides age-related inequality, the statistics also indicated regional inequality in the early 1960s, as the darkest areas in mortality were found in eastern and northern Finland. Even gendered inequalities were noticed as, due to the inclusive maternity and child health clinics, the majority of young women were integrated into health services and health education, while most of the young men had no regular health check-ups after leaving school and military service.[43] Furthermore, analyses of morbidity indicated that the nation of 4.6 million people had more than 1 million chronic patients and that the number of working-age people retired because of ill health was exceptionally high in international comparison.[44] Basically, the high death rates and the plenitude of untreated chronic diseases were seen as the results of a lack of both health care services and compensation for medical costs. Numbers of medical staff and hospital beds were below the average European standard. As Finland was among the last European countries without compulsory national health insurance in the early 1960s, households had to pay for the majority of medical costs.[45]

While the planning of health insurance was not explicitly linked to the discourse on *kansanterveys*,[46] the seminal book *Social Policy for the Sixties* (1961), written with the contribution of leading officials and scientists to guide the development of Finnish society, considered public health as deeply related to social policy. The book emphasised not only the availability of health care services, but also considered affordability as an essential factor in promoting public health. By introducing the concept 'health care rights of the citizen' (*terveydenhoidolliset kansalaisoikeudet*), the book clearly pointed out the responsibility of the government in providing equal access to health services. As social equality, economic growth and democracy were seen as closely interrelated factors in the development of modern society, inequalities in health were characterised as both morally unacceptable and economically detrimental. Ground-breakingly, investments in health were thought to increase economic growth as they enabled inactive people to become active members of society.[47]

The concept of *kansanterveys* reflected new ideals of universalism and equality in the distribution of health.[48] After more than ten years of planning, the new ideology was put into practice as the Public Health Act (*kansanterveyslaki*) was passed in 1972. The title of the law is officially translated as 'Primary Health Care Act', but ideologically telling is the literal translation: 'Act on the health of the nation/people'. Given the conceptual focus on public health in this volume, I will refer to the Act as the Public Health Act so as to retain the original Finnish formulation. Within a comparative international context, the Act is known for its combination of public health, preventive medicine and primary medical care.[49] For citizens, the most visible reform was that the Act obliged all local government authorities to establish municipal health centres for the provision of primary health care. Based on the model of the successful maternity and child health clinics, regular health surveillance with check-ups and health education was defined as the primary task of the centres.[50]

In addition to the aim of establishing equal access to health care, another goal was to reduce poverty and sickness. Despite the implementation of National Health Insurance – which granted sickness allowances to all citizens aged 16–64 (from 1964) and covered a share of medical costs (from 1967) – low-income families could not afford to pay doctors' fees. The Public Health Act made curative outpatient medical treatment in health centres free of charge for all citizens, and the principle was put into practice in 1981. Even though all political parties supported the Act, it was left-wing politicians in particular who campaigned for cost-free health care, and the issue of the charges split political opinion.[51]

The interconnectedness of *kansanterveys* and *kansantauti* was strengthened as the prevention and treatment of 'especially significant' diseases called *kansantauti* was defined as one of the main tasks of the Public Health Act.[52] In 1965, the National Board of Health emphasised the need for integrating the work of NGOs against cancer and rheumatism with the work of the government.[53] Marja-Liisa Honkasalo has pointed out that the nationwide programme for the prevention of cardiovascular diseases (1972–1997), named the North Karelia Project after the 'darkest area' of health in eastern Finland, created widespread awareness of risk for citizens (see also Chapter 11 by Johannes Kananen in this volume). Significantly, the identification of lifestyle-related risk factors – smoking, alcohol, sugar, fat and lack of physical exercise – made chronic ailments such as cardiovascular diseases preventable. Characteristically, in the nationwide campaign against heart disease, the high incidence was described as a mass epidemic. The rhetoric, as well as the interaction of homes, civic organisations and government, was adopted from previous hygiene and TB campaigns.[54]

The National Board of Health categorised the burning issues of mental problems, accidents and degenerative diseases of the ageing population as 'new *kansantauti*' in the late 1960s. Furthermore, it stated that: "We have to admit that the ways to beat . . . the above-mentioned *kansantauti* are not adequately known."[55] As the epidemiological profile had changed, complicated factors linked to people's social environment were found to cause diseases.[56] In particular, Finland's rapid structural shift from an agrarian country to an industrialised and urbanised one entailed changing living conditions with breaks in social patterns and traditions in the 1960s.[57] This signified a broadened view of health: besides medicine, social sciences gained ground in defining health. The traditional academic terminology was also reformed. In the late 1960s and early 1970s, the professorship of *hygiene* which was established in 1890 and the disciplines of *social hygiene* and *social medicine* were substituted by a new discipline: *public health science* (*kansanterveystiede*).[58]

The new social emphasis on health was linked to the cultural and political radicalism of the late 1960s. The new radical generation employed in health administration contributed to the exceptionally close connection between academic research and politics. The focus on health services alone was regarded as ineffective in improving the health of the nation in the 1970s. The new administrators thought it was important to include the target of improving health in all sectors of society – for example, in housing, environmental policy and taxation. This broadened the focus on public health beyond the scope of the Public Health Act. New legislation on occupational safety, road safety and smoking restrictions was enacted in the 1970s.[59]

Despite the new requirements for healthy lifestyles, the debate during the 1970s emphasised individual autonomy: "We have to be able to realise the right to health without coercion . . . Everyone must be given enough basic information on health so that they can choose such a prospect of health as they want."[60] In general, coercive measures were deemed acceptable only when the individual was not capable of making decisions or was a danger to others. The repeal of the coercive orders in the legislation on marriage (1969) and sterilisation (1970), the liberal-isation of abortion law (1970) and the restriction of compulsion in mental institutions were concrete efforts to reach the new goal.[61]

The aim of the Public Health Act was to create an integrated, comprehensive health care system that would treat all citizens equally. In spite of the strong push for equality, the new policy created exclusive tensions. Rural areas were prioritised in the construction of health centres because private services were thought to compensate for the lack of public health care in urban areas. The costs of private services were partly reimbursed by the National Health Insurance, but equality was undermined by the fact that the poorest could not afford to use them. Even though dental care was included in the services of health centres, it was initially accessible only to children due to limited resources. Dental care for adults began in health centres in 1977, but was subject to a fee. Availability increased rather slowly as more than 90 per cent of adults went to private dentists. As a result, almost a quarter of the adult population in the late 1970s had lost all their teeth.[62]

Regardless of the aim to include all age groups, the priority was to maintain the good results achieved in child health clinics by focusing on teenagers and working-age people.[63] Furthermore, the focus on preventative measures made the needs of hospitalised chronic patients a matter of secondary importance. The administrative position between medicine and social affairs slowed reforms, and the backwardness of the long-term care of elderly chronic patients remained a problem in the 1980s.[64]

The rise and fall of *kansanterveys*?

The Finnish concept of *kansanterveys* culminated in the provision of universal health care services. The free maternal and child health clinics (from 1944 onwards) as well as municipal health centres with low user fees (1972–1980) and free appointments since 1981 realised the ideas of universalism, equality and public responsibility for health. However, the shifting meanings of *kansanterveys* also created changing hierarchies and exclusive tensions among citizens. Even though the concept suggested that its scope was the whole nation already in the 1920s–1930s, the focus at that time was particularly care for mothers and children. Despite the emphasis on positive population policy, the exclusive practices of racial hygiene were not abandoned until the 1970s. Non-infectious chronic diseases escaped the attention of public health until they were defined as *kansantauti* in the 1960s. As a result, the needs of the adult population were given priority in the 1970s.

Because of the aim to promote regional equality, the building of health centres focused on rural areas with the poorest availability of health services in the 1970s. At the same time, a separate occupational health care system with access to curative treatment was provided by employers, partly financed by National Health Insurance, in order to remedy urban wage-workers' health problems. Thus, the parallel existence of public, occupational and private health care was consolidated. The problematic nature of the system became apparent in the 1990s. As user fees were re-established at health centres during the economic depression in 1993, curative treatment was available free of charge only to employed people with access to occupational health care and to children in the public health care system. As a result, access to health care depended to an increasing extent on socioeconomic status.[65] Especially in cities, health centres deteriorated and became poorly resourced services, mainly used by people in the lowest income groups.[66] Being an embodiment of the concept of *kansanterveys*, the changed character of health centres now also suggested a changed meaning of *kansa*. Instead of referring to all citizens, one could interpret that the concept again encompassed merely the lower classes and, as such, no longer reflected the universalistic idea of equality.

Since the 1980s, the Finnish concept of *kansanterveystyö* (public health work) was gradually replaced by new terms adopted from international vocabulary: primary health care and health promotion.[67] Without the connection to the collective concept of *kansa*, the new terminology carried a more individualistic view of health, focusing on individual access to treatment. Finally, the ongoing reform of Finnish health care and social services (2015–2019) not only repeals the Public Health Act of 1972 and restructures the service organisation created in the 1920–1970s, but also abandons the concepts of *kansanterveys* and *kansantauti*. Instead of *kansa*, the new draft laws use terms such as *väestö* (population), *as akas* (customer) and *asks* (resident).[68] Thus, the strong connection between health and the collective entity of *kansa* which linked nation, citizenship and belonging appears to be a specific historical feature which no longer has relevance in the changing economic, political and social environment of the twenty-first century.

Notes

1 Decree on the National Board of Health 188/1944. Kansanterveyslaki (66/1972); in English, Primary Health Care Act 66/1972; Decree on Primary Health Care 205/1972; Minna Harjula, *Terveyden jäljillä: suomalainen terveyspolitiikka 1900-luvulla* (Tampere: TUP, 2007).
2 Ilkka Liikanen, 'Kansa', in *Käsitteet liikkeessä: Suomen poliittisen kulttuurin käsitehistoria*, ed. Matti Hyvärinen et al. (Tampere: Vastapaino, 2003), 257–307; Elina

Nivala, 'Kunnon kansalainen yhteiskunnan kasvatuksellisena ihanteena', in *Hyvä ihminen ja kunnon kansalainen: Johdatus kansalaisuuuden sosiaalipedagogiikkaan*, ed. Leena Kurki and Elina Nivala (Tampere: TUP, 2006), 25–115, 43; Henrik Stenius, 'Kansalainen' in *Käsitteet liikkeessä: Suomen poliittisen kulttuurin käsitehistoria*, ed. Matti Hyvärinen et al. (Tampere: Vastapaino, 2003), 309–62; Kari Palonen, 'Eurooppalaiset poliittiset käsitteet suomalaisissa pelitiloissa', in *Käsitteet liikkeessä: Suomen poliittisen kulttuurin käsitehistoria*, ed. Matti Hyvärinen et al. (Tampere: Vastapaino, 2003), 569–87,581–2; Ilpo Helén and Mikko Jauho, eds, *Kansalaisuus ja kansanterveys* (Helsinki: Gaudeamus, 2003).

3   On *folkhälsa* among Swedish-speaking Finns, see Markku Mattila, *Kansamme parhaaksi: Rotuhygienia Suomessa vuoden 1935 sterilisointilakiin asti* (Helsinki: SHS, 1999).

4   The analysis of the early use of the concept *kansanterveys* is based on systematic search results of the following digitised sources: full text database of Finnish newspapers and journals, accessed through DIGI: *Kansalliskirjaston digitoidut aineistot* – the Finnish National Library's Digital Collections (http://digi.kansalliskirjasto.fi/?language=en); full text database of *Duodecim* (http://vanhaversio.duodecimlehti.fi/web/guest/ haku?p_p_id=Article_WAR_DL6_Articleportlet&p_p_lifecycle=0&_Article_WAR_ DL6_Articleportlet_viewType=searchArticle); reference database of Finnish national bibliography *Fennica* (https://fennica.linneanet.fi/vwebv/searchBasic?sk=en_FI).

5   M. O-B. 'Terveysoppi', in *Tietosanakirja IX* (Helsinki: Otava, 1917), 1452–3.

6   Minna Harjula, *Hoitoonpääsyn hierarkiat: Terveyskansalaisuus ja terveyspalvelut Suomessa 1900-luvulla* (Tampere: TUP, 2015), 31–67, 117–37.

7   The comparison is based on the number of articles including the concept in *Terveydenhoitolehti* and *Duodecim* until 1920. A volume of *Terveydenhoitolehti* included approximately 240 pages, while *Duodecim* usually ranged from 300 up to 640 pages. *Terveydenhoitolehti* was accessed through DIGI, and *Duodecim* through its website (see note 4).

8   'British Medical Journal', *British Medical Journal*, 50, no. 1 (1899): 1353; 'Reviews', *British Medical Journal*, 55 no. 2 (1904): 1321.

9   In newspapers in 1895, periodicals 1898, *Duodecim* 1902 and *National Bibliography* 1906.

10 *Duodecimin sanaluettelo Suomen lääkäreille* (Helsinki: Duodecim, 1888); *Duodecimin sanaluettelo Suomen lääkäreille* (Helsinki: Duodecim, 1898); *Duodecimin sanaluettelo Suomen lääkäreille* (Helsinki: Duodecim, 1909).

11 *Suomen kielen perussanakirja: A–K*, Kotimaisten kielten tutkimuskeskuksen julkaisuja 35 (Helsinki: Valtion painatuskeskus, 1990), 392; 'Yleistietoa kansantaudeista', *Terveyden ja hyvinvoinnin laitos*, 28 April 2015 (www.thl.fi/fi/web/kansantaudit/ yleistietoa-kansantaudeista).

12 'Kolme yhteiskunnan vihollista', *Terveydenhoitolehti* 10, no. 9 (1898): 134. Cf. Taav. Laitinen, 'Tarttuvista taudeista', *Terveydenhoitolehti* 10, no. 12 (1898): 180.

13 Yrjö Levander, 'Piirteitä kulkutautien luonteesta, historiasta ja vastustamisesta', *Terveydenhoitolehti* 29, no. 7–9 (1917): 113.

14 Leo Noro, *Sosiaalilääketieteen perusteet* (Porvoo: WSOY, 1957), 59; Erkki Varpela, 'Helsingin sydän- ja verisuonitautikuolleisuudesta', *Duodecim* 75, no. 1 (1959): 20; 'Verenpainetaudin lääkehoito', *Duodecim* 98, no. 2 (1982): 122.

15 The analysis of *kansantauti* is based on the full text database of *Duodecim* 1903–2000. The database was searched exhaustively using the keywords 'kansantau*', 'kansansairau*' and 'kansan tau*'. Both *tauti* and *sairaus* are synonyms of disease in Finnish, but the concept of *kansansairaus* was used only occasionally in 1973–2000. Articles which discuss *kansantauti* abroad or in historical contexts before the twentieth century were not included. www.duodecimlehti.fi/web/guest/haku?p_p_id=Article_ WAR_DL6_Articleportlet&p_p_lifecycle=0&_Article_WAR_DL6_Articleportlet_ viewType=searchArticle.

16 Decree 188/1944.

17 Harjula, *Hoitoonpääsyn hierarkiat*, 31–67; Riitta Oittinen, 'Leipää, suojaa ja valoa: Työläisnainen-lehti työkansan terveyden puolestapuhujana', in *Kansalaisuus ja kansanterveys*, ed. Ilpo Helén and Mikko Jauho (Helsinki: Gaudeamus, 2003), 175–95.

18 Christine Brecht and Sybilla Nikolow, 'Displaying the invisible: Volkskrankheiten on exhibition in imperial Germany', *Studies in History and Philosophy of Biological and Biomedical Sciences* 31, no. 4 (2000): 517–19.

19 For example, 'Taistelu keuhkotautia vastaan', *Rauman lehti* 5 December 1896, no. 98; 'Keuhkotauti eli keuhkotuberkuloosi ja sen syyt', *Uusi Aura* 13 January 1905 no. 10A.

20 N. J. Arppe, 'Terveydenhoito ja työväenkysymys', *Terveydenhoitolehti* 19, no. 3 (1907): 38.

21 'Eräs kansallinen työmaa', *Helsingin Sanomat* 28 September 1905 no. 225.

22 Mattila, *Kansamme parhaaksi*; Harjula, *Hoitoonpääsyn hierarkiat*, 117–23.

23 Brecht and Nikolow, 'Displaying the invisible', 518–19.

24 *Komiteanmietintö 1927:11. Kunnallisille mielisairaaloille ja tuberkuloosia sairastavien hoitolaitoksille sekä tuberkuloosin vastustamistyöhön annettavan valtionavun perustamiseksi* (Helsinki, 1927), 22, 27; DIGI. On TB: Mikko Jauho, *Kansanterveysongelman synty: Tuberkuloosi ja terveyden hallinta Suomessa ennen toista maailmansotaa* (Helsinki: Tutkijaliitto, 2007).

25 The concept was introduced in Finnish newspapers and journals in 1909–1910, DIGI.

26 Ilpo Helén, *Äidin elämän politiikka: Naissukupuolisuus, valta ja itsesuhde Suomessa 1880-luvulta 1960-luvulle* (Helsinki: Gaudeamus, 1997); Mattila, *Kansamme parhaaksi*; Harjula, *Terveyden jäljillä*, 55–73.

27 Decree 188/1944, § 8.

28 Mattila, *Kansamme parhaaksi*; Severi Savonen, *Kansanterveystyötä tehostamaan! Maalaiskuntien yleisen terveydenhoidon ohjelma.* (Helsinki: Otava, 1941); Severi Savonen, 'Suomen kansanterveystyön ohjelma', *Suomen Lääkäriliiton Aikakauslehti* 21, no. 2 (1942): 39–52; Severi Savonen, 'Kansanterveystyö väestöpoliittisena tekijänä', *Suomen Lääkäriliiton Aikakauslehti* 21, no. 2 (1942): 52–60.

29 Harjula, *Hoitoonpääsyn hierarkiat*, 123–7, 131–4.

30 Savonen, 'Suomen kansanterveystyön ohjelma', 39–41, 47–8; Harjula, *Hoitoonpääsyn hierarkiat*, 131–7; Allan Tiitta, *Collecium Medicum: Lääkintöhallitus 1878–1991* (Helsinki: Terveyden ja hyvinvoinnin laitos, 2009); Jauho, *Kansanterveysongelman synty*, 187–90.

31 Savonen, *Kansanterveystyötä tehostamaan*, 7, 54; 'Kaupunkien ja kuntien lukumäärät 1917–2017', Kunnat.net (2017), www.kunnat.net/fi/tietopankit/tilastot/aluejaot/kuntien-lukumaara/Sivut/default.aspx.

32 Suvi Nieminen, Lea Henriksson and Sirpa Wrede, 'Periferian isännistä terveyspoliittisiksi toimijoiksi. Kunnallismieskasvatus osana maaseudun kansanterveystyön rakentamista', *Sosiologia* 41, no. 1 (2004): 14–27.

33 Harjula, *Hoitoonpääsyn hierarkiat*, 138–76.

34 Ibid., 150–54, 188–99.

35 *Komiteanmietintö 1939:9: Maaseudun terveydenhoito-olot ja niiden kehittäminen* (Helsinki, 1939), 46; Harjula, *Hoitoonpääsyn hierarkiat*, 68–78, 138–49.

36 Ida Blom, 'Contagion and cultural perceptions of accepted behaviour: Tuberculosis and venereal diseases in Scandinavia c.1900–c.1950', *Hygiea Internationalis* 6, no. 2 (2007): 121–33; Harjula, *Hoitoonpääsyn hierarkiat*, 203–13, 230–31.

37 Decree 188/1944, § 8; *Duodecim*, www.duodecimlehti.fi/web/guest/haku?p_p_id=Article_WAR_DL6_Articleportlet&p_p_lifecycle=0&_Article_WAR_DL6_Articleportlet_viewType=searchArticle.

38 Savonen, 'Suomen kansanterveystyön ohjelma', 46.

39 Savonen, 'Kansanterveystyö väestöpoliittisena tekijänä', 53.

40 Marja-Liisa Honkasalo, *Reikä sydämessä: Sairaus pohjoiskarjalaisessa maisemassa* (Tampere: Vastapaino, 2008), 92–3.

41 Pekka Kuusi, *60-luvun sosiaalipolitiikka* (Porvoo: WSOY, 1961); Harjula, *Terveyden jäljillä*, 74–82; Seppo Koskinen and Tuija Martelin, 'Kuolleisuus', in *Suomen väestö*,

ed. Seppo Koskinen et al. (Helsinki: Gaudeamus, 2007), 169–238; Väinö Kannisto, 'Mikä lyhentää elinaikaamme?' *Kansantaloudellinen aikakauskirja* 40 (1945): 377–83.

42 *Komiteanmietintö 1965: B 72. Kansanterveyskomitean mietintö* (Helsinki, 1965), 6–8.

43 Official Statistics of Finland (SVT) XI: 64 1961 (Helsinki: Lääkintöhallitus, 1964), 15; Kuusi, *60-luvun sosiaalipolitiikka*, 265–6, 285.

44 Government Bill 98/1971.

45 Kuusi, *60-luvun sosiaalipolitiikka*, 256–61, 267–73; Harjula, *Terveyden jäljillä*, 82–4, 94–6.

46 *Komiteanmietintö 1959:6. Sairausvakuutuskomitean mietintö* (Helsinki, 1959); *Komiteanmietintö 1961:39 mon. Sairausvakuutuskomitean mietintö. Ehdotus sairausvakuutuslaiksi* (Helsinki, 1961); Yrjö Mattila, *Suuria käännekohtia vai tasaista kehitystä? Tutkimus Suomen terveydenhuollon suuntaviivoista* (Helsinki: Kelan tutkimusosasto, 2011), 113–32, 135–9, 144–51, 322; Heikki Niemelä, *Yhteisvastuuta ja valinnanvapautta: Sairausvakuutus 50 vuotta* (Helsinki: Kelan tutkimusosasto, 2014), 128.

47 Kuusi, *60-luvun sosiaalipolitiikka*; Harjula, *Terveyden jäljillä*, 74–82.

48 Primary Health Care Act 66/1972; *Kansanterveyslaki* 66/1972; *Elämisen laatu: Yhteiskuntapolitiikan tavoitteita ja niiden mittaamista tutkiva jaosto, liite 1* (Helsinki: Talousneuvosto, 1972), 9; *Komiteanmietintö 1971: A 25. Sosiaalihuollon periaatekomitean mietintö I. Yleiset periaatteet.* (Helsinki, 1971), 10, 22; Harjula, *Hoitoonpääsyn hierarkiat*, 256–90.

49 'Käsitemäärittelyjä', *Stakes*, http://info.stakes.fi/kansanterveystyo/FI/kasitteista/index. htm (an archived version of the page, 15 June 2010).

50 Harjula, *Hoitoonpääsyn hierarkiat*, 259–65.

51 Kuusi, *60-luvun sosiaalipolitiikka*; Harjula, *Hoitoonpääsyn hierarkiat*, 268–90; Mattila, *Suuria käännekohtia*,144–55.

52 Decree on Primary Health Care 205/1972, § 1.

53 SVT XI:68, *Yleinen terveyden- ja sairaanhoito 1965* (Helsinki: Lääkintöhallitus, 1967), 80, 87–90.

54 Honkasalo, *Reikä sydämessä*, 17–22, 35–9, 93; Pekka Puska et al., 'Background, principles, implementation, and general experiences of the North Karelia Project', *Global Heart* 11, no. 2 (2016): 173–8; *Terveydenhuollon ohjelma vuosille 1975–1979* (Helsinki: Lääkintöhallitus, 1974), 12.

55 The National Board of Health used *kansansairaus* as a synonym for *kansantauti*. SVT XI: 72–73, *Yleinen terveyden- ja sairaanhoito 1969–1970* (Helsinki: Lääkintöhallitus, 1974), 21.

56 Kari Puro, *Terveyspolitiikan perusteet* (Helsinki: Tammi, 1973); 'Elämisen laatu: Yhteiskuntapolitiikan tavoitteita ja niiden mittaamista tutkiva jaosto. Liite 1', in *Terveyspolitiikan tavoitteita tutkivan työryhmän raportti* (Helsinki: Talousneuvosto, 1972).

57 Heikki Waris, *Muuttuva suomalainen yhteiskunta* (Porvoo: WSOY, 1974).

58 Ranja Aukee, *Vanhasta uuteen sosiaalilääketieteeseen: Suomalaisen sosiaalilääketieteen muotoutuminen 1800-luvun lopulta vuosituhannen vaihteeseen* (Tampere: Tampere University Press, 2013), 23–89; Ilari Rantasalo, 'Hygieniasta kansanterveystieteeseen', *Helsingin yliopisto, kansanterveystieteen osasto* (2006), www.hjelt.helsinki.fi/laitos/ historia/rantasalo.html.

59 *Komiteanmietintö 1971: A 25*, 29; Puro, *Terveyspolitiikan perusteet*; Harjula, *Terveyden jäljillä*, 102–32.

60 Osmo Kaipainen, *Kansa kaikki kärsinyt: Onko terveys kauppatavara vai oikeus* (Hämeenlinna: Karisto, 1969), 44.

61 Harjula, *Hoitoonpääsyn hierarkiat*, 240–46.

62 Ibid., 259–67; *Valtakunnallinen suunnitelma kansanterveystyön järjestämisestä vuosina 1981–85* (Helsinki: Sosiaali- ja terveysministeriö, 1980), 29.

63 *Terveydenhuollon ohjelma vuosille 1975–79*, 5.
64 *Valtakunnallinen suunnitelma kansanterveystyön järjestämisestä vuosina 1980–1984* (Helsinki: Sosiaali- ja terveysministeriö, 1979), 45. Harjula, *Hoitoonpääsyn hierarkiat*, 167–76, 261–2.
65 Juha Teperi et al., *The Finnish Health Care System: A Value-Based Perspective* (Helsinki: Sitra, 2009); Harjula, *Hoitoonpääsyn hierarkiat*, 313–52.
66 For example, Anniina Alaoutinen, *Hyvinvoinnin tukiverkko koetuksella: Helsingin palveluvirastojen toiminta kaupunginosien eriytymisen ehkäisemiseksi* (Helsinki: Helsingin kaupungin tietokeskus, 2010).
67 Matti Rimpelä, 'Vaarantaako kansallinen terveyshanke kansan terveyden?', in *Näkökulmia 2000-luvun terveyspolitiikkaan: Stakesin asiantuntijoiden puheenvuoroja*, ed. Matti Rimpelä and Eeva Ollila (Helsinki: Stakes, 2004), 58–90; Matti Rimpelä, 'Terveyspolitiikan uusi kieli: Joutavatko kansanterveyslain käsitteet historiaan?' *Yhteiskuntapolitiikka* 70, no. 1 (2005): 54–62.
68 Finnish Government, *Health, Social Services and Regional Government Reform* (2017), http://alueuudistus.fi/en/frontpage.

6 The people's health, the nation's health, the world's health

Folkhälsa and folkehelse in the writings of Axel Höjer and Karl Evang

Annika Berg and Teemu Ryymin

In 1947, the Norwegian Chief Medical Officer, Karl Evang, translated part of the charter of the soon-to-be-established World Health Organization (WHO) – "The achievement of any State in the promotion and protection of health is of value to all" – to a Scandinavian audience as follows: "Enhver stats positive resultater i arbeidet for å fremme *folkehelsen* er av verdi også for andre stater."[1] The same year, his Swedish colleague, Axel Höjer, stated in a government White Book on the future organisation of health care in Sweden that: "Föremålet för denna vård, *folkhälsan*, är ett hela folkets intresse" ("The object of this care, the people's health, is an interest of the whole people.")[2]

Both *folkehelse* and *folkhälsa* are often translated to English as 'public health'. For instance, *Folkehelseinstituttet* is translated as 'The Norwegian Institute of Public Health', while the Swedish *Folkhälsomyndigheten* is translated as 'The Public Health Agency of Sweden'. But the similarities may be deceiving. Do these terms, *folkhälsa, folkehelse* and *public health*, really carry the same meanings?

In this chapter, we will explore historical uses of the words *folkhälsa* and *folkehelse* in the writings of Axel Höjer (1890–1974) and Karl Evang (1902–1981), who were long-standing Chief Medical Officers in Sweden and Norway, respectively.

An ardent socialist in his youth with a strong affinity for German-influenced social medicine, Evang served as the leader of the country's publicly owned health services from 1938 to 1972, only interrupted by an involuntary exile in the UK and the US during the German occupation of Norway in 1940–1945.[3] The Health Directorate, which Evang led, presided over a countrywide system of state-appointed medical officers of health. They were responsible for public health in their districts, and also provided primary medical care for the population, particularly in rural areas. In addition, the Directorate was in charge of the country's psychiatric institutions, pharmacies and oral health care, as well as working against tuberculosis (TB) and addressing hygiene issues. It controlled the country's somatic hospitals, which were, however, owned by municipalities, counties and a variety of private actors. While formally under the Department of Social Affairs, the Directorate – and its leader – had a great influence on the forming and implementation of Norwegian health policy in the post-war decades.[4]

Höjer, a Social Democrat in regular conflict with the conservative leadership of the Swedish medical corps, held the corresponding position in Sweden 1935–1952, as Director General of the Royal Medical Board. The Board was a central administrative authority (i.e., it operated under the Ministry of Social Affairs but was not part of the Ministry) responsible for supervising the lion's share of health care in Sweden.[5] Its Director General was able to act highly independently, both in relation to the government and in relation to his own subordinates.[6] After retiring from the Medical Board in 1952, Höjer – who had a long-time engagement in international cooperation – began a new career in the emerging field of development assistance.[7]

Höjer and Evang were both prolific writers, and strongly involved in discussions – at home and abroad – on the meanings and goals of health and health care. Evang, who was among the founders of the WHO, also contributed to the organisation's extensive definition of health from 1946: "Health is a state of complete physical, mental and social well-being and not merely the absence of disease or infirmity."[8]

In the following, we will investigate and compare the usages and understandings of *folkehelse/folkhälsa* in Höjer's and Evang's works: How did they use and understand the concepts? How did they evolve over time? And how, if at all, did their conceptions differ from each other?

Höjer before 1935: Children's health and civic responsibility as keys to the health of the people

Before he became head of the Royal Medical Board in 1935, Axel Höjer ran a medical practice in a poor suburb of Stockholm, completed a doctoral thesis in nutritional science, taught at the University of Lund as an associate professor in hygiene, and served as Medical Officer of Health in Malmö, Sweden's third largest city.

Returning to Sweden in early 1920 after a transformative year spent in post-war France and England, Axel Höjer and his wife Signe, a young nurse and aspiring social worker, chose to settle in Hagalund, an impoverished neighbourhood in the outskirts of Stockholm. There, besides running the medical practice, they concentrated on child health care, reforming an old French-style 'milk drop' or milk distribution centre into a small network of infant clinics inspired by British models. These clinics would later serve as the model for a nationwide, publicly funded system of children's health care centres, instituted during Höjer's time at the Royal Medical Board and still running today.[9]

The decision to prioritise children's, and especially infants', health care was largely strategic. Höjer clarified from the very start that he saw children's health as the key to improving the health status of the whole population – *folkhälsan*: "Over the past twenty years, public opinion has increasingly come to understand how important it is for *folkhälsan* that conditions for mothers and infants are rationally organised."[10]

Infant mortality and child morbidity rates were high in vulnerable areas such as Hagalund. In line with this, Höjer saw infant health care as a rational place to start in order to create a truly preventive health care system. While poor families were targeted in the pilot project, his first proposal for a nationwide system (published in 1923) was based on the idea that the system would reach *all* mothers and children (and receive public funding).[11]

The young Axel Höjer undeniably connected to classic social hygiene in several ways – for example in his use of concepts such as 'inferiority', 'human material', inspection, surveillance, etc. He also spoke of himself as a 'social hygienist'.[12] However, there were also many elements in his thinking that pointed towards social medicine in a more modern sense.[13] More specifically, Höjer urged society (or the state) to take a greater responsibility not only for preventive health care, but also for issues like housing, maternity benefits and a general distribution of wealth as preconditions for health.[14]

In Höjer's mind, and in line with more general Social Democratic ideas of social solidarity, when the level and quality of publicly provided social services (e.g., health care) increased, individuals were increasingly expected to subordinate themselves to the collective best, which was also assumed to be their own best in most – but not all – cases. In this process, people were to be educated and made responsible for themselves. By way of various educational initiatives, people would be granted *medicinsk medborgarkunskap* (approximately, 'medical citizen/ civic knowledge'), which was also the title of a book published in the late 1920s by Axel Höjer and forensic pathologist Einar Sjövall. Quite explicitly, the goal of this educational process was the establishment of a kind of medical citizenship, which implied both rights and obligations.[15]

Political citizenship was still much of a male privilege in the late 1920s, although Swedish women had gained suffrage in the national elections of 1921. However, according to a sort kind of maternalistic logic, Höjer associated *medical citizenship* primarily with women, in their capacity as mothers. Under the supervision of doctors, mothers were assigned a large part of the responsibility for safeguarding the health of themselves and their children, and thus by extension the health of the whole population.[16]

While medical citizenship was essentially female, it was also subject to certain conditions. Great responsibility was placed on mothers, a responsibility justified in terms of nature and biology. Yet childrearing and nurturing were, somewhat paradoxically, not seen as talents that came naturally to women. Therefore, the state would not only intervene at the systems level, with biopolitical measures such as breastfeeding premiums and compensation for loss of wages, but also at the individual level through education and supervision of mothers. The more disciplinary interventions were justified by a belief that women simply did not have the sufficient skills to meet the maternalistic demands of society.[17]

Highlighting the importance of children's health and procreation was also in line with Axel Höjer's formulation of an ultimate goal in the preservation or creation of a viable *släkte* – a widely encompassing concept. Actually, in Linnaean terms *släkte* is the equivalent of genus – that is, the taxonomical level above species (here: *Homo* and not just *Homo sapiens*). Höjer, it seems, used it as an approximate synonym for the human race. He also spoke of 'humanity', in almost religious terms: in the 1920s Höjer spoke of a secular religion of humanity that would include (nearly) all humankind and revolve around the mystery of regeneration.[18]

Höjer was also concerned about the national population. Moderately pronatalist at the time, he argued that the regulation of the number of children, and hence of the size and composition of the population, was an issue related to health. Health care reforms must, he argued, be accompanied by reforms that ensured families had adequate housing and sufficient levels of income for having more children. Regulating the number of children, he claimed, was a concern for individual hygiene as well as social hygiene.[19] In line with this, he argued for an upheaval of the prevailing law against contraceptive propaganda in order to prevent illegal abortions and facilitate family planning. Away from the public eye, he also lectured on the use of contraceptives.[20] However, Höjer's interest in the future of *släktet* and the population also included a eugenic interest, which focused on the prevention of specific diseases in order to improve public health and thus increase social efficiency and productivity. In this context, he could also talk about 'race', although not in an ethnically divisive sense. In Höjer's mind, to secure the future health of humankind, the collective good must prevail over individual rights, and especially so regarding mental development. Thus, people whose genetic makeup severely threatened the collective good must not have the right to reproduce.[21]

To sum up: in the 1920s and early 1930s, Axel Höjer often discussed health in connection to *folk* as well as in connection to related concepts such as *släkte, ras* (race) and *befolkning* (population). At times, he also used the term *folkhälsa*. But the road to approach health in a collective sense was still largely conceptualised in terms of social hygiene and – most importantly – child health care, comprised of collective measures in combination with education of the citizens, and particularly the female citizens in their capacity as mothers.

Folkehelse and Evang before the Second World War

Based on the bibliography of Karl Evang, it seems he did not use the term *folkehelse* in the titles of his pre-World War II writings.[22] The key concept for him at this time was *socialmedisin* (social medicine): Evang was concerned with the health of the *befolkning* (population) or *folk*, by which he was referring to the working class, the unemployed, the poor or other marginalised groups.[23] He propagated selective measures aimed at bettering the health and living conditions of such groups. For instance, in a publication from 1927 entitled *Ny folkesykdom* (A New Peoples' Disease) he dealt with abortion practices. In that book, he used the term *folk* as synonymous with working-class women.[24]

In his contribution to a series of public broadcasting lectures published in 1938 as *Socialhygiene og folkehelse*, Evang did not use the term *folkehelse* at all.[25] His chapter dealt with 'social medical perspectives for the future' (*socialmedisinske fremtidsperspektiver*). He defined *socialmedisin* in a Grotjahnian sense as "that part of medical science that deals with . . . the societal roots of disease", contrasting it with curative, individualistically oriented medicine that was provided, for instance, in hospitals.[26] When he wrote about the target group for social medicine, he used the term *befolkningen*.

Folkehelse was, however, far from an unknown concept in early twentieth-century Norway. It was used in at least in two ways: first, in a German-influenced sense denoting the people's health, emphasising individual responsibility and the healing power of nature; second, as a translation of the Anglo-American term *public health*, emphasising the responsibility of the medical profession to protect the people's health by scientific, particularly laboratory, means. In the first sense, the concept appeared in publications such as the journal *Folkehelsen*, which appeared from 1916. This journal was published by Norske Kvinners Sanitetsforening (the Norwegian Women's Sanitary Association), a voluntary organisation working in the fields of hygiene and health. In 1920, a recently established organisation called Folkehelseforeningen (the Folkehelse Association) also used the same title for its publication.[27] This association promoted ideas such as personal hygiene, public baths and proper nutrition, mixing ideas from holistic natural healing (*naturheilkunde*) and conventional medicine:[28]

> Our work will thus not be directed towards specific issues, but towards anything we deem crooked and wrong [*vrangt og skakt*] in our people's current daily life. We will first and foremost invoke nature's own healing powers, in the form of light, air and water, and a suitable daily bread in true accordance with the best traditions of the art of medicine.[29]

In this context, *folkehelse* denoted the (Norwegian) *people's moral and physical health* and *efforts to strengthen* it. One of the physicians involved, Dr Einar Møinichen (1873–1961), who also ran his own *Naturheil* institution, promoted *folkehelsearbeid (folkehelse* work) along these lines at the national congress of the Norwegian Medical Association in 1920. He defined *folkehelse* as 'the people's health and vitality'.[30]

However, the medical establishment used the same term as a translation of the Anglo-American term 'public health', emphasising science and laboratory medicine instead of individual responsibility and nature. In 1929, the government-owned State Vaccine and Serum Institute was renamed Statens folkehelseinstitutt after a suggestion by the Chief Medical Officer (1927–1930), Karl Wilhem Wefring.[31] Wefring, who had good contacts with the US Rockefeller Foundation (RF), which also provided an endowment to fund a new building for the institute, was clearly influenced by an American understanding of *public health*. This understanding emphasised 'hygienic work' against diseases such as tuberculosis (TB), as well as sanitation and organisational questions.[32] The International Health Division of the RF endowed numerous similar public health institutes in North America and Europe, aiming to "transplant American models of public health" to other countries.[33] From this perspective, central means to promote public health included environmental sanitation, suppression of community infections either by early detection or by the use of vaccines and immune sera, personal hygiene and early diagnosis of health problems. These methods were also central in the RF-funded 'hygiene courses' for state medical officers in Norway established in 1930.[34] In his inaugural speech for the new institute, Wefring did not comment on the new name of the institute – but stated:

Not only do I hope and believe, but am certain, that the scientific and practical work that is carried out [at the institute], now and in the future, will be a main arsenal and a main bastion in the fight against all influences detrimental to a people's health, in all their chequered multiplicity – in air, in water, in soil, in foodstuffs and stimulants. One might say about a human's life course, from the cradle to the grave, that it is in danger, wherever it goes, when it comes to life and health. To remove some of the most dangerous stumbling rocks – precisely this is the programme for public health [*offentlig hygiene*; literally, 'public hygiene'].[35]

The established usage of *folkehelse* in these twin senses, then, did not fit easily with Evang's emphasis on social medicine. This probably explains the marginality of the concept in his pre-Second World War writings.

A matter of concern for society: Director General Axel Höjer's views on the health of the people

In 1935 – three years into the reign of Social Democracy in Sweden and one year after the publication of Alva and Gunnar Myrdal's pivotal *Crisis in the Population Question* – Axel Höjer was empowered to promote health on a national level as the new Director General of the Royal Medical Board. Also in practice, he expanded his target from children to the entire population, and to the organisation of health care more generally. At the same time, he started to speak more frequently of *folkhälsa*, thereby putting the health status of the entire Swedish people into focus.

Of course, this expanded focus was in line with his job description. But it was also linked to a highly progress-oriented view of history where the role of preventive health care was seen as part of a natural, almost predetermined, development.[36] By the early 1950s, Höjer claimed in front of the World Health Assembly that Sweden had reached the stage where children's health care would no longer be prioritised. Instead, child health care was to be integrated into health care programmes catering to all members of society. Karl Evang, who had initiated the discussion, argued in a similar way.[37]

However, expanding the concept of health was not just about the inclusion of all citizens – children and adults, rich and poor – in a project aimed at the whole population. Höjer also began to express himself more ambitiously about the *content* and *meaning* of health. As early as the late 1930s, he spoke of both mental and physical health as goals for preventive work; and after the war he also included social health among these goals, as did the WHO in its new and ambitious health definition (to whose formulation Evang, as noted, had contributed).[38] Moreover, Höjer argued that social progress, in combination with advances in medical science, promised to increase the *level* of health to a virtually ideal standard: Höjer claimed that he saw 'complete health' as an increasingly realistic goal.

In 1938, a few years after taking office as Director General, Höjer wrote a text, aimed at an international audience, which ended with a section about health as *the* national goal. People's health and health care, Höjer wrote (separating the two concepts, just as he did in Swedish), could not possibly be disconnected from issues such as housing, prevention of alcohol abuse, poor relief and social security. At the same time, he argued, health – at least in its broadest sense – was such a crucial condition for human well-being that it could be used as a yardstick of social progress overall: "Could such provisions be made for the people that everyone could preserve full physical and mental health, we would be successful in our political strivings in general."[39]

Höjer believed that if Sweden applied policy measures backed up by scientific findings in the area of preventive medicine, it would be able to get rid of "the handicap of illness and economic disability" within as little as five to ten years. This would both improve the nation's living conditions and make it use its resources to the full, and people from every social class would participate in the pursuit of health in a democratic manner. Höjer founded this faith upon a belief that "the basic condition for efficient labor and for happiness in one's own life is complete physical and mental health". It was also based on a notion that the Swedish people had begun to see illness and premature death as a "shame and a reproach". Höjer believed he was able to claim that Swedish people:

> at present are, by and large, inspired by one guiding thought: no matter how living conditions, working conditions, geographic locations, milieu, and race may vary, a modern state must seek to achieve one thing - the assurance of complete health to each and every one of its citizens.[40]

Under such conditions, it would be very easy to involve the population in the promotion of their own health. Höjer was also happy to note that Swedish politicians had, apparently, "begun to take to heart the words of the old Disraeli that the care of the people's health must be the prime interest of every politician".[41]

Höjer's grandiose plans were somewhat hampered by the outbreak of the Second World War. The conflict affected Sweden deeply, even if the country was never occupied or directly involved in combat. In principle, however, Höjer's eagerness to pursue full health as a national goal or even a human right remained unfazed. And, though he primarily focused on people's health in a nation-bound sense in his role as Chief Medical Officer, he pointed out that people worldwide, in democratic as well as in non-democratic countries, had increasingly begun to see themselves and others as "parts of a humanity, in which every individual and every family demand that the advances of science should come to their advantage". All over the world, he claimed, the "effectually far-reaching, perhaps even revolutionary, principle about everyone's right to full health is making itself heard with strength".[42]

In a 1944 *Festschrift* to Gustaf Möller, Minister for Social Affairs, Höjer claimed that although the immediate task of medical science was to heal the sick, its future task was an even greater one: namely, to abolish disease itself.[43]

Höjer saw basic health care measures such as hygiene, good eating habits and healthy dwellings as instrumental for a healthy population. At the same time, his belief in the attainability of 'full' health led to demands for a large-scale expansion of the health care system, with more doctors and a stronger focus on prevention. It was, according to Höjer, two main developments that motivated the expansion of health care: first, "[s]cientific progress, which makes it possible to achieve much better results, with healthier and therefore happier, more work efficient and more joyful people"; second, the democratic breakthrough, which had put everyone, and not just a few, in the position where they could require access to front-line medical treatment.[44]

In anticipation of a future where people could escape any illness whatsoever through a healthy and 'natural' way of living, Höjer believed it rational to focus on tracking human disease in the bud.[45] By way of a new, nationwide system of health centres, operating on different levels and targeting every part of the population, regular and thorough health checks would be executed to track diseases before they became too expensive and difficult to treat. Monitoring would be deployed at different life stages, and was also meant to include more proactive measures for health promotion.[46]

This elevation of ambitions was most strongly reflected in the government committee report on outpatient medical care that Axel Höjer regarded as his 'testament'.[47] Here, *folkhälsan* was emphasised as the ultimate goal of publicly organised health care, the pursuit of which was in the interest of the whole population.[48] The report, published in 1948, built on a five-year investigation. While focusing on national health, it relied heavily on transnational comparisons.[49] The American so-called Parran plan (1944) was an important influence, and the committee also referred to a number of British sources of inspiration – from the interwar Peckham Experiment to the Beveridge Report (1942) and the government's White Paper *A National Health Service* (1944).[50] Höjer's report was strongly contested by a dominant conservative faction of the Swedish medical corps, and the Social Democratic government resisted it too. In a longer perspective, however, the ideas presented in the report would be largely realised through the expansion and reformation of the Swedish health care system. However, and somewhat ironically, the idea of regular, mandatory health checks for all citizens, which Höjer himself regarded as fundamental, was excluded in the process of implementation.[51]

The report stated that the overall state of health in Sweden – as measured in terms of mortality, infant mortality and life expectancy – had improved significantly over the past 200 years, and also in comparison with other countries. However, the fact that people's health had improved did not mean that it had reached its optimum level. Exploratory health checks had shown that the national health statistics omitted, and thereby concealed, many diseases that significantly reduced health and well-being. Here, the report discussed both individual and collective aspects of ill health, pointing at reduced life satisfaction and work capacity as well as economic strain on both the individual and society.[52]

According to Höjer and his committee, a large part of "the ill health that had caused these figures" could have been avoided by way of a "sufficiently early and sufficiently good medical care".[53] Therefore, the report claimed, the capacity of the health care system must be significantly increased. In addition, both medical treatment itself and its funding and administration must be rationalised. The committee asserted that all it did was follow "the general trend of development of social medicine in Sweden". To follow this natural line of development meant that health care must be organised according to certain basic principles:

> [that] all necessary medical care should be made available to everyone in need thereof, at no special cost at the time when the care is given; that the public should take responsibility for the implementation of this request through an expanded and regulated organisation; that in this [organisation], general health care, hospital care and preventive personal health controls should be coordinated with each other and with outpatient medical care; and that outpatient medical care – which, in our country, has largely been left to doctors themselves and their private initiatives, particularly with regard to general medical care in the cities and specialised care in both urban and rural areas – should be expanded and regulated by way of the public sector.[54]

The idea that *det allmänna* ('the common', that is, public authorities) should take the responsibility for health and medical services was motivated by their importance for 'the whole people and society'. According to Höjer, everyone, regardless of political colour, must agree that society should protect their natural resources rather than meddle in 'personal business'. On this basis, and by defining people's health and work capacity as a prime natural resource rather than a personal matter, he and his committee framed health care as society's most urgent task.[55]

In principle, since *folkhälsan* was "a matter of interest for the entire people", health care should be organised by the state.[56] In practice, however, the report recommended that the organisation of health care – including a new, nationwide network of health centres – should be delegated to the most suitable level of public administration.[57] When Axel Höjer defended the committee's conclusions, he reasoned in line with the same kind of liberal welfare rationality, where decentralisation and coordination were seen as tools in a rational and efficient organisation of public health care.[58]

Axel Höjer's definition of health care as a public interest was also associated with a Marxist view on social justice. All segments of the population would be granted access to health care services according to need. Neither poor nor rich would be disadvantaged, and nor would people living in remote areas. The costs of health care, however, would be distributed in relation to wealth; that is, as Höjer saw it, costs would be shared between citizens in a spirit of solidarity.[59]

All these reforms would create a substantial demand for more doctors. To meet this demand, the investigation suggested medical education in Swedish universities should be expanded to cater to twice as many students as before.[60] In addition, the investigation recommended a limited import of doctors from abroad.[61] Eventually, the new health care organisation would also require full-time salaries and regulated working hours for doctors.[62] However, Höjer's investigation underlined that the reforms would also require a new kind of doctor, one who could combine an understanding of the fundamental factors affecting population health with top-notch scientific knowledge.[63] Training these new doctors, who would unite the roles of scientist and social worker without losing the medical authority of their predecessors, would require fundamental reforms of medical education, integrating a range of social science subjects into the curriculum of medical schools. Educational institutions for nurses and other health care personnel would require similar reforms, the report stated.[64]

Höjer's talk about modern doctors as social scientists is significant. It shows that his strategies for *folkhälsa* must be seen in light of the establishment of academic social sciences in Sweden, his frequent contacts with the Swedish elite of social scientists as well as with representatives of international social medicine, and his and his wife Signe's early contacts with English social reformers. Swedish Social Democrats in general too put deep trust in the emerging social sciences. From Axel Höjer's own perspective, the point of promoting *folkhälsa* and social medicine was not to promote biological explanations of social phenomena, but to bring social, social scientific and, to some extent, socialist perspectives into the medical field. Höjer and his opponents could cordially agree on this, if not on much else.[65]

An earlier example of Höjer's desire to include medicine (in a broader sense) within the emerging field of the social sciences can be seen in the mid-1930s' discussion on the establishment of a national institute for *folkhälsa* and social hygiene, and whether it would be most suitable to institute this as part of the Royal Medical Board (as Axel Höjer argued) or as a more multidisciplinary institution under the Ministry of Social Affairs (which was where it finally ended up). The disagreement over the location of the new institute shows that Höjer, already at that time, was keen to redefine the meaning of medical expertise so that this expertise could include the methods of social science and the policies of social redistribution of resources that he himself wanted to advocate (even if its result was that the Medical Board lost grip of parts of the public health project that Höjer would like to have kept under his umbrella). The discussions do not indicate that any of the participants perceived a fundamental breach between social hygiene and *folkhälsa*, but rather that one was perceived as a means to reach the other.[66] The decision to name the institute *Statens institut för folkhälsan* rather than *Statens institut för social hygien* (State Institute for Social Hygiene) may however have been influenced by the explicitly expressed hope that the institute would receive some funding from the Rockefeller Foundation as part of the latter's international mission to fund institutes for public health.[67] Later on though, when referring to public health in the American sense of the word, Höjer consistently used the term *hälsovård* (health care) rather than *folkhälsa*.[68]

As Höjer's ambitions grew, he gradually shifted his primary attention from the individual to the public sector, although he still emphasised that the individual's and the public sector's responsibility for the people's health were two sides of the same coin, and that rights were coupled with responsibilities.[69] This shift is also reflected in the complete revision of *Medicinsk medborgarkunskap*, which was published in 1945 under the title *Folkhälsan som samhällsangelägenhet* (People's health as a matter of societal concern).[70] The title reflected the core message that the state and the public sector must do their best to create conditions for the full health of each citizen.

However, when the public sector had done what it could, it had the right to demand things in return from its citizens; or, as Höjer expressed it in 1949:

> If we who are older and in power do what is required of us, then, but only then, we have the right to say to the youth: 'Look. We are in some difficulty. We need your help. We ask for sacrifices from you. Look at the goal: a healthy people. Is not it worthwhile that we all contribute to achieve that?'[71]

In some of his writings, he suggested that great personal sacrifices might be necessary. Therefore, "[w]hat is rational for the family and therefore for the people, must also be made rational for the individual". Habitual thoughts and patterns of behaviour had to be changed.[72]

These drastic formulations should be seen in light of Höjer beginning genuinely to regard full physical and mental health as a realistic goal. The imagined attain-ability of this goal implied higher demands on individuals, at least in the long run. In combination, advances in medical science, new infrastructures for communication, and the expansion and improvement of health care paved the way for a society where the old social-liberal principle about helping people to help themselves could transform into a perception of the individuals' *duty* to help themselves.[73]

Höjer had great faith in the majority's ability to control and conduct their own development in the right direction – that is, towards *folkhälsa*. However, he combined this faith with an increased emphasis on a direct disciplining of certain categories of people. This was because scientific progress was thought to have increased the chances of identifying individuals who were unable to provide for the health of themselves and their offspring, either through destructive behaviour or through faulty genetic makeup, and who were thereby also thought to threaten the people as a collective. Leaning on science, society could justify its right to intervene against such individuals, for instance through the sterilisation laws introduced in Sweden in 1934 and 1941. In *Folkhälsan som samhällsangelägenhet*, Einar Sjövall and Axel Höjer lent their support to the legislation, and even suggested that it should be complemented by systematic registration of people who ought to be sterilised, for example by way of health controls of the sort suggested by Höjer in the report on open medical care.[74]

Regardless of his strong emphasis on health being conditioned by the environ-ment, Höjer thus acknowledged a continuing need for eugenic measures. This attitude was far from incompatible with his growing ambitions for the general health of the population. In some respects, it can even be seen as a *consequence* of these higher ambitions. Höjer did not necessarily consider the right to health to be coupled with the right to reproduce.

Höjer reckoned the elimination of bad genes would take a long time, and might never be accomplished. Nevertheless, the people of the future would not settle for imperfection. Rather soon, Höjer thought, they would also start to devote them-selves to positive eugenics in the strict sense – or, in other words, breeding. Unlike before, Höjer now almost seemed to welcome this development, assuming that it could soon be based on science:

A more purposeful creation of a healthier *släkte* will likely be part of the general health care discussions before very long. When reaching a greater scientific maturity and depth, positive eugenics opens up vertiginous perspectives.[75]

In practice, Höjer's visions of *folkhälsa* as full health for all, in combination with a utilitarian view on social solidarity, meant that the people as a whole were prioritised at some expense of people who were regarded as unable to live a full, worthy life. During the 1940s, the Medical Board argued strongly for the sterilisation of people who were categorised as mentally deficient.[76]

Like Karl Evang, Axel Höjer began to speak increasingly and appreciatively about social medicine in the 1940s, especially after visiting the US in 1947 and 1948. However, and significantly, he spoke about social medicine either as a practice or as an ideology – that is, not as a synonym for *folkhälsa* in his own sense of the word as the goal of health care.[77]

Folkehelse for Evang during and after the war: The nation's health

Evang was highly influenced by the contemporaneous developments in health policy and administrative medicine in the UK and the US during the war.[78] After returning to a liberated Norway, he singled out the UK's Beveridge Report (1942) and government White Paper *A National Health Service* (1944), as well as the US Wagner proposals (1939, 1943 and 1945), as important influences on his own plans for the future development of Norway's health services.[79]

Evang developed his plans (1943–1944) in the form of draft papers for the exiled Norwegian government in London. In contrast to his pre-war writings, he ascribed the term *folkehelse* a special meaning in his draft from 1944 entitled 'Plan for folkehelse og helsestellet i Norge'.[80] Evang's use of *folkehelse* was probably influenced by the White Paper *A National Health Service*, in particular.

Evang addressed the first peacetime national congress of the Norwegian Medical Association in September 1945 with a speech later published as 'Noen aktuelle oppgaver ved gjenreisingen av den norske folkehelsen og det norske helsevesen' – which could be translated as 'Some present tasks for the reconstruction of the Norwegian nation's health and the Norwegian health services'.[81] His use of the notion of *folkehelse* denoted *the nation's health status*.[82] He highlighted issues such as certain health problems and the state of nourishment among the population; in contrast to his earlier work, however, he used the term 'population' in the sense of the *whole nation* – 'the Norwegian people' (*det norske folk*), not only disadvantaged groups or the working class.[83] Thus, while the meaning of *folkhälsa* in Axel Höjer's usage had evolved from the health of mother and child to that of the entire population, Evang's usage of *folkehelse* shifted from class to nation.

However, Evang also referred to a complex system consisting of both the nation's health status *and* the health services aspiring to maintaining and enhancing this status. On this point, Evang and Höjer differ: the latter distinguished between *folkhälsa* and *hälsovård*, while the former included both in the concept of *folkehelse*. Evang expressed this wider understanding of *folkehelse* at the outset of his speech, where he presented "some words on the health status of the Norwegian people at the end of the war":

> German and Nazi misrule and terror have, among other things, expressed themselves in the disintegration of important elements of the Norwegian health services during the five years of occupation. Medical materials of every sort have to a great extent been exhausted or destroyed. The health of the population is weakened through the years of mal- and undernourishment, the lack of medicines and hospitals, firewood, clothing and housing. Certain epidemic diseases, tuberculosis and other illnesses have got a grip on the population that was unknown in the pre-war years.[84]

Evang's use of *folkehelse* denoting both the nation's health status and the health services thus engaged a somewhat different semantic field compared with the pre-Second World War usages of the notion. Rather than referring to the people's health and vitality, or to hygiene, sanitation and prevention of contagious epidemic diseases (i.e. public health in the Anglo-American sense of the word), on the one hand, it pointed to the health status of the nation as measured by numerous indicators (mortality, weight and height development, nourishment status and so on); on the other hand, it pointed to the full range of comprehensive, publicly provided health services.

Evang developed this wide understanding of *folkehelse* also in a popularised version of his reconstruction plan, published in 1947 as *Gjenreising av folkehelsa i Norge* (The reconstruction of *folkehelsa* in Norway), where he discussed the nation's health status.[85] In addition, he considered a wide variety of curative, preventive and administrative health measures that were to enhance *folkehelse*. For instance, the measures he proposed in order to reconstruct the nation's health (*folkehelsa*) ranged from the rebuilding and reorganisation of hospitals, via specific measures to deal with TB, venereal diseases (VD), cancer, mental health problems and rheumatism, to measures to strengthen the population's nourishment status, the building of mother-and-child centres, education of nurses – and the reorganisation of the administration of the health services. In 1952, he described "the fantastic development" of *folkehelsen* during the last fifty years – and again used the term to encompass both the nation's health status and the health services.[86]

After the war, Karl Evang's focus shifted from class to nation. This shift was reflected in his usage of the concept of *folkehelse* in the sense of the nation's health. Trond Nordby has discussed the shift, and attributed Evang's new ideas of the nation to his experience of war.[87] However, as noted above, Evang also drew on the influential Beveridge Report, and subsequent White Paper, *A National Health Service*. The latter aspired to a comprehensive health service 'for all': in order to "ensure that everybody in the country . . . shall have equal opportunity to benefit from the best and most up-to-date medical and allied services available", a national health service was necessary.[88] In his report, Lord Beveridge used notions such as "the health of the people" as well as "medical treatment of the nation" in connection with plans for "comprehensive health and rehabilitation services".[89] Likewise, both the US Wagner Bill (1939), which would have made it possible for US states to establish systems of compulsory health insurance, and the Wagner-Murray-Dingell Bill (introduced in 1943 and revised, unsuccessfully, in 1945) utilised the concept of 'national health', drawing on earlier attempts by President Roosevelt to establish 'a national health program'.[90]

After the 1950s, the concept of *folkehelse* figures only sporadically in Evang's publications. For instance, in his 1965 book on the use and misuse of medicine (aimed at the general public), he used the notion only once – denoting the population's health status. He used the concept in a similar way in his 1972 book on drugs, youth and society.[91] In his seminal book from 1974, social medicine was once again the core concept.

Public health and *folkehelse*

Karl Evang was inspired by the Anglo-American discourse and development in several respects. It may be argued that his use of the concept *folkehelsen* in the immediate post-war years – to denote mainly the nation's health status and the system for maintaining it – was derived from Anglo-American concepts and notions of national health. The English concept *public health*, on the other hand, had a distinct meaning for Evang: it referred to a specialised field of medical knowledge and practice. *Public health* was, in other words, something that could (and should) contribute to *folkehelsen*, and was also part of the apparatus to maintain it; but they were by no means identical. The tendency to translate *folkehelse* straightforwardly as 'public health' thus obfuscates that Evang attributed different meanings to the English and Norwegian concepts. The fact that some scholars translate 'public health' as *folkehelse* in connection with Evang, and that translations of Evang's texts to English often do the same, gives rise to conceptual confusion.[92] In this section, we instead differentiate between these concepts and use italics to denote the English historical concept *public health*, as used by Evang.

In 1953, Evang stated in the *Journal of the Norwegian Medical Association* that the Scandinavian languages lacked altogether a term that would sufficiently cover the English term *public health*, and proceeded to differentiate between three versions of it:[93]

- a continental (German) variety, emphasising judicial/police expertise, forensic medicine and pathology, contagious epidemic diseases, 'social' diseases such as TB and VD, as well as the interpretation and implementation of medical acts and regulations;
- an Anglo-American version, emphasising public health as a medical affair, focusing on epidemiology in a wide sense – health education as well as environmental, workplace and foodstuff hygiene, and mother-and-child health issues;

- and, finally, a 'Slavic' (Russian) sense, characterised by a holistic under-standing of health work prioritising the government's responsibility in the field of health.[94]

According to Evang, 'public health' in the Scandinavian countries contained elements of all three varieties, albeit in different mixes.

He also proposed a nine-point preliminary definition of 'public health' as 'social and administrative medicine', consisting of:

1)   general promotion of health through heightening of living standards;
2)   preventive medicine;
3)   curative and palliative medicine;
4)   rehabilitation;
5)   measures aimed at 'biological minus variants' that could not be rehabilitated, such as certain groups of the elderly, 'retards', epileptics, the blind, deaf and 'strongly handicapped';
6)   health control of presumed healthy population groups;
7)   health statistics;
8)   education of health personnel; and
9)   international cooperation on the field of health.[95]

Evang criticised earlier definitions of the term for lacking a focus on the need for an organisation or administrative apparatus to plan 'public health' work – what was needed was 'a general staff' for 'public health'.[96]

In part, this definition reflected well-established practices in the medical services that Evang headed. For instance, he had already in the pre-war period supported eugenic measures, such as sterilisation aimed at "biological minus variants", even though he explicitly distanced himself from racialised variants of eugenics.[97] In other words, while Evang's uses of *public health* and *folkehelse* certainly overlapped to some degree, they nevertheless pointed to different things.

The promotion of *public health* became one of Evang's main goals within the new World Health Organization.[98] Evang, who had been involved in the establish-ment of the WHO, chaired the organisation's programme committee at the First World Health Assembly in 1948, and was President of the Second World Health Assembly in 1949.[99] He served on the organisation's executive board (1948–1949), and in 1951 was elected chairman of the WHO Expert Committee on Public-Health Administration, where he promoted his vision of *public health*.[100]

From the nation's health to world health: Axel Höjer after 1952

At least since the late 1930s, Axel Höjer had embraced a vision of full health for all, or nearly all, of the Swedish people. When he started working at an international level, he broadened this vision of *folkhälsa*, people's health, also in regard to the other part of the concept – that is, the people. He now began to talk about health in a global sense too.

Axel Höjer had been actively involved in international health cooperation already during the interwar period. On becoming Director General of the Medical Board in 1935, he almost immediately got engaged in the work of the League of Nations' Health Organization.[101]

After the war, Höjer led the Swedish delegation at the WHO's first five annual World Health Assemblies. For most of that time he was also one of 18 members of the WHO Executive Board.[102] In the WHO, Höjer worked closely with Karl Evang and the other Nordic delegates. This collaboration helped Höjer succeed Evang as a member of the Executive Board in 1949 when Evang's term of office expired.[103]

Höjer was enthusiastic about the WHO, especially in the beginning. Small states were able to make their voices heard, he said, and "many prominent women" played an important role in the discussions. According to Höjer, the various delegations did their best not to let political differences hinder worldwide collaboration for better health – or, more precisely, better world health:

> The problems are very different, for instance, in Sweden and in India or in Liberia. If Sweden can help in the work for a better world health [*världshälsa*], we will not just fulfil a simple human obligation: we will also learn a lot, both in the medical and other fields. I have participated in a lot of congresses but have never before felt so clearly that the world now stands in transition between two stages: the old one of competition, when people came together to see what benefits they could usurp at the expense of others; and the coming one, when it will become obvious that the whole world, and we ourselves alike, will do best by trying to help each other as best we can. It is through health care and social welfare that the world is about to learn this seemingly simple, yet so difficult lesson.[104]

Here, while Höjer used the word *världshälsa* to refer to the health of the people in a global sense, he also associated the concept with a duty that fell to Sweden and other nations, as well as with an infrastructure for collecting and disseminating knowledge. Höjer also argued that health care aiming at the promotion of world health was a means for bringing humanity to peace and cooperation.

After retiring from the Royal Medical Board in 1952, Höjer continued to work for the WHO in India and Africa. Axel and Signe Höjer's international commitment also continued after their return to Sweden in the 1960s, when they engaged in NGO campaigns against leprosy and nuclear armament, and promoted Swedish development aid to the Third World.

When, during his years in international work, Höjer widened his notion of people's health and talked about world health as the health of the world's population, it was a change of discourse that was related to a more general change in the view of the world, and of Sweden's role in it. Both Axel and Signe Höjer emphasised that the West had a duty to bring people in the underdeveloped parts of the world into a position where they would be able to help themselves to build their own welfare states, after centuries of oppression, without reproducing old relationships of dependency.[105] Sweden, they assumed, was particularly well suited to help countries in need, not least when it came to international health work. That was because the country had escaped material damage and casualties during the war, but could still benefit from the technical progress made at that time, particularly in the field of disease control. Also, while Sweden indeed had a colonial history, it was quite distant in time and seldom discussed. And, last but not least, they underscored that the country had recently gone through a rapid process of modernisation, which could provide useful lessons for the South.[106]

In Höjer's view, sickness and health were both global phenomena, and this in itself demanded a worldwide perspective. Axel Höjer stressed that prosperity and social justice were necessary conditions for health throughout the world; but he also pointed out that this was not enough:

> In a well-planned and successful economy, it will certainly be easier to avoid infections, under- and malnutrition and other health injuries that follow in the steps of poverty and misery. But this only applies to a population that is well educated, enlightened and disciplined.[107]

For Höjer, thus, macro-scale biopolitical measures and the disciplining of individuals were fundamentally intertwined at the global level as well as at the national, and each set of technologies was seen as a condition for the other.

A strong motive behind the conceptualisation of global health – and consequently, some kind of global health care – was the old insight that diseases, and infectious diseases in particular, know no national boundaries. But Höjer stressed that while disease and ill health were threats against everyone, regardless of nationality or location, they were also phenomena that could unite people. Thus, although he sometimes bought into a somewhat exoticising tropical medicine discourse, he also displayed a distinctly different ambition in his attempts to show the universality of disease in order to create identification. For example, Höjer pointed out that diseases like leprosy, malaria and cholera were not as 'tropical' as they sometimes were portrayed – in fact, Sweden had been haunted by the very same diseases until quite recently. The big difference, according to Höjer, consisted in how far different countries had progressed in the fight against them.[108]

The talk about a community in illness related to a perception that all people were united in a common concern for everyone's full health. This interest should not be limited by national borders, or exploited by individual nations or multinational companies. Ultimately, Höjer saw world health as relying on a sense of solidarity, felt by all individuals and directed towards all other individuals in the world.[109] In other words, it depended on an expansion of social solidarity into a kind of global solidarity. This whole argument was also part of an emerging discourse of development aid.[110]

As Höjer put it, the duty (and joy) of helping out in the fight for full *världshälsa* was also motivated by scientific advances making that fight technically possible – particularly in the field of preventive health care.[111]

According to Höjer, the great obstacle to secure *världshälsa* was economic. At the same time, he considered that obstacle avoidable. Höjer never portrayed health care policy, nationally or internationally, as a choice between different methods of health promotion. Instead, as he saw it, the real opposition stood between investments in health care and investments in the military sector.[112] To put military efforts against social efforts was an old rhetorical tactic, which had been used extensively in the women's peace movement, among others.[113] Höjer had also used it himself as early as 1928 in a speech to the Social-Democratic Party Congress.[114] The difference was that he now applied this argument to global health care.[115]

At the same time, Höjer criticised the WHO for dodging responsibility in critical issues. The organisation's apolitical stance had prevented it from speaking out against nuclear weapons, and contributed to the difficulty in formulating a position on family planning. In the future, he said, the WHO would have to abandon its policy to never act politically. The issue of *folkhälsa* was deeply and unavoidably political, and it became even more political when considered on a global scale.[116]

In connection to world health, Höjer repeatedly appealed to the Swedes' sense of solidarity. He did this not only while encouraging people to donate money through NGOs such as Save the Children, but also when trying to make them willing to, eventually, finance development aid through their income tax.[117] However, the Swedish Social Democratic vision of social solidarity had traditionally been based on a notion of reciprocity; rights were connected to plights. As we have seen, Axel Höjer very clearly reaffirmed this notion when discussing *folkhälsa* from a national perspective. In contrast, his vision of global solidarity did not include a similar sense of reciprocity. Höjer could talk about the importance of anchoring decisions and cooperating with aid recipients, but he hardly ever spoke about *demands* that could be placed on Third World people, as citizens of a global community. Strikingly too, he did not apply eugenic arguments in his discussions of the Third World. Moreover, he never raised the issue of fighting corruption as a prerequisite for global health, although he clearly identified corruption, communalism and nepotism as fundamental structural problems in countries such as India.

This silence regarding reciprocal duties and necessary sacrifices from people in the post-colonial world may be partly explained by the audiences – national and international – that Höjer addressed and the frameworks that he worked within. In any case, it indicates that despite all his rhetoric about *världshälsa*, Höjer still perceived full health on a global level as a rather far-off goal.

Concluding remarks

In the decades after the First World War, both Karl Evang and Axel Höjer prioritised health promotion among selected groups: the poor, the marginalised, the working class (Evang); children (and mothers) (Höjer). Both expressed themselves using terms such as 'social hygiene' and, sometimes, 'social medicine'. Höjer also used the notion of *folkhälsa* already in the 1920s. In contrast, the use of *folkehelse* was marginal in Evang's writings even during the Second World War. We have argued that this may be understood in the context of other established uses of the notion in Norway. Such established notions included, on the one hand, a German-influenced understanding of the people's moral and physical health, and, on the other, an Anglo-American understanding of (scientific) public health work.

In the 1930s and 1940s, Evang and Höjer reconsidered earlier ideas about the target groups of health promotion. From the mid-1930s, Höjer became increasingly concerned about the whole Swedish population when talking about *folkhälsa*. As of 1944, Evang took the notion of *folkehelse* in use when discussing the nation's health – influenced not least by British ideas of national health.

In spite of Höjer and Evang sharing many fundamental principles pertaining to the aims, means and scope of health care during the post-war period, some crucial differences in their usage of *folkhälsa/folkehelse* may be identified. From 1944 onwards, Evang tended to use the term *folkehelse* to denote both the nation's health status and the health apparatus to maintain it, while Höjer differentiated between *folkhälsa* (to denote the people's health status) and *hälsovård* (referring to the practices intended to promote *folkhälsa*, including social hygiene, social medicine and public health in the Anglo-American sense of the word, and the institutionalisation of such practices). One reason for Evang's conflation of health status and health care may be that he and many others considered the Norwegian health services and the health of the population severely damaged by the exigencies of war and occupation, and in dire need of reconstruction. The situation in non-occupied Sweden was less urgent compared to Norway.

In the 1950s and 1960s, Höjer further broadened his ideas about the target group of public health care to include the whole global community, although his vision of complete health for all people in all countries as the goal of global health care was arguably more utopian than his vision of complete health for the Swedish people. Interestingly, when moving on to talk about *världshälsa* rather than *folkhälsa*, Höjer also became more prone to conflate goals and means (health and health care) in the manner Evang used to do when talking about *folkhälsa* in a Norwegian context.

Unlike Höjer, Evang continued to work as Chief Medical Officer in his native country until the early 1970s. However, although thus keeping an active and leading role in the field of national health care, Evang used the concept of *folkehelse* less frequently from the 1950s onward.

Despite their differences, Höjer and Evang shared an understanding of *public health* in the Anglo-American/German sense as something highly distinct from *folkhälsa/folkehelse*. For Evang, public health was a branch of medical science encompassing social and administrative medicine, while Höjer consistently translated the US term 'public health' as *hälsovård* (health care) rather than *folkhälsa*.

To conclude, these two examples serve to show that the tendency to treat concepts like public health, people's health and national health as interchangeable across different linguistic and historical contexts deprives them of their historical meaning – and thus makes it difficult to understand what actors such as Höjer and Evang really meant when they spoke about *folkhälsa* or *folkehelse*.

Notes

1 Karl Evang, 'Det internasjonale helsearbeid', *Nordisk Medicin* 36, no. 44 (1947): 2172–8, 2176 (emphasis added).

2 Statens offentliga utredningar (State public reports; hereafter SOU) 1948:14, *Den öppna läkarvården i riket: Utredning och förslag*: 271 (emphasis added). The report was completed in 1947 but published in 1948.

3 On Evang, see Trond Nordby, *Karl Evang: En biografi* (Oslo: Aschehoug, 1989); Siv Frøydis Berg, *Den unge Karl Evang og utvidelsen av helsebegrepet: En idéhistorisk fortelling om sosialmedisinens fremvekst i norsk mellomkrigstid* (Oslo: Solum, 2002); Aina Schiøtz, *Folkets helse: Landets styrke 1850–2003* (Oslo: Universitetsforlaget, 2003).

4 On the system see Schiøtz, *Folkets helse*, 309–47.

5 On the organisation and responsibilities of the Medical Board and its predecessors, see Erik Björkquist and Ivar Flygare, 'Den centrala medicinalförvaltningen', in *Medicinalväsendet i Sverige 1813–1962: Utgiven med anledning av Kungl. Medicinalstyrelsens 300-årsjubileum*, ed. Wolfram Kock (Stockholm: Nordiska bokhandelns förlag, 1963); Annika Berg, *Den gränslösa hälsan: Signe och Axel Höjer, folkhälsan och expertisen* (Uppsala: Acta Universitatis Upsaliensis, 2009), 207–11.

6 Roger Qvarsell, 'Att räkna sjuka och friska: Medicinalstyrelsen som socialvetenskaplig entreprenör', in *Samhällets linneaner. Kartläggning och förståelse i samhällsvetenskapernas historia*, ed. Bengt Erik Bengtsson and Roger Qvarsell (Stockholm: Carlssons, 200), 123–59, 123–5.

7 On Höjer, see Berg, *Den gränslösa hälsan*; Annika Berg, 'Power, knowledge and acknowledgement of expertise: Signe and Axel Höjer's strategies to launch public health ideas, 1919–1970', in *In Experts We Trust: Knowledge, Politics and Bureaucracy in Nordic Welfare States*, ed. Åsa Lundqvist and Klaus Petersen (Odense: University of Southern Denmark Press, 2010), 181–221.

8 *Constitution of the World Health Organization* (2006), www.who.int/governance/eb/who_constitution_en.pdf; cf. Nordby, *Karl Evang*, 137–44; Berg, *Den unge Karl Evang*.

9 More on this in Berg, *Den gränslösa hälsan*.

10 Axel Höjer, 'Något om barnmorskeväsendet i England: Intryck från en studieresa där sept–dec 1919', *Jordemodern* 33 (1920): 209.

11 Axel Höjer, Hjalmar Fries, Carl Gustaf Hulting, Adolf Lichtenstein and Gotthilf Stéenhoff, 'Betänkande rörande övervakning av späda barn: Till pediatriska sektionen av Läkaresällskapet', *Hygiea* 85 (1923): 573, 581–2. Cf. Nikolas Rose, 'Medicine, history and the present', in *Reassessing Foucault: Power, Medicine and the Body*, ed. Roy Porter and Colin Jones (London: Routledge, 1994), 48–72, 65–6; Michel Foucault, 'The politics of health in the eighteenth century', in *Power/Knowledge: Selected Interviews and Other Writings 1972–1977*, ed. Michel Foucault and Colin Gordon (New York: Pantheon, 1980), 166–82, 172–5.

12 Axel Höjer, 'Barns hälso- och sjukvård', in *Tidens läkarbok*, ed. Gunnar Dahlberg (Stockholm: Tiden, 1926), 303–4; Axel Höjer, 'Den s. k. preventivlagens otidsenlighet', *Tiden* 20 (1927): 83–4; Axel Höjer, 'Reseberättelse, inkommen till Medicinalstyrelsen 5/10 1920, d:nr 1703/1920 M', in Medicinalbyrån, E III. 1920, archives of the Royal Board of Medicine in the Swedish National Archives, Stockholm; Axel Höjer, 'Något om engelsk barna- och modersvård', *Vårdarebladet* 10 (1920): 30; Höjer et al., 'Betänkande rörande övervakning av späda barn', 570–82; Axel Höjer, Sven Tunberg, Gunnar Myrdal, Georg Andrén, Nils von Hofsten, Sven Wicksell, Gustaf Åkerman and Arvid Runestam, *Debatt i befolkningsfrågan* (Stockholm: Kooperativa förbundet, 1935): 34.

13 Cf. Karin Johannisson, 'Folkhälsa. Det svenska projektet från 1900 till 2: a världskriget', *Lychnos: Årsbok för idéhistoria och vetenskapshistoria 1991* (Uppsala: Lärdomshistoriska samfundet, 1991): 139–95, 169; Dorothy Porter and Roy Porter, 'What was social medicine? An historiographical essay', *Journal of Historical Sociology* 1 (1988): 90–106; Paul Weindling, 'Social medicine at the League of Nations

and the International Labour Office compared', in *International Health Organisations and Movements, 1918–1939*, ed. Paul Weindling (Cambridge: Cambridge University Press, 1995), 134–53, 135–6; Michel Foucault, 'The birth of social medicine', in *Essential works of Foucault, 1954–1984: Vol. 3, Power*, ed. Paul Rabinow, James D. Faubion and Robert Hurley (New York: New Press, 2000): 134–56.

14 In the 1920s, Höjer became more concerned with the impact of the outer environment, particularly nutrition and housing, on people's health. Einar Sjövall and Axel Höjer, *Medicinsk medborgarkunskap* (Stockholm: Bonnier, 1929), 55–88. This part of the book was written by Höjer, according to a letter by Einar Sjövall in Signe and Axel Höjer's archives in the National Archives, Stockholm (SAHA), 2a vol. 2.

15 Sjövall and Höjer, *Medicinsk medborgarkunskap*, 287–97.

16 See e.g. Sjövall and Höjer, *Medicinsk medborgarkunskap*, 32–54, 295; Axel Höjer, 'Hygieniska synpunkter på barnantalets reglering', *Tiden* 21 (1928): 15–24. Cf. Kjell Östberg, *Efter rösträtten: Kvinnors utrymme efter det demokratiska genombrottet* (Stockholm and Stehag: Brutus Östlings Bokförlag Symposion, 1997).

17 Axel Höjer, 'Om "Mjölkdroppar" som övervakningsställen för späda barn', *Hygienisk revy* 12 (1923): 59.

18 Berg, *Den gränslösa hölsan*, 151-6.

19 Höjer, 'Hygieniska synpunkter', 16-18.

20 Berg, *Den gränslösa hälsan*, 127, 157.

21 Sjövall and Höjer, *Medicinsk medborgarkunskap*, 20–28, 31–2, cit. on p. 26; Höjer, 'Hygieniska synpunkter', 16-18.

22 Cf. Nordby, *Karl Evang*, 333-58.

23 Berg, *Den unge Karl Evang*, 38-9; Nordby, *Karl Evang*, 172.

24 Berg, *Den unge Karl Evang*, 55.

25 Karl Evang, 'Socialmedisinske fremtidsperspektiver', in *Socialhygiene og folkehelse*, ed. Sverre Kjølstad et al. (Oslo: Stenersens, 1938), 69-80.

26 Ibid., 74.

27 Harald L. Tveterås, *Norske tidsskrifter: Bibliografi over periodiske skrifter i Norge inntil 1920* (Oslo: Universitetsbiblioteket, 1940), 38.

28 'Program', in *Folkehelseforeningen* 1, no. 2 (1920): 10.

29 Cf. the manifesto of the association, published in *Meddelelser fra Den norske nationalforening mot tuberkulosen* 9, no. 37 (1919): 109–10, 110.

30 Einar Møinichen, 'Linjerne for folkehelsearbeidet', *Tidsskrift for Den norske lægeforening* 40 (1920): 720–24, 722. On the German tradition of *Volksgensundheit*, and its relation to *naturheilkunde*, see Avi Sharma, *We Lived for the Body: Natural Medicine and Public Health in Imperial Germany* (DeKalb, IL: NIU Press, 2014); Cornelia Regin, *Selbsthilfe und Gesundheitspolitik: Die Naturheilbewegung im Kaiserreich (1889 bis 1914)* (Stuttgart: Steiner, 1995).

31 *Stortingsproposisjon* [Norway's National Budget] *Nr. 1 (1929)*, ch. 453 and 2451, 1.

32 See for instance Karl Wilhelm Wefring, 'Ordningen av vort offentlige lægevesen', *Tidsskrift for Den norske lægeforening* 48 (1928): 965–80, 970, 979, 980; Karl Wilhelm Wefring, 'Endring i Sundhetsloven av 16. mai 1860', *Tidsskrift for Den norske lægeforening* 50 (1930): 487–90, 487. According to Paul Weindling, "[t]he American approach to public health . . . combined organizational questions, health education, and the practicalities of sanitary technologies with high-powered laboratory research on vaccines and pathogens". Paul Weindling, 'American Foundations and the Internationalizing of Public Health', in *Shifting Boundaries of Public Health: Europe in the Twentieth Century*, ed. Susan Gross Solomon, Lion Murard and Patrick Zylberman (Rochester: University of Rochester Press, 2008), 63–86, 68.

33 Paul Weindling, 'Public health and political stabilisation: The Rockefeller Foundation in Central and Eastern Europe between the two World Wars', *Minerva* 31, no. 3 (1993): 253–67, 255; cf. John Farley, *To Cast Out Disease: A History of the International*

Health Division of the Rockefeller Foundation (1913–1951) (Oxford: Oxford University Press, 1993); Elisabeth Fee, 'Designing schools of public health for the United States', in *A History of Education in Public Health: Health that Mocks the Doctors' Rules*, ed. Elisabeth Fee and Roy M. Acheson (Oxford: Oxford University Press, 1991), 155–94, 187–8.

34 Cf. Karl Wilhelm Wefring, 'Fysikateksamen. Kurser i hygiene for offentilge læger', *Tidsskrift for Den norske lægeforening* 50 (1930): 543–7.

35 Karl Wilhelm Wefring, 'Statens institutt for folkehelsen', *Tidsskrift for Den norske lægeforening* 49 (1929): 965–72, 971.

36 Axel Höjer, *Hälsovård och läkarvård: I går – i dag – i morgon* (Stockholm: KF, 1949), 12–13, 115. Cf. Åsa Linderborg, *Socialdemokraterna skriver historia: Historieskrivning som ideologisk maktresurs 1892–2000* (Stockholm: Atlas, 2001), 461–3.

37 *Fifth World Health Assembly, Geneva, 5 to 22 May 1952: Resolutions and Decisions; Plenary Meetings, Verbatim Records; Committees, Minutes and Reports; International Sanitary Regulations, Reservations; Annexes* (Geneva: World Health Organization, 1952), 226.

38 Axel Höjer, 'Public health and medical care', in *Some Aspects of Swedish Social Welfare*, ed. J. Axel Höjer, Otto R. Wangson and Tor Jerneman (Stockholm: Royal Swedish Commission/New York's World Fair, 1939), 3–41, 40–41; SOU 1948:14, 107–9, 203, 253–4, 292.

39 Höjer, 'Public health and medical care', 41.

40 Ibid.

41 Ibid., 40.

42 Axel Höjer, 'Aktuella socialmedicinska uppgifter', in *Socialmedicinsk tidskrift* 18 (1941): 129–37,150–55, 130.

43 Axel Höjer, 'Reformkrav och framtidsvyer inom hälso- och sjukvård', in *Ett genombrott: Den svenska socialpolitiken, utvecklingslinjer och framtidsmål. Festskrift till Gustaf Möller den 6 juni 1944* (Stockholm: Tiden, 1944), 343–70, 343.

44 Höjer, *Hälsovård och läkarvård*, 51–2, cit. on p. 51; Axel Höjer, 'Demokratisk sjukvård', *Morgon-Tidningen* 5 April 1948.

45 Höjer, *Hälsovård och läkarvård*, 43; Höjer, 'Demokratisk sjukvård'; SOU 1948:14, 215–17, 253–4, 387, cit. p. 254. Cf. Höjer, 'Reformkrav och framtidsvyer', 357.

46 Höjer, *Hälsovård och läkarvård*, 34–68; SOU 1948:14, 285, 292, 318, 321–2. Cf. Axel Höjer, 'Ur J. Axel Höjers minnen' (unabridged memoirs), in *J. Axel Höjers arkiv* [archives of J. Axel Höjer], Swedish National Archives, Stockholm, 583–609; Axel Höjer, 'Den öppna läkarvården', *Sveriges landstings tidskrift* 36, no. 1 (1949): 1–8, 5.

47 SOU 1948:14. In Swedish, the word *testamente* signifies a bequest or will in the juridical sense, besides being a word with strong biblical connotations.

48 SOU 1948:14, 271.

49 Ibid.

50 Ibid., 167–76, 185–92, 195–7, 208.

51 Berg, *Den gränslösa hälsan*, chapter 2:3.

52 SOU 1948:14, 17–22, cit. p. 17.

53 Ibid., 23.

54 Ibid., 241.

55 Ibid.

56 Ibid.

57 Ibid., 271–84, 311–14. See also Höjer, *Hälsovård och läkarvård*, 85–90; Höjer, 'Den öppna läkarvården', 4. Cf. Peter Garpenby, *The State and the Medical Profession: A Cross-National Comparison of the Health Policy Arena in the United Kingdom and Sweden, 1945–1985* (Linköping: Linköpings universitet, 1989), 159–66.

58 Höjer, 'Den öppna läkarvården', 3–5.

59 SOU 1948:14, 241.

60 Ibid., 263, 309, 390, 392; Höjer, 'Den öppna läkarvården', 3; Höjer, *Hälsovård och läkarvård*, 81–2, 112.
61 SOU 1948:14, 310–11; Höjer, *Hälsovård och läkarvård*, 74; Höjer, 'Den öppna läkarvården', 3; Höjer, 'Ur J. Axel Höjers minnen', 527–30.
62 SOU 1948:14, 221–4, 232–4, 315-18.
63 Ibid., 293.
64 Ibid., 107–9, 216, 390.
65 Cf. Berg, *Den gränslösa hälsan*, 273-4.
66 For a more elaborate discussion on this debate, see Berg, *Den gränslösa hälsan*, 209–11. Cf. SOU 1937:31; Johannisson, 'Folkhälsa', 180.
67 SOU 1937:31, 6, 19, 22, 68, 75, 78. Höjer, too, held hope in "a Public Health institute which, after the model of other Rockefeller institutions, would, among its main tasks, undertake the training of public health officers". Höjer, 'Public health and medical care', 35–6, cit. on p. 35.
68 See e.g. Höjer's narratives about his long, Rockefeller Foundation-sponsored roundtrip in the USA and Canada in 1947–1948, or his subsequent propaganda for a Nordic, Rockefeller-type of public health school. Axel Höjer, 'Amerikansk medicin', *Sveriges landstings tidskrift* 35 (1948): 25–31; Axel Höjer, *En läkares väg. Från Visby till Vietnam* (Stockholm: Bonniers, 1975), 200–204; cf. Höjer, 'Public health and medical care'.
69 Höjer, 'Aktuella socialmedicinska uppgifter', 130.
70 Axel Höjer and Einar Sjövall, *Folkhälsan som samhällsangelägenhet* (Stockholm: Albert Bonniers, 1945), 5–7. Cf. Sjövall and Höjer, *Medicinsk medborgarkunskap* (1929, with new editions in 1930 and 1936).
71 Höjer, *Hälsovård och läkarvård*, 116; Cf. also Axel Höjer, 'Våra folksjukdomar och kampen mot dem', in *Ett friskare folk. Typföredrag till hälsokampanjen 1945* (Stockholm: Sveriges Läkarförbund, 1946), 90–91.
72 Axel Höjer, 'En läkares syn på befolkningsfrågorna', *Svenska läkartidningen* 38 (1941): 2253–8. Cf. Signild Vallgårda, *Folkesundhed som politik. Danmark og Sverige fra 1930 til i dag* (Aarhus: Aarhus University Press/Magtudredningen, 2003), 35; Berg, *Den gränslösa hälsan*, 282.
73 Cf. Nikolas Rose, 'Government, authority and expertise in advanced liberalism', *Economy and Society* 22 (1993): 283–99, 296.
74 Höjer and Sjövall, *Folkhälsan som samhällsangelägenhet*, 7, 78–81.
75 Höjer, 'Reformkrav och framtidsvyer', 346–7, cit. on p. 347.
76 Cf. Mattias Tydén, *Från politik till praktik. De svenska steriliseringslagarna 1935–1975* (Stockholm: Almqvist & Wiksell International, 2002), 320.
77 Berg, *Den gränslösa hälsan*, 268-74.
78 Eg. Nordby, *Karl Evang*, 119–21.
79 Karl Evang, 'Noen aktuelle oppgaver ved gjenreisningen av den norske folkehelsen og det norske helsevesen', *Tidsskrift for Den norske lægeforening* 65 (1945): 266–71, 267.
80 'Utkast til en plan for folkehelse og helsestell i Norge etter krigen', Helsedirektoratet i London, Da. #0166, 13.80, National Archives of Norway (RA); 'Norsk helsestell og norske helseproblem', Helsedirektoratet i London, Da. #0031, Medisinaldirektør Evang: Helseplaner, RA. Cf. Nordby, *Karl Evang*, 118, n. 63; 125, n. 87; 126.
81 Evang, 'Noen aktuelle oppgaver', 266–71.
82 Ibid., 269, 270, 271.
83 Ibid., 268. He also wrote about "vårt folkelegeme", that is, "our national body" (p. 266).
84 Ibid., 266.
85 Karl Evang, *Gjenreising av folkehelsa i Norge* (Oslo: Fabritius, 1947), 13, 25, 29.
86 Karl Evang, 'Helsestellets utvikling i Norge gjennom 50 år', *Sosialt Arbeid* 26 (1952): 58–63.
87 Nordby, *Karl Evang*, 114–15.

88 *A National Health Service: Presented by the Minister of Health and the Secretary of State for Scotland to Parliament by Command of His Majesty* (London: Ministry of Health/Department of Health for Scotland, 1944).

89 William Beveridge, *Social Insurance and Allied Services: Presented to Parliament by Command of His Majesty November 1942.* HMSO CMND 6404.

90 Cf. e.g., Paul Starr, *The Social Transformation of American Medicine: The Rise of a Sovereign Profession and the Making of a Vast Industry* (New York: Basic Books, 1983).

91 Karl Evang, *Bruk og misbruk av legemidler. En almenfattelig fremstilling* (Oslo: Tiden, 1965), 13; Karl Evang, *Narkotika, generasjonene og samfunnet* (Oslo: Tiden, 1972), 7.

92 Ole Berg, 'Den evangske orden og dens forvitring', *Michael* 10 (2013): 149–97, 158, 169. See also Karl Evang, *Health Services in Norway* (Oslo: Norwegian Joint Committee on International Social Policy, 1960), 169, 172.

93 Karl Evang, "Public health'. Sosial og administrativ medisin', *Tidsskrift for Den norske lægeforening* 73 (1953): 767–7, 768. See also Karl Evang, 'Utdannelse for offentlig lægearbeid', *Tidsskrift for Den norske lægeforening* 68 (1948): 249–52, 250.

94 Evang, 'Public health', 768–9. Cf. Nordby, *Karl Evang*, 143 and Berg, 'Den evangske orden', 169.

95 Evang, 'Public health', 770–72.

96 Ibid., 772.

97 Per Haave, *Sterilisering av tatere 1934–1977. En historisk undersøkelse av lov og praksis* (Oslo: Norges forskningsråd, 2000), 335–44; Schiøtz, *Landets styrke*, 231.

98 Nordby, *Karl Evang*, 159–60.

99 *The First Ten Years of the World Health Organization* (Geneva: World Health Organization, 1958), 482–8.

100 *Expert Committee on Public-Health Administration. First Report. WHO Technical Report Series No. 55* (Geneva: WHO, 1952), 6.

101 Berg, *Den gränslösa hälsan*, 348–53.

102 The board met a few times a year to prepare a general programme proposal and set the agenda for the next World Health Assembly. Bror Rexed, *Sverige och WHO i 40 år* (Stockholm: Socialdepartementet and Socialstyrelsen, 1988), 13–14; *WHO: What it Is, What it Does* (Geneva: WHO, 1988), 20; *The First Ten Years*, 495. During the third World Health Assembly (May 1950) Höjer was also chair of the programme committee that discussed the draft programme prepared by the board before it was presented to the entire assembly. *Third World Health Assembly, Geneva, 8 to 27 May 1950: Resolutions and Decisions; Plenary Meetings, Verbatim Records; Committees, Minutes and Reports; Annexes* (Geneva: WHO, 1950).

103 *Second World Health Assembly, Rome, 13 June to 2 July 1949: Discussions and Resolutions; Plenary Meetings, Verbatim Records; Committees, Minutes and Reports; Annexes* (Geneva: WHO, 1949), 109–17. Cf. Rexed, *Sverige och WHO*, 13–14; *The First Ten Years*, 73, 92–3. Höjer was also eager to highlight his cooperation with the Indian delegation. Höjer, 'Ur J. Axel Höjers minnen', 665.

104 Axel Höjer, 'Världshälsovårdskonferensen och dess arbete. Tvenne radioanföranden den 13 och 20 juli', *Hygienisk revy* 37 (1948): 203.

105 Axel Höjer, 'Det tysta ropet från urskogen', *Sociala meddelanden* (1958): 733–52.

106 Berg, *Den gränslösa hälsan*, 426-7, 462-4.

107 Axel Höjer, 'En dröm som kan bli verklighet', *Vårt Röda Kors* 13, no. 3 (1958): 10.

108 Axel Höjer, 'Gigantiska uppgifter för hälsovården i Indien', *Sundsvalls tidning*, 20 July 1953.

109 Axel Höjer, 'Present day interdependence', SAHA, 2b vol. 3; Axel Höjer, 'En friskare värld', *Världshorisont* 17, no. 9/10 (1963): 13–14.

110 Höjer, 'En världsdel vaknar', SAHA, 2a vol. 1: 23. See also eg. Höjer, 'Det tysta ropet', 750–51.

111 Höjer, 'En dröm', 8.
112 *Third World Health Assembly*, 319–20; Axel Höjer, 'Peace and health', *Journal of the Trivandrum Medical College* 1, no. 1 (1952): 8–10; Axel Höjer, 'Report on Ghana 13: Draft', SAHA, 4b vol 4: 16–17; Höjer, 'En friskare värld', 14.
113 See, e.g., Irene Andersson, *Kvinnor mot krig. Aktioner och nätverk för fred 1914–1940* (Lund: Historiska institutionen vid Lunds universitet, 2001), 306.
114 *Protokoll från Sverges* [sic] *Socialdemokratiska Arbetarepartis trettonde kongress i Stockholm den 3–9 juni 1928* (Stockholm: SAP, 1928), 214–15.
115 He also criticised the USA's and USSR's expensive space initiatives on the same grounds. Höjer, 'Present day interdependence', xiv; Höjer, 'En friskare värld', 14.
116 Höjer, 'Ur J. Axel Höjers minnen', 727–9. Cf. Höjer, 'Report on Ghana 13: Draft', 16–17.
117 Axel Höjer, *Liv och död i det nya Indien* (Stockholm: Svenska FN-föreningen Mellanfolkligt samarbete, 1955), 15–16; Höjer, 'Det tysta ropet', 750–51; 'Generaldirektör Höjer vill ha en ökad U-hjälp', *Sydsvenska Dagbladet Snällposten*, 26 April 1965; Axel Höjer, 'En procent av den taxerade inkomsten till u-land?', *Farmaceutisk revy* 66 (1967): 350–55.

7 Cherishing the health of the people:

Finnish non-governmental expert organisations as constructors of public health and the 'people'

Sophy Bergenheim

Introduction

In addition to the connotations and meaning of concepts varying from one language to another, concepts are understood and used differently depending on the time, context and actor. In this chapter, I illustrate how the concepts of *folkhälsa* and *kansanterveys* have been utilised in various ways in a historical context, in the 1940s and 1950s, and by two similar actors: Samfundet Folkhälsan i svenska Finland, or Folkhälsan for short (the Public Health Association of Swedish Finland)[1] and Väestöliitto (the Finnish Population and Family Welfare League).[2]

Folkhälsan was established in 1921 for promoting the 'life force' of the Swedish-speaking Finns. It was led by medical experts and public health nurses, and the association's activities primarily consisted of medical research and various forms of social and health care for the Swedish-speaking population. Väestöliitto was founded in 1941, after the Finno-Soviet Winter War (1939–1941), as an umbrella organisation for individuals and associations interested in population policy. Its purpose was to spread information on and promote policies for population policy. The organisation was officially unaffiliated, but its leading figures had strong ties to centre-right and conservative parties.

In this chapter, I study how the Swedish-speaking actors of Folkhälsan and the Finnish-speaking actors of Väestöliitto understood public health (i.e., *folkhälsa* or *kansanterveys*, respectively). The Nordic etymology of the concept (and the name Folkhälsan) encourages the focus to be directed to the actors' conceptions of, firstly, the people (*folk*, *kansa*); secondly, health (*hälsa*, *terveys*); and, thirdly, 'people's health' (*folkhälsa*, *kansanterveys*). I thus address the following questions: According to Folkhälsan and Väestöliitto, who constituted the people and who did not; who were included and who were excluded? What was defined as 'health' (or the opposite), by whom and on what grounds? What did 'people's health' encompass?

I address these questions by analysing how Folkhälsan and Väestöliitto constructed and framed issues and phenomena as (public) health-related problems and, respectively, ideals. This approach allows us to examine historical interpretations and connotations related to these key concepts, and encourages a sensitivity towards their historicity and political nature. Furthermore, the selection of study subjects sheds light on the role of non-governmental organisations (NGOs) as policy actors and experts. This chapter thereby also contributes to the discussion regarding policy processes and knowledge production.

I am dealing with two actors operating in different languages, which poses some extra challenges for distinguishing between historical and analytical concepts. To keep the distinction as clear as possible, in addition to using the key concepts in Swedish and Finnish (*folk/kansa*, *hälsa/terveys*, *folkhälsa/kansanterveys*), I denote similarities in the Finnish and Swedish historical concepts through the italicised English terms *people*, *health* and *people's health*. When providing a more analytical account of these concepts or placing them in a broader frame or discussion, I use English concepts without italicisation, the established 'public health' or the more unconventional 'people's health' for better reflecting the Nordic etymology.

Folkhälsan and Väestöliitto

Folkhälsan was established in 1921 as the successor to the racial hygienic Florin Commission (1912–1921). From the Commission, Folkhälsan inherited the task of conducting anthropological and medical research on the Swedish-speaking population of Finland. Both the Florin Commission and Folkhälsan were products of their time: the early twentieth century saw the spread and establishment of racial hygienic research, policies and practices in Finland. Folkhälsan sought to foster 'good Swedes' in Finland in order to improve the life force and hamper the 'degeneration' of the Swedish-speaking population. As Folkhälsan's brochure *Vår Hustavla* from 1921 declared: "No inferior Swedes shall be found in this country!"[3] (In the original Swedish, the word 'inferior' would literally translate to 'bad', with connotations of poor quality, *dålig: Det får ej finnas dåliga svenskar i detta land!*)

This aspiration was connected to the political situation in Finland: the newly independent (1917) country struggled to find its societal, political and constitutional form. In 1918, Finland descended into a brutal civil war in which the bourgeois Whites won over the socialist Reds. The 1920s and 1930s saw bitter language feuds. The Swedish-speaking bourgeois elite, which Folkhälsan's actors also represented, feared political and cultural oppression on the part of the Finnish-speaking majority, and therefore sought to strengthen the composition and status of the Finland-Swedish population. This objective was also fuelled by class-based fears: the Swedish-speaking working class and small-scale farmers were to be educated and controlled in accordance with bourgeois values in order to prevent further social unrest. For Folkhälsan, racial hygiene and public health were part of a small-scale nation-building process – namely, the construction the Finland-Swedish *folk*.[4]

The founders and leaders of Folkhälsan were medical scientists in fields such as hygiene, physiology, pathological anatomy and neuropathology. Ossian Schauman, specialised in internal medicine, led the Florin Commission and was the first chair of Folkhälsan until his death in 1922. He worked closely with Harry Federley, a professor of genetics and internationally renowned scientist. Federley was the leading figure of Folkhälsan until his death in 1951: as the association's secretary (1921–1937) and as chair (1937–1951). He was a strong proponent of racial hygiene. In 1929, he led the committee that prepared the Finnish sterilisation law (enacted in 1935), and in which he had a strong influence.

Väestöliitto was founded in 1941 as a non-governmental umbrella organisation for associations involved in population policy. Its objective was to elevate the number and quality of the population. Similarly to Folkhälsan, this goal was fuelled by an 'underdog trauma'. The Winter War (1939–1940) and Continuation War (1941–1944) against the Soviet Union led to an alarming notion that the Finnish population was too small considering Finland's geopolitical vulnerability, neighbouring a powerful and hostile country.

The member associations of Väestöliitto included social and health policy organisations and politically engaged associations, both left- and right-wing, the latter often with a nationalist stance. Officially, Väestöliitto was not affiliated to any party. However, several of its board members and executive managers were affiliated to nationalist organisations and/or the centre-right Agrarian League and the conservative Coalition Party. Väestöliitto was thus a conservative organisation. It also engaged in close governmental collaboration, and its board included two representatives of the Ministry of Social Affairs, which gave it a half-governmental position despite its official non-governmental status.

Väestöliitto's executive managers and board members (whom I refer to when speaking of 'Väestöliitto') consisted of professionals representing various fields of expertise. V.J. Sukselainen – one of the people behind the establishment of Väestöliitto, and its long-standing chair (1941–1971) – held degrees in sociology and economics. In addition, he was a politician: in 1945–1964, he was the leader of the Agrarian League (as of 1965, the Centre Party) and twice served as Prime Minister, among other roles. Long-standing (1943–1965) executive manager Heikki von Hertzen was a Master of Law trained on the bench. In addition, he was a notable figure within Finnish housing policy, and acted as chair of the Finnish Housing Foundation (1951–1976). Other important figures in Väestöliitto during the 1940s and 1950s included vice-chairs Aarno Turunen and Elsa Enäjärvi-Haavio. Turunen was a professor of gynaecology and obstetrics, and one of the people behind the blood service of the Finnish Red Cross. Enäjärvi-Haavio was the first Finnish woman to obtain a doctoral degree in folkloristics, as well as the first female adjunct professor of the discipline.[5] She was affiliated to the conservative National Coalition Party, and actively involved with the Finnish non-governmental sector and with cultural policy. Within Väestöliitto, she was the primary figure behind its home aid activities.

People's health, racial hygiene and population policy

As noted in the introductory chapter, public health has been intertwined with several fields and policies, such as racial hygiene, family policy and population policy. Folkhälsan and Väestöliitto illustrate this point clearly, as well as the fluidity of these fields and concepts.

For Folkhälsan, *folkhälsa* served as an all-encompassing umbrella concept. The hegemonic status of the concept is not reflected, however, in its prevalence in the association's material but, rather, in its absence. In Folkhälsan's annual reports and minutes from the 1940s and 1950s, the concept *folkhälsa* is hardly ever used. To the actors of Folkhälsan, the concept was self-evidently ubiquitous in the association's activities. Everything the organisation did was regarded as furthering *folkhälsa* – the concept was, after all, even the key word in its name.

In newspaper stories, directed at a broader public, the representatives of Folkhälsan (often Harry Federley) coupled *folkhälsa* with care for physical and mental health and the hereditary disposition of the Swedish-speaking *folk* (sometimes also referred to as *befolkning*, population) – in other words, racial hygiene or *arvshygien* (hereditary hygiene). While the term 'racial hygiene' was, in general, gradually abandoned in post-war Finland, the idea remained strong in Folkhälsan.

However, in 1946, Federley criticised how some racial hygienists – namely, the Nazis – had gone too far and had tarnished "the sound idea" behind racial hygiene. As a result, the scientific discipline had been rendered disreputable "even among the genuine geneticists, who had wished to keep their science [racial hygiene] free from politics and all kinds of mundane currents of the human society". The solution was to turn to the concept of *arvshygien*, heredity hygiene. According to Federley, it was a more accurate representation of what the discipline encompassed, "namely, the care for the inherited dispositions, regardless of race".[6] In Federley's view, the problem was first and foremost rhetoric: the term *rashygien* had been tarnished, but 'genuine' racial hygiene was merely science and did not involve any political goals. In other words, he did not contest the idea of race itself. On the contrary, Federley attempted to depoliticise it by transferring the socio-political dimension of race into the seemingly objective and value-free sphere of medical scientific rhetoric and framing.[7]

Väestöliitto operated with a slightly different vocabulary. As an organisation specialising in population policy, it treated population policy as its umbrella concept and theme. The core issue of Väestöliitto was the 'population question', an unproblematised understanding that the Finnish population (*väestö*) was too small and that population growth was heading for a halt. Väestöliitto's ultimate formulation read: "The population question in Finland is, in short, a question of *our people's [kansa] survival*" (original emphasis).[8] According to Väestöliitto's programme, the answer to the 'population question' was to elevate the quantity as well as the quality of the population. The quantitative goals were defined very explicitly: ideally, families were to have "at least" six children, and four at the very least. The long-term objective was to double the population to 8 million (a number which to this day has never been achieved).[9]

In 1945, Väestöliitto established a distinct department for *kansanterveys*. In its action plan, it described its purpose as focusing on issues concerning the number and quality of the Finnish *kansa* from a "health care, medical, race theory and heredity perspective". Quantity-related topics included maternal and child health care issues such as sexually transmitted diseases (STDs), abortions, pregnancy and childbirth, etc. Questions concerning quality, for their part, focused on "matters that have an influence on the quality of the entire *kansa* from one generation to the next". Such matters included, among others, hereditary diseases, hereditary mental illnesses and "abnormal states" – in particular, feeble-mindedness, sterilisation and castration and the "medical causes behind criminality".[10] In early 1941, the goal of sterilising individuals with criminal or medical dispositions, which also risked rendering their offspring "asocial", was described as "improving the race" and the "composition of the society" (in Finnish: *Sterilisoimisella pyritään siis rodun parantamiseen … oikein käytetyllä sterilisoimisella on yhteiskunnan kokoomusta parantava vaikutus*).[11]

Both Folkhälsan and Väestöliitto thus linked *people's health* with racial aspects and heredity. However, the organisations differed in their hierarchical framing. For Folkhälsan, *folkhälsa* was the master concept. In Väestöliitto's framing, on the other hand, *kansanterveys* was subject to population policy (even though they were intertwined and the distinction was far from clear-cut). Nevertheless, the two organisations had the same core concept(ion)s and objectives: they both strived to elevate the quantity and quality of the collective (*folk/befolkning* or *kansa/väestö*). Their agenda was based on eugenic pronatalism, which was linked to nationalism. The basic premise was that a large enough population of high quality would ensure a thriving *people* (the Finland-Swedish *folk* or the Finnish *kansa, väestö* or nation), which would be able to defend itself against external threat (the Finnish-speaking majority or the Soviet Union).

The mothers of the *people*

In line with the pronatalist premise of Folkhälsan and Väestöliitto, both organisations were vocal promoters of motherhood. They did not merely encourage reproduction, but sought to establish motherhood as the female norm – the more children, the more virtuous the woman.

In this endeavour, the organisations relied on measures that can be characterised as positive racial hygiene, such as the Mother's Reward (*moderbelöning, moderpremiering*; the latter literally means 'rewarding the mother'). The award, which was indeed labelled (somewhat anachronically) positive *arvshygien* by Harry Federley in 1946, was organised by the Florin Commission and later Folkhälsan in the 1910s–1930s. It was granted to a mother who, like her husband, came from a good Swedish-speaking family and had "at least four mentally and physically healthy and robust, well cared for 4–14-year-old children" (the age limit was subsequently raised to 17). Disqualifying family traits and illnesses included, among others, alcoholism and mental health problems. The reward was also explicitly used as a propaganda tool for educating the masses on the importance of racial hygiene. As an analogy for emphasising the importance of heredity control, Federley paralleled the breeding of humans with crop cultivation and animal breeding.[12]

After the war, Professor Fabian Langenskiöld, head of the hospitals of the Helsinki Deaconess Institute and the Invalid Foundation, proposed a new form of reward, this time in the form of a settlement support. It was designed to be an interest-free loan granted to young to-be-married Swedish-speaking couples, on condition that they fulfilled similar health, social and heritage conditions as for the Mother's Reward and pledged to stay in their (rural) place of residence. Having one child would correspond to paying back a quarter of the debt, and having four children would settle the debt completely. A divorce, on the other hand, would lead to the loan falling due immediately.[13]

In addition to pronatalist and racial hygienic aspirations, the settlement support reflects Folkhälsan's defensive minority nationalism. After the Second World War, Finland was trying to resettle 400,000 evacuees from the areas in Karelia (eastern Finland) and Lapland that were annexed by the Soviet Union. Folkhälsan's settlement support was to serve as a protective measure against the national resettlement policy. The state bought land from landowners whose holdings exceeded the areal limit, and redistributed the land to the evacuees. As the evacuees spoke Finnish or Karelian, there was a risk of Swedish losing its hegemony in Swedish-speaking municipalities. The settlement support was to encourage young Swedish-speaking couples to buy land from Swedish-speaking landowners, thereby keeping the majority land ownership and language Swedish. The settlement support was, however, never adopted in practice.

Väestöliitto celebrated motherhood in a similar vein as Folkhälsan. As of 1941, Väestöliitto organised a national Mother's Day event in order to "emphasise the meaning of motherhood and the maternal calling for individuals as well as the entire *kansakunta* [nation, people]".[14] The idea gained widespread support and the presidential couple attended the events. In 1947, Mother's Day became an official flag-raising day. In addition to Mother's Day celebrations, Väestöliitto organised the event *Kodin viikko* (Week of the Home), which celebrated family life and provided family-related education and information. In 1944, Väestöliitto proposed awarding mothers of large families with official badges of honour in recognition of their important work in raising new generations. The first mothers were decorated by the President of Finland at *Kodin viikko* in 1946, and, as of 1947, the ceremony became part of the national Mother's Day celebration.[15]

Väestöliitto also strongly emphasised the duty aspect of motherhood. Given that Väestöliitto coupled population growth with the survival of the people and the nation, it framed reproduction as a civic responsibility rather than a private matter. It strongly condemned the 'child limit', i.e., voluntary refraining from reproduction, which was seen as a transgression against the nation and society itself. As an illustrating example, during the establishing phase of Väestöliitto, a division dedicated to *kansanterveys* framed the reproductive and childrearing woman as the female equivalent of the (male) soldier, performing her national duty in defending her country: "Giving birth is the most valuable national service a woman can do for her country, and it is by no means effortless or danger-free."[16] According to Väestöliitto, the entire 'population question' was a result of short-sighted and selfish individuals (i.e., women) failing to fulfil their reproductive duty.

Whereas individuals were seen as obliged to procreate, Väestöliitto argued that the state also had a responsibility towards its citizens in making the fulfilment of this duty as safe as possible. In the late 1930s and early 1940s, the majority of women gave birth at home (1939: 72 per cent; 1944: 55 per cent), and many births took place without any medical assistance (1939: 28 per cent; 1944: 15 per cent).[17] This was reflected in high maternal mortality rates. In the early 1940s, over 400 women per 100,000 live births died due to pregnancy- and birth-related complications. Infant mortality was likewise high: over 60 children per 1,000 live births died during their first year.[18] In comparison, in early 1940s' Sweden, maternal mortality was under 200 per 100,000 live-born children. Sweden's infant mortality rate, for its part, had dropped to under 30 per 1,000 live-born children by 1942.[19] (In 2015, maternal and infant mortality in Finland was 2 per 100,000 live births and 1.7 per 1,000 live births, respectively.[20])

Reducing health and medical risks related to pregnancy, childbirth and infancy were among the core quantity-related *kansanterveys* objectives of Väestöliitto. In order to address these phenomena, Väestöliitto advocated, among others, prenatal services, maternal hospitals and maternal care, and maternity and child welfare clinics, as well as child care education for mothers.[21]

So-called criminal abortions (abortions were illegal until the first abortion law in 1950[22]) were a particularly concerning *kansanterveys* issue for Väestöliitto. The organisation argued that the practice was so widespread that it had a negative impact on population growth. Moreover, according to Väestöliitto, most criminal abortions were dangerous procedures that caused serious injuries and disabilities, often infertility.[23] In Väestöliitto's population policy framing, abortions were thus condemnable for two main reasons. Firstly, they were a breach of the civic duty of reproduction and motherhood. Secondly, criminal abortions that rendered women sterile created a multiplicative negative effect by permanently preventing new generations from being born.

Marriage, the nuclear family and fertility control

In the late 1940s, similar actors teamed up to offer marriage counselling for Finnish- and Swedish-speaking married couples. In 1947, Väestöliitto established its first marriage counselling centre, whose services focused primarily on health-related issues, whereas the Church offered spiritual guidance in marital conflicts.[24] Throughout the 1940s and 1950s, Väestöliitto's marriage counselling was explicitly labelled *kansanterveys* work in the organisation's annual reports. In line with the organisation's population policy-driven *kansanterveys* framing, the counselling centres approached quantity as well as quality from a medical, hereditary and eugenic perspective.

In 1950, Folkhälsan took its cue from Väestöliitto and established a Swedish marriage counselling centre in collaboration with the Association for Swedish Parish Work in Finland and the Swedish Population Association, albeit without a strict division of roles. The Swedish counselling centre offered both health-related and therapeutic counselling, as well as legal, economic and hereditary advice. The focus, however, was on therapy and psychological counselling, particularly in resolving marital conflicts.[25]

The marriage counselling centres of both Väestöliitto and Folkhälsan served as apparatuses for normalising the nuclear family and male breadwinner model. Services were, by definition, delimited to married couples, and the shared objective of the organisations was to promote happy marriages, which would naturally generate offspring. The pronatalism of both Väestöliitto and Folkhälsan had thus eased on the alarmed, duty-emphasising tone in the 1950s. Instead, they strived to construct marriage and clear gender roles as a desirable family model that entailed stability and happiness. In other words, the associations had not given up on their pronatalist aspirations, but pursued them through conservative-bourgeois gender roles that associated womanhood, motherhood, marriage and domestic life with happiness.

The two organisations' means of promoting these ideas, however, differed some-what in accordance with their differences in approach and emphasis on marriage counselling. Alongside its focus on health and medical aspects, Väestöliitto approached the issue from a corporeal angle; more precisely, through fertility control. In the 1940s and 1950s, Väestöliitto was a pioneer in researching, developing and promoting contraceptives.[26] The prevention of fertilisation might appear to clash with pronatalist aspirations, but, as Ilpo Helén has pointed out, Väestöliitto linked family planning and contraception to the matrimonial norm and the nuclear family. The organisation regarded pregnancy-related fear and anxiety as causing sexual reluctance and creating negative associations towards family life, which reduced marital happiness.[27] "Happy families" with control over their reproduction, on the other hand, would eventually lead to an increasing birth rate and "a viable and healthy society".[28]

Given that sexual desire and contraceptives were reserved for marriage, only marriage counselling centres gave advice on fertility control. Contraception in the hands of single women, meanwhile, was deemed immoral, as it encouraged sexual promiscuity. Unwanted pregnancies should therefore be prevented not through fertility control, but through moral rigour: sexual continence and moral education.[29]

Väestöliitto's anti-abortion endeavours were associated with a similar normat-ive differentiation between married and unmarried women. 'Criminal abortions' had been a central concern since the early days of Väestöliitto, and it had actively participated in the preparation work of the first abortion law, which came into force in 1950. The legislation only allowed abortions on strict medical, ethical, social or eugenic grounds.[30] In 1951, the government gave Väestöliitto the task of implementing abortion-prevention work in the entire country through its national network of social counselling centres, and of establishing social support measures.[31]

The reception and treatment of unmarried and married women facing an unexpected pregnancy differed substantially at the social counselling centres. Married women were educated on fertility control and guided towards private counselling at the marriage counselling centres. They were also granted abortions more often. "Lone mothers", on the other hand, received no information on contraception, and were persuaded to keep the child. Nurses were not to intimidate or threaten their patients, but the "pertinent information" given did include the "fact" that an abortion terminated a life and stressed the risk of infertility associated with illegal abortions.[32] Single women were also granted abortions primarily on eugenic grounds, in which case a condition for abortion was sterilisation.[33]

The policies reflect the pronatalist, conservative and racial hygienic priorities of Väestöliitto. Within the frame of marital life, fertility control ultimately promoted procreation. However, in the hands of single women, it encouraged immoral behaviour and refraining from reproduction. Therefore, if a single woman found herself facing an unexpected pregnancy, the smaller moral concession was to welcome her offspring as an unorthodox addition to the population; unless, of course, the child was suspected of possessing undesired qualities, in which case it was best to permanently prevent such qualities from spreading.

While Folkhälsan also provided counselling in similar health and medical matters (e.g., fertility control, heredity and issues related to sexual relations), it had a stronger focus on emotional and relationship issues. As noted earlier, counselling and therapy were the most important types of service offered by Swedish Marriage Counselling. In 1952, Folkhälsan introduced a new form of activity that also focused on improving the emotional relationship and companionship of couples – namely, "marriage schools". These offered lectures on various themes related to marital life, such as "happiness and responsibilities in marriage", economic and legal pers-pectives, and child-raising, as well as "marital life from a medical perspective" (i.e., family planning).[34]

Like Väestöliitto, Folkhälsan delimited fertility control to marital relationships and the nuclear family, although the demarcation between married couples and unmarried women was significantly subtler. This was partially due to Folkhälsan's stronger emphasis on psychological and emotional issues. In addition, Folkhälsan had not acquired a similar half-governmental task or status as Väestöliitto, which had created opportunities or incentives for the latter to pursue clear-cut policies. Nevertheless, Folkhälsan also provided fertility control counselling exclusively for married couples and married women. Folkhälsan thus shared similar premises and priorities with Väestöliitto. Pronatalist goals prevailed, but not at any cost. The objective was to foster and normalise happy nuclear families, for instance through marriage schools that taught them how to act and perform properly in a marriage.

Physical, mental and moral heredity

Both Folkhälsan and Väestöliitto spoke of quality and degeneration. For both organisations, heredity concerned not only biological or physical qualities, but also mental and moral capabilities. Accordingly, the ultimate goal was to get individuals with physically, mentally and morally desired characteristics to procreate. These conceptions were intertwined with classist notions and anti-Malthusianism.

According to nineteenth-century neo-Malthusian theories, poverty among the working class was the consequence of overpopulation; more precisely, of excessively high birth rates. The promoted solution was family planning and birth control in order to keep the number of children per family at a sustainable level. Harry Federley, however, argued in 1918 that neo-Malthusian ideas were at the root of degeneration. It was precisely the genetically superior who were capable of distinguishing between procreation and eroticism, and thereby capable of family planning, whereas the genetically inferior (in which he included the proletariat) procreated uncontrollably. Federley's comment was related to the Civil War, which he interpreted as a rebellion of the genetically inferior against their superiors.[35] Ironically, Federley's arguments were not essentially contradicting neo-Malthusian ideas. Neo-Malthusianists advocated the regulation of reproduction among the working class in order to avoid pressure for resource distribution; in other words, they worked in favour of the bourgeoisie and private ownership. From the perspective of Federley and other right-wing racial hygienists (including many active figures in Folkhälsan), however, the idea had backfired.

Väestöliitto, in contrast to neo-Malthusianists, directed the focus precisely to the distribution of resources. According to Väestöliitto, poverty or unemployment did not stem from too large a population or too many workers, but from the economic organisation of society.[36] However, the organisation also perceived it as problematic that "people of more limited means" carried the heaviest burden of procreation, whereas the upper socio-economic classes had limited the number of children born into the family.[37] In the long run, this would lead to degeneration, as the proportion of the better endowed diminished. However, lower class and poverty did not automatically count as degenerative traits. While Väestöliitto put the greatest blame for the 'population question' on the upper socio-economic classes, it also advocated numerous social and economic reforms for supporting low-income families, working mothers, etc.

While Väestöliitto's population policy framing was not explicitly adversarial in terms of class, the organisation did harbour normative class-based conceptions. These were visible in the services it provided, such as the marriage and social counselling centres, and the social reforms it promoted. For example, family taxation and housing policy reforms proposed and pursued by Väestöliitto were designed to encourage and facilitate the male breadwinner and housewife model and a bourgeois lifestyle. Thus, while increasing birth rates were welcomed throughout the class society, the expansion of some classes was more preferable than others, and the nuclear family was seen as the moral backbone of a healthy society.

In the course of time, Folkhälsan's classist notions eased, but did not vanish. Similarly to Väestöliitto, class-based preferences were reflected in the Mother's Reward, marriage counselling and so forth. Karin Spoof, who ran Folkhälsan's mental hygiene clinics in Helsinki and Turku, delivered a more explicit expression. She identified blue-collar professions and industrial-urban environments, along with bilingualism (i.e., mixed marriages), as sources of mental disturbances.[38]

Mental health problems and criminality – often seen as interlinked – were an issue for Folkhälsan and Väestöliitto alike. They both perceived the feeble-minded and mentally ill as asocial creatures that had a morally and mentally detrimental effect on the composition of society due to their inclination to delinquency and sexual promiscuity (prostitution, sex crimes), as well as dependency. Furthermore, they passed these qualities on to their offspring, which not only caused human suffering but also contributed to the degeneration of the society/race. In line with this reasoning, both organisations advocated hindering the procreation of individuals with such undesired dispositions through "the safety valve of society", as Federley called it: sterilisation.[39] In 1950, the sterilisation legislation was indeed reformed. The new laws, the Sterilisation Act and the Castration Act, were even stricter than their predecessors, leading to a peak in compulsory sterilisations in 1956–1963.[40]

From positive and negative racial hygiene to positive and negative people's health

The research period of this chapter renders Folkhälsan and Väestöliitto different types of study subject from a conceptual history perspective. In the 1940s, Väestöliitto was being founded, whereas Folkhälsan (and its predecessor, the Florin Commission) had already been active for two to three decades. An organisation kicking off its activities, like Väestöliitto, defines its goals, its activities and itself – and, in that process, its key concepts – in a significantly more explicit manner compared to an already established organisation, such as Folkhälsan. Normative and conceptual development, on the other hand, is not documented as explicitly and unambiguously as new activities or deliberate turning points, since the change is self-evident to contemporary actors. The actors' terminology (i.e., the words they use), however, might remain largely the same – as in the case of Folkhälsan. This composition poses some (intriguing) challenges to a conceptual historian trying to trace developments, meanings and comparisons of historical concepts while avoiding anachronic interpretations.

In this endeavour, I have turned to the work of Finnish historian Markku Mattila, who has outlined a categorisation of practical racial hygiene in Finland ca. 1880–1935 (Figure 7.1).

I have used Mattila's categorisation for analysing Folkhälsan's and Väestöliitto's public health discourse(s) of the 1940s and 1950s and for comparing it with the racial hygiene discourse until the 1930s. In this categorisation and analysis, I use the term 'people's health' (non-italicised, as it is an analytical concept), which reflects the etymological-conceptual basis of the Finnish and Swedish concepts better than the English term 'public health'.

Before proceeding to the new categorisation (shown in Figure 7.2), I will elaborate on its key concepts. 'Race' is replaced by 'people' (*folk, kansa*). In comparison to the notion of a Finland-Swedish anthropological race during the 1920s–1930s, in the 1940s–1950s, Folkhälsan's understanding of people (*folk*) was determined by Finland-Swedishness. It was derived from the notions of a socio-cultural minority group that shared specific characteristics (language, ethnicity, etc.) that set it apart from the rest of the Finnish population (the Finnish-speaking population in particular). In Folkhälsan, these characteristics were seen to be closely linked to heredity – indeed, they were not necessarily distinguishable at all. Väestöliitto, on the other hand, had a much broader and ambiguous understanding of *kansa*: it was synonymous with the even more prominent key

	ANTHROPOLOGICAL RACIAL HYGIENE	MEDICAL RACIAL HYGIENE	POPULATION POLICY RACIAL HYGIENE	Target of action
POSITIVE RACIAL HYGIENE	– elevating the birth rate of (one's own) anthropological race – cultivating (one's own) anthropological race	– practical public health work – practical care for mother and child (prenatal, maternal and child care)	– promoting the birth of fit individuals (through legislation) – care for the mother, child and family (through legislation) – (legislative) public health work	THE BIOLOGICALLY FIT
NEGATIVE RACIAL HYGIENE	– preventing the mixing of races – race segregation – marital impediments	– treatment of the hereditarily flawed – sterilisation and castration – segregation – marital impediments – abortions	– denying unfit families social benefits – imposing marital impediments	THE BIOLOGICALLY UNFIT
Rationale for categorising the body of people	PHYSICAL ANTHROPOLOGY Craniometry etc.	HEREDITY-BASED CRITERIA Flaws, illnesses, mental state, etc.		
What 'race' referred to	ANTHROPOLOGICAL RACE	THE POPULATION		

Figure 7.1 Division of practical racial hygiene into different sections (1880s–1930s). From Mattila, *Kansamme parhaaksi*, 16, reproduced by permission of the author; the English translation is mine and approved by the author.

concept *väestö* (population), which referred to the entire population of Finland, without any explicit demarcations.

I have transformed the other key concept of Mattila's categorisation, 'hygiene', into 'health' (*hälsa, terveys*), which respectively transforms 'racial hygiene' into 'people's health'. In Folkhälsan's understanding of people's health (*folkhälsa*) in the 1940s–1950s, Finland-Swedishness, medical people's health and population policy were not clearly distinguishable, separate ideas or policies. Rather, Finland-Swedishness acted as a main frame for medical and population policy. This is a significant difference compared to the categorisation of Mattila, in which anthropological racial hygiene was a distinctively separate category. For Väestöliitto, the Finland-Swedish factor was, of course, no factor at all – as noted above, it did not (explicitly) acknowledge any cultural or ethnic subgroups.

According to Minna Harjula, in post-war Finland, racial hygiene was replaced by new concepts and discourses such as public health and population policy.[41] The

	FOLKHÄLSAN	VÄESTÖLIITTO		Target of action
	FINLAND-SWEDISH PEOPLE'S HEALTH	MEDICAL PEOPLE'S HEALTH	POPULATION POLICY PEOPLE'S HEALTH	
POSITIVE PEOPLE'S HEALTH	– elevating the birth rate of the Finland-Swedish population – encouraging fit individuals to procreate – promoting marriage between Swedish-speaking Finns	– practical people's health work – practical care for mother and child (prenatal, maternal and child care) – people's health education	– promoting the birth of fit individuals (through legislation) – care for the mother, child and family (through legislation) – (legislative) people's health work	THE SOCIO-BIOLOGICALLY FIT
NEGATIVE PEOPLE'S HEALTH	– promoting sterilisation of unfit individuals – denying unfit individuals and families benefits or privileges	– treatment of the hereditarily flawed – sterilisation and castration – marital impediments – abortions	– denying unfit families social benefits – imposing marital impediments	THE SOCIO-BIOLOGICALLY UNFIT
Rationale for categorising the body of people	SOCIO-CULTURAL CHARACTERISTICS Language, ethnicity, cultural heritage, place of domicile, etc.	HEREDITY-BASED CRITERIA Flaws, illnesses, mental state, etc.		
What 'people' referred to	THE FINLAND-SWEDISH POPULATION	THE ENTIRE POPULATION		

Figure 7.2 Division of people's health into different sections (1940s–1950s).

conceptions and discourses of Väestöliitto and Folkhälsan, however, do not follow this general development – and the two organisations themselves differed in their use of the concepts. The evolution from racial hygiene to public health was a slow process. More precisely, it was not a clear-cut switch from one concept to another, but a development of shifting meanings. Notions of race and racial hygiene not only prevailed in concepts like public health, but also coexisted with them. In other words, in line with the periodisation outlined in the introductory chapter, the post-war period was a conceptual transition period.

This is demonstrated in the categorisations in Figures 7.1 and 7.2, which show that racial hygiene of the early twentieth century and people's health of the 1940–1950s shared many premises, ideals and objectives. Both were normative ideas, and both can be classified through definitions of positive and negative.

Post-war positive people's health sought to identify and normalise a specific medical, social and moral ideal. Similarly to Mattila's categorisation, the target of action still consisted of the biologically fit individuals – with my addition of the criteria for social fitness. Both Folkhälsan and Väestöliitto targeted individuals who fit their socio-biological norms through various positive measures, ranging from education and medical counselling to legislation and economic support. The organisations shared a similar understanding of the socio-biological norm: married, middle-class couples (women, in particular) of fertile age who were in good mental and physical health and free from hereditary diseases, and who were willing and able to procreate. They were overall upright citizens, preferably abstainers and churchgoers as well as residents of rural areas.

In addition, for Folkhälsan, the social factor intrinsically included the socio-cultural factor, i.e., Finland-Swedishness. While Väestöliitto did not explicitly discuss minorities or language issues, it should be noted that its conceptions of desired qualities implicitly created exclusive criteria. By portraying markedly bourgeois characteristics (the nuclear family and the male breadwinner model) and a non-nomadic rural lifestyle as the ideal, it simultaneously defined minorities like the Sami or Roma as undesired.

Negative people's health, respectively, sought to identify as well as prevent and eliminate undesired socio-biological characteristics that both organisations perceived as irremediable and/or hereditary. Such characteristics included, e.g., alcoholism, delinquency, congenital disabilities or illnesses (such as epilepsy or deafness) and mental health issues (for instance, feeble-mindedness or schizophrenia). The target consisted, in other words, of the socio-biologically unfit. Also in this case, the targets of Folkhälsan were within the socio-cultural realm of Finland-Swedishness – it sought to cultivate the population of Swedish-speaking Finns rather than target unfit, non-Finland-Swedish individuals.

In regard to medical people's health and population policy, not that much had changed. The organisations put more weight on education than before, but almost all forms of negative as well as positive racial hygiene were still present as negative and positive people's health in the 1940s–1950s. The activities of Väestöliitto encompassed more or less all of these forms. For the part of Folkhälsan, its activities were a mix of medical people's health and an adaptation of population policy for a minority population.

Conclusions

Who are the *people*? For Folkhälsan and Väestöliitto, it meant different things. For Folkhälsan, *folk* meant the Swedish-speaking population in Finland: a minority that shared a socio-cultural and ethnic heritage and language. Väestöliitto, on the other hand, spoke of *kansa* as the entire population of Finland, with no acknowledgement of socio-cultural minorities. However, the framing of *kansa* created normative criteria that implicitly excluded not only 'unfit' individuals, but also 'unfit' minorities.

Both Folkhälsan and Väestöliitto had an 'underdog trauma', which had an impact on their conceptions of the people, of health and of people's health. The representatives of Folkhälsan had experienced the political and cultural threat of a minority in relation to the Finnish-speaking majority, particularly in the 1910s–1930s. Against this background, the members of this organisation thought it essential to prevent the degeneration of the Finland-Swedish population. The founders of Väestöliitto, on the other hand, had been alarmed by the 'population question', which acquired a particular geopolitical note due to the Winter and Continuation Wars against the Soviet Union.[42]

These traumas, however, manifested themselves somewhat differently in the conceptions of the two organisations. Even though the cultural and political position of the Swedish-speaking Finns was not threatened in a similar manner as in the early twentieth century, the social, physical and cultural degeneration of the minority remained an alarming scenario. In addition, the racial hygienic legacy of Folkhälsan was still clearly visible in the 1940s–1950s. It maintained a strong emphasis on heredity, and it sought to further and normalise a specific social, cultural and physical Finland-Swedish ideal.

Folkhälsan was not particularly behind its time in its racial hygienic ethos, however. While Folkhälsan and Väestöliitto differed on a rhetoric level – Folkhälsan stuck to its 'hygiene' concepts and *rashygien*/*arvshygien*, whereas Väestöliitto primarily spoke of *kansanterveys* and population policy – the conceptions of Väestöliitto also followed racial hygienic ideas. After all, the target of both organisations was to elevate the quantity and quality of the people. The main difference between Väestöliitto and Folkhälsan was that Väestöliitto understood *kansanterveys* to be part of population policy, which was the central, ubiquitous theme in the activities of the organisation. At the same time, Väestöliitto linked its conception of population policy to a broader, geopolitical and societal perspective and nation-state nationalism. For Folkhälsan, on the other hand, population policy and *rashygien* intertwined without any particular hierarchy. Instead, they were understood through the (often unexpressed) master concept *folkhälsa*, which was intrinsically linked to the primary frame of Finland-Swedishness. Respectively, Folkhälsan inextricably linked people's health and 'minority nationalism'.

Despite these differences, both associations shared a normative understanding of the social, cultural and health ideal and, respectively, of undesired traits and individuals. In other words, the conception of *people* included inclusive and exclusive norms. The idea that undesired characteristics were socially or physically inherited was central in the construction of exclusive norms. It was a future-orientated idea: it was designed not only to prevent the inevitable exclusion and misery of future generations with poor social and physical qualities, but also, first and foremost, to ensure that the *people*, as a collective, would thrive.

Given that both organisations and their representatives were respected as public health and population policy experts, they possessed a significant amount of power, and their normative conceptions were likewise powerful. Folkhälsan and Väestöliitto used their power position in various ways; from top-down educational work and various positive measures to participating in (eugenic) legislative work. The primary target of both organisations (in a positive and negative sense) was women – mothers – and their fertile and reproductive bodies. The organisations did, indeed, share the exact same objective: to ensure that fit mothers contributed to the growth of the people with as many fit children as possible. This was to ensure the survival of 'Us', the 'people', in the face of the threat of the 'Other'.

Notes

1 Due to the length of the official Swedish name and of its English translation, I will use the short version 'Folkhälsan' in this chapter.
2 Due to the long English name, I will use the Finnish name 'Väestöliitto' in this chapter.
3 Harry Federley, 'Samfundet Folkhälsans tillkomst och utveckling', in *Samfundet Folkhälsan i Svenska Finland 1921–1946: Festskrift utgiven med anledning av Samfundets 25-års jubileum*, by Samfundet Folkhälsan (Helsinki: Frenckellska Tryckeri Aktiebolaget, 1946), 7–54. *Vår Hustavla* is reprinted in, e.g., Henrik Meinander, *Nationalstaten: Finlands svenskhet 1922–2015* (Helsinki: Svenska litteratursällskapet i Finland, 2016). For academic accounts of racial hygiene among the Swedish-speaking Finns (the Florin Commission, Folkhälsan, Harry Federley and other representatives of Folkhälsan, etc.), see, e.g., Marjatta Hietala, 'From race hygiene to sterilization: The eugenics movement in Finland', in *Eugenics and the Welfare State: Sterilization Policy in Denmark, Sweden, Norway, and Finland*, ed. Gunnar Broberg and Nils Roll-Hansen (East Lansing: Michigan State University Press, 2005), 195–258; Markku Mattila, *Kansamme parhaaksi: Rotuhygienia Suomessa vuoden 1935 sterilointilakiin asti* (Helsinki: Suomen Historiallinen Seura, 1999).
4 For a comprehensive history of the Swedish-speaking population in Finland and its identity-building, see Max Engman, *Språkfrågan: Finlandssvenskhetens uppkomst 1812–1922* (Helsinki: Svenska litteratursällskapet i Finland, 2016); Meinander, *Nationalstaten*. Class-based, racial hygienic aspirations and conceptions following the civil war are also discussed in Chapter 4 by Ainur Elmgren.
5 In Finnish: *dosentti* (the title of Docent).
6 Harry Federley, 'Samfundets moderpremiering och dess syfte', in *Samfundet Folkhälsan i svenska Finland 1921–1946: Festskrift utgiven med anledning av Samfundets 25-års jubileum*, by Samfundet Folkhälsan (Helsinki: Frenckellska Tryckeri Aktiebolaget, 1946), 127–35, 128.
7 See Chapter 11 by Johannes Kananen in this volume for an account of a similar attempt to depoliticise public health through a medical framing.
8 Väestöliitto, *Väestöliitto 1941: Ohjelma. Säännöt* (Helsinki: Väestöliitto, 1942), 18.
9 Ibid. For a more detailed analysis of the population policy framing of Väestöliitto, see Sophy Bergenheim, '"The population question is, in short, a question of our people's survival": Reframing population policy in 1940s Finland', in *Reforms and Resources*, ed. Martin Dackling et al. (Aalborg: Aalborg University Press, 2017), 109–42.
10 Väestöliitto, Minutes dated 4 Jan 1945 (board meeting). Appendix 1: Action plan for Väestöliitto's public health department, Archive of Väestöliitto.
11 Väestöliitto, Minutes dated 8 Jan 1941 (meeting of the Central Commission on Population Policy). Appendix C: Experts' report of the Public Health Division to the CCPP, Archive of Väestöliitto.
12 Federley, 'Samfundets moderpremiering', 131.

13 Folkhälsan, Minutes dated 3 Oct 1945 (meeting of the board and the practical-hygienic section). Appendix H: Promemoria gällande fortsatt mödrapremiering (av Fabian Langenskiöld), Archive of Folkhälsan.
14 Väestöliitto, *Toimintakertomus 1943* (Helsinki: Väestöliitto, 1944), 27.
15 Armas Nieminen, 'Viisi vuotta toimintaa terveen väestönkehityksen sekä kodin, perheen ja lasten yhteiskunnan hyväksi', in *Väestöpolitiikkamme taustaa ja tehtäviä: Väestöliiton vuosikirja I*, by Väestöliitto (Porvoo and Helsinki: WSOY, 1946), 86–115, 103–4.
16 Väestöliitto, Minutes dated 8 Jan 1941, Appendix C.
17 Heikki Pitkänen, 'Äitiyshuollosta', *Duodecim* 79, no. 24 (1963): 1003–10.
18 Max Roser, 'Maternal mortality', *OurWorldInData.org* (2017), https://ourworldindata. org/maternal-mortality/ (accessed 29 Aug 2017); Statistics Finland, 'Infant mortality in 1751–2016', *Findicator* (2017), http://findikaattori.fi/en/table/45 (accessed 29 Aug 2017).
19 Roser, 'Maternal mortality'; Max Roser, 'Child mortality', *OurWorldInData.org* (2017), https://ourworldindata.org/child-mortality/ (accessed 29 Aug 2017).
20 Official Statistics of Finland, 'Deaths by underlying cause of death (ICD-10, 3-character level), age and gender 1998–2018', *Causes of Death* (e-publication) (Helsinki: Statistics Finland, 2017), http://pxnet2.stat.fi/PXWeb/pxweb/en/StatFin/StatFin__ter__ksyyt/050_ksyyt_tau_105.px/ (accessed 29 Aug 2017); Official Statistics of Finland, 'Appendix table 3: Mortality during infant and perinatal period 1987–2015', *Causes of Death* (e-publication) (Helsinki: Statistics Finland, 2017), www.stat.fi/til/ksyyt/2015/ksyyt_2015_2016-12-30_tau_005_en.html (accessed 29 Aug 2017).
21 Väestöliitto, *Väestöliitto 1941*, 24–7; Väestöliitto, Minutes dated 4 Jan 1945 (board meeting), Appendix 1.
22 Act on Induced Abortion 82/1950.
23 E.g., Väestöliitto, *Väestöliitto 1941*, 28.
24 Väestöliitto, Minutes dated 10 Feb 1954 (board meeting). Appendix 7: Terveydenhoitolehti, Avioliitto ja koti, 31–4, Archive of Väestöliitto.
25 Samfundet Folkhälsan, *Samfundet Folkhälsan i svenska Finland: Förhandlingar 1950* (Helsinki: Tilgmanns tryckeri, 1951), 19–20.
26 Aura Pasila, 'Early history of the oral contraceptive pill in Finland: Diffusion of the new contraceptive and fertility patterns', *Finnish Yearbook of Population Research* 46, no. 1 (2011): 49–70, 54–5.
27 Ilpo Helén, *Äidin elämän politiikka: Naissukupuolisuus, valta ja itsesuhde Suomessa 1880-luvulta 1960-luvulle* (Helsinki: Gaudeamus, 1997), 237–8, 250.
28 Väestöliitto, *Kodin, perheen ja lasten yhteiskunta: Kansalaistietoa väestökysymyksestä* (Helsinki: Väestöliitto, 1946), 3.
29 Helén, *Äidin elämän politiikka*, 237–8, 250.
30 Act on Induced Abortion 82/1950.
31 Väestöliitto, *Annual Report 1951*, Archive of Väestöliitto.
32 Helén, *Äidin elämän politiikka*, 244–8, quotations on p. 247.
33 Miina Keski-Petäjä, *Aborttitoiveet ja abortintorjunta: Raskaudenkeskeytyksen hakeminen 1950–60-lukujen Suomessa* (Helsinki: Väestöliitto, 2012).
34 Samfundet Folkhälsan, *Samfundet Folkhälsan i svenska Finland: Vad vi gjorde 1952* (Helsinki: Tilgmanns tryckeri, 1953), 22.
35 Mattila, *Kansamme parhaaksi*, 103.
36 Väestöliitto, Minutes dated 18 Dec 1940 (meeting of the Central Commission on Population Policy). Appendix A1 (dated 20 Dec 1940 [*sic*]): Letter describing future activities, Archive of Väestöliitto.
37 Väestöliitto, Minutes dated 9 Dec 1940 (consultation meeting). Appendix A (dated 19 Nov 1940): Letter sent by the Association of Finnish Culture and Identity to Finnish social and health policy associations regarding collaboration in population policy issues, Archive of Väestöliitto; Väestöliitto, Minutes dated 18 Dec 1940, Appendix A1.

38   Karin A. Spoof, 'Folkhälsans mentalhygieniska verksamhet', in *Samfundet Folkhälsan i svenska Finland 1921–1946: Festskrift utgiven med anledning av Samfundets 25-års jubileum*, by Samfundet Folkhälsan (Helsinki: Frenckellska Tryckeri Aktiebolaget, 1946), 118–26.

39   See, e.g., Federley, 'Samfundets moderpremiering', 129; Väestöliitto, Minutes dated 8 Jan 1941, Appendix C; the reform of the sterilisation legislation was mentioned in all Väestöliitto's annual reports and action plans in the 1940s.

40   Mattila, *Kansamme parhaaksi*, 337.

41   Minna Harjula, *Terveyden jäljillä: Suomalainen terveyspolitiikka 1900-luvulla* (Tampere: Tampere University Press, 2007), 54–6; see also Chapter 5 by Minna Harjula in this volume.

42   For further analyses of the impact of war on public health and welfare state development, see, e.g., Helene Laurent, 'War and the emerging social state: Social policy, public health and citizenship in wartime Finland', in *Finland in World War II: History, Memory, Interpretations*, ed. Tiina Kinnunen and Ville Kivimäki (Leiden: Brill, 2012), 315–54; Pauli Kettunen, 'Wars, nation and the welfare state in Finland', in *Warfare and Welfare: Military Conflict and Welfare State Development in Western Countries*, ed. Herbert Obinger et al. (Oxford: Oxford University Press, forthcoming).

8 Public health categories in the making of citizenship

The case of refugees and Roma in Sweden

Norma Montesino and
Ida Ohlsson Al Fakir

Introduction

Medical knowledge and public health policies have had crucial roles in the construction of normality; they have provided concepts, categories and practices that have been used in the construction of social deviance. Taking this circumstance as a point of departure, this chapter studies *socialt handikapp* (social disability), a concept developed within the area of public health and eventually used in the description and practical dealing with social problems in the aftermath of the Second World War. The aim is to show the authoritative and instrumental role this concept has had in forming the perceptions of social deviance and in the managing of individuals and groups perceived as social deviants.

During the post-war decades, the boundaries between 'deserving' and 'undeserving' poor – citizens and aliens – shifted. New groups of poor and aliens, who until then had been defined as unworthy of benefits, were now considered worthy of social support and citizenship status.[1] The shifting status of these groups within the welfare administration – i.e., the boundary change – was legitimised and handled with conceptual tools that were originally used to differentiate healthy citizens from the sick. This entry of the undeserving into deserving categories created new spaces in which categorical divisions became relative and negotiable. In this chapter, we argue that knowledge, concepts and practices from the area of public health played crucial roles in this relativising and redrawing of boundaries. Medical knowledge provided the conceptual instruments (basic categories, arguments, terms, etc.) for the legitimisation and expansion of a social project that promised to change situations and diagnoses earlier perceived as definitive and non-negotiable, and make them treatable and possible to change. These processes were part of a general social development in which new forms of expert knowledge entered the international arena. In the following, we discuss these processes by focusing on the particular case of Sweden.

The time under study – 1945–1980 – represents a unique period in the history of the Swedish welfare state. In the context of war-torn Europe, Sweden's favourable economic and political situation enabled comprehensive social policy planning and expansion. The country's rich natural assets and intact heavy industries were important resources for international reconstruction. However, an expansion of production demanded a growing workforce. This was achieved mainly through international labour migration and the incorporation of women into the national labour market. Adult participation in the regulated labour market and, connected to this, increased interest in the integration of new groups into the active labour force became priorities of Swedish post-war welfare policies. Developing the conceptual and practical tools to identify, take care of, treat and rehabilitate those who were classified as unable to work was among the main goals of these new policies.

Since the beginning of the twentieth century, establishing the boundaries between the able-bodied and the disabled had developed as an area of knowledge and intervention within the field of public health.[2] Scientific knowledge was developed that legitimised policies entitling citizens classified as disabled to a minimal level of protection. After the Second World War, however, the category of disability became central in the expanding welfare policies and practices destined to transform individuals outside the regulated labour market into productive workers. The use of disability as an instrument in such welfare work changed the boundaries between deserving and undeserving citizens, and between unwanted aliens and potential citizens.

Through the international work led by the United Nations, the category of disability became part of an institutionalised vocabulary, and the concept of rehabilitation became a useful tool to solve thorny aspects of the international 'refugee question'.[3] In Sweden, the availability of resources made it possible to invest in research and practices in the area of public health (including fields such as epidemiology and social medicine), and thereby to create new expertise for the social area, which in turn was a prerequisite for the expanding social policies. In this context, *socialt handikapp* became a category as well as a conceptual instrument that was practical in many different institutional settings: it 'travelled' from the area of public health to social work, from medical practices to practices focused on individuals and groups perceived as social deviants.

Our empirical focus is on the post-war handling of a group of Roma people settled in Sweden since the end of the nineteenth century, and a group of European stateless refugees received in Sweden within international selected refugee quotas. This Roma group and the arriving refugees were identified as new target groups of Swedish social policies. However, we sustain the universal applicability of these processes: the cases of Roma and refugees discussed here illustrate general processes initiated after the war in which individuals and groups earlier perceived as outsiders should, in line with the new policies, be treated as potential members of the national population. By using the case study of Swedish post-war welfare interventions, we will contribute to the understanding of how public health concepts and categories were used in the construction of citizenship and its alterities. This allows us to reinterpret the processes that in a delimited time period moved, changed or extended the boundaries of belonging.

In the next section, we contextualise these processes theoretically in a framework according to which citizenship is a dynamic process. The making of citizenship encompasses different areas that provide arguments for the constitution of different kinds of citizenship. We suggest that concepts and practices from the area of public health legitimised the incorporation of new groups. The following section focuses on the role of the disability category in welfare policy and on the specific social dimension this category assumed after the Second World War. The ensuing two sections discuss how this category worked in the concrete policies developed in relation to the reception of refugees and the incorporation of Roma groups into the Swedish population. A summary and a concluding discussion end the chapter.

Shifting borders of deviance

Boundaries and borders are fundamental mechanisms in the production of belonging and otherness.[4] They are (re)formulated and (re)invented in representations and categories and through practices. Shifting categorical borders create and recreate arguments for membership, perceptions about and relations between citizens, almost-citizens and non-citizens. Borders and their associated practices are thus crucial tools in the shaping of citizenship, otherness and positions in between.[5] In this chapter, we have been theoretically inspired by the dynamic approach developed by Bridget Anderson, who rejects the established binaries citizens–non-citizens, deserving–undeserving and included–excluded, and instead points to *the historically contingent boundary-making processes*. During such processes, certain groups are constructed and approached as deserving of membership, while others are totally rejected at the border, or partially stopped at various gates within the welfare system. In Anderson's analysis, the citizen category carries both formal/legal and symbolic/ relational characteristics; the former dimension represents some factual reality and the latter refers to the negotiable parts of this reality. Whereas formal citizenship corresponds to the juridical level of the state, membership in the community (the nation) prescribes adherence to certain values and virtues. The focus of this chapter is the role of public health categories in the process of citizen-making after the Second World War.

To illustrate how boundary-making processes may work, Anderson has created the analytical figures of the Non-Citizen and the Failed Citizen, which are shaped in relation to the Good Citizen, who populates the community of value or the imagined community – i.e., the nation.[6] The values and virtues that characterise the Good Citizen are defined both from the outside and the inside – that is, in relation to the Non-Citizen as well as the Failed Citizen. The two latter categories constitute the undeserving poor. The figure of the Failed Citizen represents the 'internal others', those who are considered incapable of or unworthy of full membership. For people who are formally members of the nation-state but do not always live up to the ideal of the liberal sovereign self (i.e., rational, self-owning and economically independent), there is another useful metaphor: the Tolerated Citizen. These are not-quite-good-enough citizens, formally part of the population yet on the margins of the community (of value).[7] Anderson describes the dynamic of these configurations and the instable and arbitrary state of inclusion, which means that historically Tolerated Citizens can easily become Failed Citizens, and

Failed Citizens at certain moments in history have been perceived and treated as outsiders. In this context, we describe how concepts and categories used in the area of public health became instrumental in the social boundary changing processes that occurred after the Second World War. Hence, we focus on a specific and delimited period in the history of public health, a period when causes of disease and social marginalisation were placed on a collective level, outside of the individual.[8] The state assumed the social responsibility to cure and counteract such conditions and positions. However, as we discuss in this chapter, these processes also had consequences that could be stigmatising for the individual.

The empirical material for our analysis has been collected in previous research projects.[9] However, inspired by Anderson, we develop our earlier conclusions by placing a stronger emphasis on governmental rationalities – i.e., the function of public health in the governing of the population – and, more specifically, the role played by the disability category in the construction of new parameters of inclusion after the Second World War. In doing so, we identify the new dimensions that the disability concept assumed as it was transferred from the area of public health to the social field.

The source material consists of policy documents, research material, corres-pondence and other types of contemporary records that illustrate national and international policies and practices developed concerning groups perceived as socially deviant during and after the Second World War. During this period, some refugees interned in international refugee camps in different European countries and a group of approximately 800 Roma people (so-called *svenska zigenare*, 'Swedish Gypsies'), who had been living in Sweden since the late nineteenth century, were formally recognised as members of the Swedish population. It was the classification by national and international experts of these groups as *socialt handikappade* (socially disabled) that conditioned and legitimised the new policy. The processes that were initiated by the Swedish authorities aimed towards a transformation of these 'newcomers' into Swedish citizens. However, being classi-fied as *socialt handikappade* implied that they supposedly lacked the conditions and properties to handle this transformation on their own. Experts and professionals became the gatekeepers who formulated new criteria and created new scales for the differentiations of disability. These criteria expanded their field of expertise and the space for new interventions.

Framing disability

When causes of disease were localised outside of the individual in the nineteenth century, a temporality of the state of sickness was established.[10] Prevention, treatment and rehabilitation became central concepts that structured and gave meaning to the new institutionalised medical practices developed to handle disease. These processes changed the status of the sick and the socio-political meaning of sickness and disability. Furthermore, they influenced the perceptions and representations of the poor as well as (later) policies concerning those perceived as aliens.[11] Hence, the development of the concept of disability also changed ideas and practices concerning dependency, making it an explicit part of public health policies and practices. Dependency – a key concept in welfare distribution – has since the early twentieth century been conceived as a *lack* of resources or properties necessary for salaried work.[12]

Using Anderson's differentiated citizen figures, we argue that concepts and practices from the area of public health have been used in order to provide arguments for distinguishing the Failed Citizens from the Tolerated Citizens, and Non-Citizens from citizens. Medical categories such as disability have contributed to the construction of dependency as deviance while at the same time providing arguments to support demands on public responsibility for the national poor. Disability and disease were conceptualised as 'lacks' on the individual level, which exempted individuals from the obligation to work.[13] These different types of 'lacks' provide legitimacy to activities targeting Tolerated and Failed Citizens. Differentiations and categorisations take place on different scales, both at the level of the individual and at policy level. Being categorised as disabled was a condition for certain welfare benefits after the Second World War. Individuals classified as disabled could be exempted from the obligation to work and become part of what Deborah Stone has conceptualised as the need-based distributive system. Hence, she argues, categorising individuals as disabled provided a solution to a redistribution dilemma of the welfare state. Stone's elaborated theoretical framework places the disability category right in the centre of twentieth-century welfare policies. As social insurances tied to participation in the labour market were established, disability became the administrative category that entitled "its members to particular privileges in the form of social aid and exemptions from certain obligations of citizenship".[14] Originally, the disability category had a rather limited scope, including only physically handicapped citizens – e.g., war invalids and victims of industrial accidents. Within the framework of public health, however, a considerably wider definition including both psychological/mental and social causes of handicap was developed by welfare experts working with groups considered to be on the margins of established society.[15] This new approach created a conceptual space for developing new policies targeting groups previously perceived as undeserving.[16]

Social disability: A Swedish case

The use of the disability category in the conceptualisation of social problems justified new expertise and interventions, and thus implied a further expansion of the social area. Social medicine was scientifically and socio-politically an important vehicle in this development.[17] Physicians and medical officers in the field became social policy experts, adding a social dimension to the understanding of deviance and arguing for the inclusion of new groups.[18] Notably, the Swedish physicians Gunnar Inghe and John Takman linked social conditions and traits to the medical definition of disability.[19] They often worked in close collaboration with social workers: women represented social knowledge, whereas men provided medical expertise.[20] These experts became authoritative voices in developing new forms of social knowledge.

Thus, from the previously dominant focus on the *medical* aspects of the disabling condition of individuals, the disability category was redefined to include *social* aspects. Hence, *socialt handikapp* was related to diverse criteria such as age (children and the elderly poor), family situation (families with several children, single mothers), education (illiteracy), cultural belonging (minorities or non-European poor), etc. It was in this process of blurring boundaries that the incorporation of the new Roma and refugee citizens occurred in Sweden. Metaphorically, they were moved from the status of Non-Citizens or Failed Citizens to the status of Tolerated Citizens.

Within the established administrative order, these new citizens became the responsibility of the social welfare services, i.e., the organisations formed to manage *socially disabled* citizens. In Sweden during the early post-war decades, such policies were primarily developed and implemented as part of the expansive administration of the labour market, which included extensive vocational training programmes.[21] The basic classification principles for entitlement to assistance were age and (poor) health, but the fundamental condition for being included in any classification system at all was territorial belonging. This membership criterion was modified after the Second World War, when the category of *socialt handikapp* provided concrete arguments for the admission of new – in the sense of either newly arrived or newly recognised – citizens considered socially deviant. The negative representations of those previously described as undeserving poor were replaced by less derogatory classifications, which legitimised both the Swedish policies towards Roma groups (within the framework of the contemporary 'Gypsy question') and the international administration of certain European refugees.[22]

These two cases, we argue, should be analysed as part of the same development, not only because they (roughly) coincide in time but also because of the common conceptualisations and activities used in the managing of groups commonly analysed separately.

Refugees: Classifications and practices

In the 1950s' international debate, the condition of 'refugeeness' was conceptualised as a legal disability. This legal definition was constructed in relation to the characteristics linked to citizenship:

> Laws concerning aliens are made with the conception of the normal, the protected alien in the mind of the law-giver. It follows that the refugee, in whose case this protection is missing, suffers from a number of legal disabilities.[23]

The link that related the category of refugee to the category of citizen was thus defined in terms of a 'lack' or 'absence' of what was understood as the principal characteristics of citizenship: first and foremost, legal protection by a nation-state and the legal responsibility of the nation-state towards its members, regardless of their whereabouts and pursuits. The refugee, however, was an alien without protection by any nation-state.[24] This *legal disability* could be negotiated on condition of the demonstration of the capacity to work. Stone identifies three fundamental dimensions that give legitimacy to the disability concept in policy work: the worthiness of the individual defined as disabled; the incapacity of this person; and the clinical methods that are used to understand and reveal this disability and incapacity.[25] The experts' definition of refugees (and Roma in Sweden) as disabled gave them a new status, and the possibility of becoming Tolerated Citizens. In a way, it was recognition of their suffering, a suffering beyond individual control. Hence, in this context, the concept of disability created – with its added social dimensions – the arguments and tools for inclusion.

The expansive potential of the disability concept can be easily identified in the study of the international and national responses to the European refugee situation after the Second World War. During this time, the international authorities had to manage the situation of around 2 million people in Europe without citizenship, i.e., stateless persons.[26] Additionally, many of them were in bad health and the majority in a situation of total dependence on the international authorities. The fear of epidemic diseases governed the immediate response of the authorities, in which medical knowledge and practice played key roles.[27] The medical staff in the international refugee camps divided refugees into two groups: the healthy and the unhealthy. They further divided the latter group into people with chronic disease and people with non-chronic disease, and sought to identify and isolate refugees with epidemic and/or contagious diseases such as tuberculosis (TB), diphtheria and typhus.[28]

These classifications played a crucial role for the organisation of the camp routines and in the regulation of the organised migration and resettlement programmes for refugees. In the management of refugees in international camps, national teams of doctors, in collaboration with international experts, selected some refugees for different resettlement programmes, thereby designating others to remain in the camps; more than 100,000 refugees in the international camps were excluded from all programmes. By 1949, this group was estimated at 173,300 individuals.[29] These refugees were people who belonged to the traditional poor relief categories: children, the sick, the elderly and the disabled – i.e., groups that lacked the capacities required for work in the regular labour market.

The basic criteria for further classification of these refugees were mainly based on medical categories, but new – social – aspects were also added. The camp authorities kept records of the interned refugees, including medical evaluations of their partial or potential capacity to work and their rehabilitation potential.[30] By the end of the 1940s, the medical records kept by the camp authorities classified the refugees using a nomenclature of "difficult cases", based on both medical and social criteria. Difficult Case A comprised of people with TB, while other chronically ill people were classified as Difficult Case D; elderly refugees were Difficult Case K, etc. These categories were described as "the hard core", consisting of *disabled refugees*.[31] Their 'disability' was differentiated according to physical, mental and social aspects.

During the 1950s, refugees classified as socially disabled became the focus of international negotiations. In the refugee camps, social disability was related to diverse criteria, all of which were associated to poverty (i.e., dependence). Hence, families with several children, the elderly, single mothers and/or unaccompanied minors, Roma families and certain small groups from non-European countries were all classified as socially disabled refugees. The international authorities negotiated the situation of these refugees and established special support for the countries that accepted them.[32] Sweden was among the countries that in 1945 committed to receive 10,000 people from different camps in Germany. A large part of these refugees was expected to be in need of medical care.[33]

In these international negotiations, new parameters for inclusion were developed. At first, medical criteria were used to provide legitimacy on a policy-level, and the nation-state provided the institutional framework for the national membership of these groups. Later, social criteria permitted the entry of those refugees that did not fit the medically defined group. The first group admitted in Sweden arrived in the beginning of the 1950s and consisted of refugees diagnosed with TB and their families; the second group consisted of elderly persons and refugee families classified as socially disabled.[34] The basic criteria to admit these refugees were their supposed incapacity, an incapacity which could have medical and/or social causes and which laid outside their individual responsibility. Subsequently during the 1950s and 1960s, new, always small, groups kept coming. According to an official investigation in 1967, 15,600 refugees were transferred to Sweden between 1950 and 1965. Amongst these, 13,500 were considered able-bodied by the medical expertise. The remaining 2,100 belonged to the quota of handicapped refugees agreed upon with the United Nations Relief and Rehabilitation Administration.[35]

Roma in Sweden: Classifications and practices

The category of disability became an entry category also in the new Swedish Roma policies developed after the Second World War.[36] These policies consisted mainly of new labour market programmes and practices concerning *svenska zigenare* (the Swedish Roma), i.e., a group of Roma who had lived in Sweden since the late nineteenth century and were entitled to Swedish citizenship in the early 1950s.

Several social and medical experts were involved in the debate on the situation of these new Swedish citizens. The group was described as socially disabled, and the experts claimed that their disability consisted of their incapacity to adapt to new ('modern') living conditions, an incapacity admittedly caused by external processes. Previously, this group had supported themselves by working in traditional and mobile occupations that, due to social, technologic, economic and cultural changes, no longer existed. The poverty and exclusion of the group was thus explained as an inevitable consequence of the progress of modern society; they were described as victims of this development. Furthermore, in the 1950s, some social welfare experts attributed the causes of their poverty to a "dying Gypsy culture" that made the Roma unable to adapt to the requirements of modern society. These representations transformed the "Gypsies" into an impoverished people without the resources to resolve their economic and social problems by themselves.[37]

Hence, the Swedish Roma were defined as socially disabled from diverse perspectives; different experts developed different dimensions in their perceptions of the group's disabilities. Social workers focused on the economic situation, and stated that Roma families were no longer self-supporting, and, accordingly, defined their alleged social disability in terms of dependence on welfare. The (predominantly male) Roma who were physically able to work were considered disabled because they could not be incorporated into the labour market due to illiteracy and an alleged inability to cope with the routines of everyday wage work. One of the arguments was that they did not have the basic knowledge required to understand their new situation.[38]

In a comprehensive and all-encompassing socio-medical investigation in the early 1960s, the social physician John Takman and a team of socio-medical experts (with men representing the medical expertise and women the social expertise) tried to measure the degree of the Roma's disabilities, and hence their rehabilitation potential. The study dealt with their health conditions (e.g., undernourishment, physical condition, disease, impairments, etc.) and their social situation (family composition, educational level, illiteracy, work experiences, living situation, etc.). The researchers also enquired about the Roma's own concerns and wishes concerning their future, i.e., their wants and needs related to health, housing, education and work. On the basis of the aggregated and processed information, Takman proposed individual- and family-orientated 'rehabilitation measures', which included modern housing, education and professional training to prepare for the adults' incorporation into the labour market and the children's incorporation into the school system.[39]

Later in the 1960s and during the 1970s, experts in the educational-psychological field added several, more detailed and specific, social disabilities to the 'Gypsy problem'. For example, focusing on the Roma family, they argued that parenthood – notably in relation to public institutions such as schools – was a role that the adult Roma were not able to fulfil without external support.[40] Roma children were also described as disabled, the argument being that they were unable to deal with normal schooling without special assistance. Stone has pointed out that the concept of disability contains a powerful dynamic of "definitional expansion", which implies that each element "is a door through which new phenomena can enter and acquire legitimacy as types of disability for official purposes".[41] Hence, the original medical category of disability could – through the added social dimension – be used to define and explain an array of (individual, educational, cultural and socio-economic) causes that, according to their analysis, hindered Roma people in becoming full citizens, i.e., living up to the ideals of the Good Citizen.[42]

Institutionalised activities

The definition of Roma and refugees as socially disabled were links in a chain of self-multiplying policies and interventions developed in different institutional settings. Initially, the social authorities had institutional responsibility for the Swedish Roma and for those refugees who could not be incorporated into the labour market, while the National Labour Market Board (AMS) was responsible for those able to work. In the late 1950s, however, the AMS assumed responsibility for the whole category of the Swedish Roma – partly because of their supposed disabilities (rehabilitation in general being under the administration of the AMS), and partly because of the prominent position of the AMS in the Swedish post-war welfare state. The AMS was a national authority established in 1948 with the explicit purpose to take a leading role in the practical realisation of the socio-political reforms of the time, of which full employment was both a means and a target.[43] The authorities contended, however, that not everybody within the group of the Swedish Roma would be able to work. Some were classified as disabled due to age, others because of health problems. In any case, examinations and expert opinions were needed to differentiate individuals in relation to their level of disability. The transfer of public health categories and practices to the social area thus gave new dynamics to the expansion and development of new forms of expertise.

Important for this development was the 1962 AMS decision to fund a socio-medical study (discussed above) of, initially, only a limited number of adult Roma. This number grew during the following years so that, in 1965, it included all (identified) members of the Swedish Roma community in Sweden.[44] The legitimisation as well as the expansion of this study was articulated in the terms and concepts of public health. On the one hand, experts argued for more comprehensive and detailed studies of the group for the sake of improving the health situation among the Roma themselves. On the other, convincing arguments of expansion were formulated with reference to population health on a more general scale.[45] Medical-genetic and epidemiological studies of so-called *social isolates* were in vogue in international science during the 1960s. The scientific experts, who already had defined the Swedish Roma as a *social isolate*, would underline this argument and link it to wider welfare state ambitions concerning the whole population. The results of these arguments were extended examinations of the Swedish Roma and more differentiated categories of social disability, despite the original ambition/claim to 'normalise' them through state-endorsed and scientifically supported interventions in the fields of housing, education and work.

During the 1970s, matters related to the Swedish Roma were moved back to the Department of Social Welfare. The reception and introduction of new groups of arriving refugees also became the responsibility of this department. By this time, the social authorities were using the concept of *handikapp* (disability) as a concept with a wide field of application. The plasticity of the category was specifically useful, it was argued, since it permitted classifications and interventions based on whatever could be identified as a ground for deviation – be it age, cultural background, language, education or otherwise.[46]

Hence, once the socio-medical experts had examined and differentiated the disabilities of adult Roma in detail in the 1960s, social workers were entrusted with the responsibility for their 'social rehabilitation'. New studies were launched, further differentiating the concept and contents of disability concerning Swedish Roma.[47] In this context, 'social rehabilitation' still signified the incorporation of adult individuals into the labour market and children into the schooling system. These tasks extended the spaces for social intervention.

The focus on *cultural difference* was further institutionalised during the 1970s when non-European refugees arrived in European countries.[48] These refugees were described as culturally and/or ethnically different by both international and national organisations. Cultural difference was subsequently defined as a social disability.[49] Legal disability related to statelessness could be negotiated if the refugee was a healthy young man, while the disability associated with Roma identity could be 'treated' by teaching and training Roma about the obligations of citizenship.[50] To achieve this goal, social workers and other staff stated that specialised knowledge was necessary, arguing that they lacked the competence to deal with the new groups. This led to the rise of *new* professional expertise, giving way to new positions and expanding research, all for the sake of 'treating disabled' newcomers. By the end of the 1970s, it was difficult to incorporate even young and healthy refugees into the labour market. The period of economic expansion was over; newly arrived refugees were routinely incorporated into the activities developed for welfare dependents, that is, in activities institutionalised in the social welfare services.[51]

In recent decades, the category of disability has been replaced with new terms that focus on the social environment that leads to the disability of individuals. The terms used in these contexts – e.g., *funktionsnedsättning* and *funktionsvariation* (functional impairment and functional variation, respectively) – are more explicitly linked to societal institutions. The new terminology thus relativises disability by focusing on a particular reduced function in relation to a conceived 'normal' functioning in society. Central to this 'normality' is, for adults, participation in the regulated labour market; one-third of the unemployed that in 2015 were registered at the employment office were coded as *funktionsnedsatta* (functionally impaired).[52] According to recent research, this development and particular use of public health concepts in the social area today can be connected to neoliberal economics, where a 'medico-economic discourse' has been developed.[53]

Put in more general terms, medical terminology has during recent decades become more influential in the construction of social problems.[54] Today, *cultural* or *ethnic difference* is subordinated to the representation of refugees and other migrants and Roma groups as socially disabled, for example by the usage of such perceived differences as a basis for the classification systems of welfare institutions.[55] Cultural difference, ethnical background and deficient Swedish language remain criteria used in the classification of social disability.

Concluding discussion

This chapter deals with the influence of public health concepts and categories in policy work in Sweden after the Second World War. The medical concept of *handikapp* (disability) became a category with great potential as it was transferred from the area of public health to a specific use in the social field. It legitimated the expansion of this field by providing conceptual and practical instruments used in new investigations and knowledge production, thus forming new spaces of inter-vention. These processes contributed to changing national migration and welfare policies on refugees and Roma groups, which is illustrated with two case studies: the management of some European refugees considered especially difficult to incorporate into mainstream society; and the handling of a Roma group formally recognised as Swedish citizens but perceived as unable to fulfil the demands of citizenship.

In these processes, social problems were conceptualised in new ways, enabling new groups to benefit from the Swedish welfare system. The boundaries that separated aliens from citizens, the undeserving from the deserving, shifted. Metaphorically speaking, it was a matter of Non-Citizens becoming Tolerated Citizens, and the subsequent development of policies and practices to transform them into Good Citizens. Repressive and openly excluding strategies were superseded by differentiated strategies developed to handle – i.e., socially relocate – individuals and groups earlier defined as deviants. The original medical category of disability was supplemented with social dimensions mainly related to working capacity in the regulated labour market. This expanded disability category added a temporal dimension – a potentiality of change – to the political-administrative management of the population; disability was a relative and 'treatable' category, hence social relocation became possible.

New conceptual boundaries thus legitimised new policies, which created activities that made membership in the community of value (i.e., the nation) a relative state. Public health categories were used in these processes of boundary change; the social dimension of disability could legitimise new social policies and practices whose implementation moved the boundaries between outsiders and citizens. However, these new boundaries also contributed to the construction of a different citizen status. The entry of the new members became an arena of nego-tiation in which different actors participated, actors who formulated new spaces of intervention. These processes have mainly been interpreted as a turning point in Swedish policies on poor strangers – i.e., inclusion of the 'undeserving'. However, as we argue elsewhere, while indeed aiming for social inclusion, the policies related to groups identified as deviants rather implied new strategies of governing deviance.[56] They were *legitimised* by the rhetoric of social inclusion; but, in reality, they produced a fabric of measures, practices and further interventions which, in the long run, have contributed to prolonging the social marginality of many refugees and Roma groups, notably *within* national borders.

These post-war processes stand in stark contrast to recent developments in Europe, where migrating Roma groups and refugees are treated as *criminals* (i.e., non-deserving) and little effort is made to protect and/or enhance their legal or social rights as citizens. Bearing this in mind, our study exposes some contradictions in Swedish post-war welfare policies. Most notably, it highlights their connection to the expansive potential of the disability concept, which enabled the construction of new excluding spaces within institutionalised forms. In the formation of these new spaces, the actors involved created and shaped identities, restraints and opportunities. Through the processes of defining and managing Roma and refugees in Sweden – the Tolerated but potentially Good Citizens – experts, officials and professionals were able to construct themselves as Good Citizens. Hence, the definition of Roma and refugees as *socialt handikappade* (socially disabled), and the institutional activities that followed suit, make visible the relational nature of the making of citizenship and the power of public health concepts and categories in the representation of social problems.

Notes

1 'Deserving' and 'undeserving' poor are empirical concepts in historical sources from the nineteenth and early twentieth century (and before). They concern the historical and fundamental distinctions made between worthy and unworthy recipients of help. Differentiations have always had to do with issues of belonging, but before national citizenship was established as the overriding token of membership, other forms of capital would be used to create and express belonging. K.D.M. Snell, *Parish and Belonging: Community, Identity and Welfare in England and Wales, 1700–1950* (Cambridge: Cambridge University Press, 2006); Bronislaw Geremek, *Den europeiska fattigdomens betydelse* (Stockholm: Nordfront, 1991). For a study of practices of belonging in Sweden, see Theresa Johnsson, *Vårt fredliga samhälle: 'lösdriveri' och försvarslöshet i Sverige under 1830-talet* (Uppsala: Acta Universitatis Upsaliensis, 2016).
2 Deborah A. Stone, *The Disabled State* (Philadelphia: Temple University Press, 1984).
3 The United Nations Relief and Rehabilitation Administration (UNRRA) came to special agreements with particular countries whereby they committed to the receipt of certain quotas of so-called disabled refugees. Louise W. Holborn, *Refugees: A Problem of Our Time: The Work of the United Nations High Commissioner for Refugees, 1951–1972. Vol. 1* (Metuchen, NJ: Scarecrow, 1975); Peter Gatrell, *The Making of the Modern Refugee* (Oxford: Oxford University Press, 2015).
4 Maribel Casas-Cortes et al., 'New keywords: Migration and borders', *Cultural Studies* 29, no.1 (2015): 55–87; Janine Dahinden, 'A plea for the "de-migranticization" of research on migration and integration', *Ethnic and Racial Studies* 39, no. 13 (2016): 2207–25.
5 Bridget L. Anderson, *Us and Them? The Dangerous Politics of Immigration Control* (Oxford: Oxford University Press, 2013), 3.
6 Ibid.; Benedict Anderson, *Imagined Communities: Reflections on the Origin and Spread of Nationalism* (London: Verso, 2006).
7 Anderson, *Us and Them?*
8 Dorothy Porter, *Health, Civilization and the State: A History of Public Health from Ancient to Modern Times* (London: Routledge, 1999).
9 The source material was previously analysed and presented in Norma Montesino, *Zigenarfrågan: Intervention och romantik* (Doctoral disseration, Lunds universitet, 2002); Norma Montesino and Malin Thor, 'Migration och folkhälsa: Hälsovårdspolitiska bedömningar i den svenska flyktingmottagningen under 1940-talets första hälft', *Historisk tidskrift* 129, no.1 (2009): 27–46; Norma Montesino, 'Social disability: Roma and refugees in Swedish welfare', *International Journal of Migration, Health and Social Care* 8, no. 3 (2012): 134–45; Ida Ohlsson Al Fakir, *Nya rum för socialt medborgarskap: Om vetenskap och politik i 'Zigenarundersökningen'– en socialmedicinsk studie av svenska romer 1962–1965* (Växjö: Linnaeus University Press, 2015); Norma Montesino and Ida Ohlsson Al Fakir, 'The prolonged inclusion of Roma groups in Swedish society', *Social Inclusion* 3, no. 5 (2015): 126–36.

10 David Armstrong, *Political Anatomy of the Body: Medical Knowledge in Britain in the Twentieth Century* (Cambridge: Cambridge University Press, 1983).
11 On changing representations of the poor in public health, see ibid.; Porter, *Health, Civilization and the State*.
12 Nancy Fraser and Linda Gordon, '"Dependency" demystified: Inscriptions of power in a keyword of the welfare state', *Social Politics* 1, no. 1 (1994): 4–31.
13 Henri-Jacques Stiker, *Corps infirmes et sociétés: Essais d'anthropologie historique* (Paris: Dunod, 2005).
14 Stone, *Disabled State*, 4.
15 In addition to Roma and refugees, these groups included an array of categories such as 'alcoholics' and 'paupers'. See John Takman, *The Gypsies in Sweden: A Socio-Medical Study* (Stockholm: Liber Förlag, 1976); Gustav Jonsson, *Det sociala arvet* (Stockholm: Tiden, 1969); Gunnar Inghe and Maj-Britt Inghe, *Den ofärdiga välfärden* (Stockholm: Tiden/Folksam, 1967); John Takman, *Socialmedicinsk vardag* (Stockholm: Wahlström & Widstrand, 1966); Gunnar Inghe, *Klientelet på ungkarlshotellen* (Stockholm: Socialvårdens planeringskommitté, Stencil, 1962); Gunnar Inghe, *Fattiga i folkhemmet: En studie av långvarigt understödda i Stockholm* (Stockholm: Stadsarkivet, 1960). Cf. Jacques Donzelot, 'The promotion of the social', in *Foucault's New Domains*, ed. Mike Gane and Terry Johnson (London: Routledge, 1993), 106–38.; Stiker, *Corps infirmes*.
16 Montesino, 'Social disability'; Ohlsson Al Fakir, *Nya rum*.
17 Ohlsson Al Fakir, *Nya rum*, 94–114; Dorothy Porter, *Health Citizenship: Essays in Social Medicine and Biomedical Politics* (Berkeley: University of California Press, 2011).
18 Ohlsson Al Fakir, *Nya rum*; Annika Berg, *Den gränslösa hälsan: Signe och Axel Höjer, folkhälsan och expertisen* (Uppsala: Uppsala universitet, 2009); Kerstin Vinterhed, *Gustav Jonsson på Skå. 2: Kampen* (Stockholm: Marieberg, 1980), 53–66, 84–7.
19 E.g., Takman, *Gypsies in Sweden*; Jonsson, *Det sociala arvet*; Inghe and Inghe, *Den ofärdiga välfärden*; Takman, *Socialmedicinsk vardag*; Inghe, *Klientelet på ungkarlshotellen*.
20 E.g., social worker Maj-Britt Inghe was married to and worked with physician Gunnar Inghe.
21 Ohlsson Al Fakir, *Nya rum*, 82–92; Montesino and Ohlsson Al Fakir, 'Prolonged inclusion'.
22 Montesino, *Zigenarfrågan*.
23 G. J. van Heuven Goedhart, 'The problem of refugees', *Académie de Droit International, Recueil des Cours, Collected Courses* 82 (1953): 261–371, 284.
24 Van Heuven, 'Problem of refugees'.
25 Stone, *Disabled State*, 172f.
26 Mark Wyman, *DP: Europe's Displaced Persons, 1945–1951* (Philadelphia: Balch Institute Press, 1989).
27 Paul Weindling, '"Belsenitis": Liberating Belsen, its hospitals, UNRRA, and selection for re-emigration, 1945–1948', *Science in Context* 19, no. 3 (2006): 401–18.
28 Holborn, *Refugees*.
29 Malcolm J. Proudfoot, *European Refugees: 1939–52: A Study in Forced Population Movement* (Evanston, IL: North Western University Press, 1956).
30 Holborn, *Refugees*.
31 Concerning the 'hard core', see ibid.; van Heuven, 'Problem of refugees'.
32 Holborn, *Refugees*; Gatrell, *Making of the Modern Refugee*.
33 Socialstyrelsens arkiv FXXa, Vol. 16.
34 Torsten Bruce, 'Problems of the sick', in *European Seminar on the Social and Economic Aspects of Refugee Integration* (Stockholm: Swedish Royal Organizing Committee, 1960).
35 Utlänningsutredningen, *Invandringen: problematik och handläggning: Utlännings-utredningens betänkande, 2*, Statens offentliga utredningar (State public reports;

hereafter SOU) 1967:18 (Stockholm, 1967). In the late 1960s and early 1970s, the authorities planned to transfer new groups of Albanians, Assyrians and Roma dwelling in displaced persons' camps.

36 Ohlsson Al Fakir, *Nya rum*.

37 Carl-Herman Tillhagen, *Zigenarna i Sverige* (Stockholm: Natur o. Kultur, 1965); *1954 års zigenarutredning, Zigenarfrågan: betänkande*, SOU 1956:43 (Stockholm, 1956).

38 John Takman, 'Socialpsykiatriska synpunkter på de svenska zigenarna', *Svenska läkartidningen* 49, no. 14 (1952): 926–34; SOU 1956:43.

39 John Takman, *Zigenarundersökningen 1962–1963. Stockholmspopulationen: En summarisk rapport* (Stockholm and Uppsala, 1963); John Takman, *Zigenarundersökningen 1962–1965: Slutrapport den 31 mars 1966* (Stockholm, 1966); Takman, *Gypsies in Sweden*; Ohlsson Al Fakir, *Nya rum*.

40 Arne Trankell and Ingrid Trankell, *Undersökning rörande möjligheterna att underlätta de skolpliktiga zigenarbarnens skolgång* (Stockholm: Stockholms Universitet, Stencil, 1965).

41 Stone, *Disabled State*, 174.

42 Arne Trankell and Ingrid Trankell, *Summarisk beskrivning av förloppet från behandlingsarbetets början: Stockholms stads- och Pedagogiska institutionens försöksprojekt för Stockholms zigenarbefolknings rehabilitering. Rapport 2* (Stockholm: Stockholms stads and Pedagogiska institutionens försöksprojekt för zigenarbefolkningens rehabilitering, 1967); Arne Trankell and Ingrid Trankell, *Effekter av behandlingsarbetet under familjebehandlingsfasen. Rapport 3* (Stockholm: Stockholms stads and Pedagogiska institutionens försöksprojekt för zigenarbefolkningens rehabilitering, 1967); Arne Trankell and Ingrid Trankell, *Förslag till samordnat aktionsprogram: Rapport 4* (Stockholm: Stockholms stads and Pedagogiska institutionens försöksprojekt för Stockholms zigenarbefolkningens rehabilitering, 1967); Arne Trankell and Ingrid Trankell, *Det samordnade aktionsprogrammet förverkligande: Initialskedet. Rapport 5* (Stockholm: Stockholms stads and Pedagogiska institutionens försöksprojekt för zigenarbefolkningens rehabilitering, 1967).

43 Bo Rothstein, *The Social Democratic State: The Swedish Model and the Bureaucratic Problem of Social Reforms* (Pittsburgh: University of Pittsburgh Press, 1996); Ohlsson Al Fakir, *Nya rum*.

44 Ohlsson Al Fakir, *Nya rum*.

45 Lars Beckman, Ragnar Berfenstam and John Takman, 'Motiveringar för fortsatt socialmedicinsk undersökning av zigenarna i Sverige' in *Zigenarundersökningen 1962– 1963. Stockholmspopulationen: En summarisk rapport*, by John Takman (Stockholm and Uppsala, 1963), s 2 f, appendix; John Takman, 'Planering av epidemiologisk undersökning: Förekomsten av Reumatoid Artrit bland zigenare i Stockholm. En epidemiologisk undersökning' (John Takmans arkiv: Zigenarundersökningen A:5. Stockholms stadsarkiv, Stockholm), memorandum.

46 Lennart Holmgren and Bo Svedberg, 'Handikapp: Begrepp med stort användningsområde', *Socialnytt*, no. 9 (1970): 50–55.

47 The Pedagogy Department formed the institutional environment for these projects, which in the late 1960s and the 1970s resulted in at least nine reports and one doctoral thesis on the nature of the problems, their solutions and the consequences of the interventions.

48 Anne Paludan, 'Refugees in Europe', *International Migration Review* 15, no. 1–2 (1981): 69–73.

49 Ali Berggren, 'Socialvårdsbyrån: Bakgrund, verksamhet och problem', *Sociala meddelanden*, no. 7–8 (1962): 593–604; Inga Bååth, 'Flyktingar', *Sociala meddelanden*, no. 6–7 (1962): 607–34.

50 On the acitivites concerning refugees, see Malin Thor, 'Arbetsmarknadsstyrelsen och kvotflyktingarna', in *Efterfrågad arbetskraft? Årsbok från forskningsprofilen Arbetsmarknad, Migration och Etniska Relationer*, ed. Svante Lundberg and Ellinor

Platzer (Växjö: Växjö University Press, 2008), 5–32. On the activities concerning Roma, see Montesino, *Zigenarfrågan*.

51 Montesino, *Social Disability*.
52 Mikael Färnbo, 'Var tredje arbetslös kodad som funktionsnedsatt', *Dagens Arena*, 27 September 2015.
53 Mikael Holmqvist, Christian Maravelias and Per Skålén, 'Identity regulation in neo-liberal societies: Constructing the "occupationally disabled" individual', *Organization* 20, no. 2 (2013): 193–211.
54 Peter Conrad, The *Medicalization of Society* (Baltimore: Johns Hopkins University Press, 2007).
55 Marita Eastmond, 'Egalitarian ambitions, construction of difference: The paradoxes of refugee integration in Sweden', *Journal of Ethnic and Migration Studies* 37, no. 2 (2011): 277–95; Mikael Holmqvist, *The Institutionalization of Social Welfare: A Study of Medicalizing Management* (New York: Routledge, 2008).
56 Montesino and Ohlsson Al Fakir, 'Prolonged inclusion'.

9 Alcohol consumption as a public health problem 1885–1992

Johan Edman

Alcohol consumption has been subject to regulation in many European countries at least since the mid-1800s. The problematic consequences of alcohol consumption, putative causes and possible solutions have been at different times described as individual or collective, and problematised as either a medical or a social issue. Alcohol misuse has been framed as a disease, as a moral defect or as rational behaviour in a dysfunctional society. Proposed solutions have included, for instance, medicines and forced labour, in addition to psychotherapy and socialist class struggle.

In this context, the activity of framing alcohol use as a challenge for public health appears almost parasitic, drawing on seemingly arbitrary references to most different aspects of the perceived problem. In this chapter, I will analyse the ways in which alcohol misuse has been presented as a public health issue by examining the first and largest international alcohol conferences during the years 1885–1992. What qualifies as a public health problem? Who are the people targeted by public health interventions?

I will briefly discuss how alcohol has been framed within the ambiguous concept of public health, and present the conferences that have produced the source material. Thereafter I will present the results of an empirical study of discussions of alcohol misuse as a public health problem in the periods 1885–1939 and 1948–1992. The chapter concludes with a summarising discussion.

Public health and the conferences

Alcohol plays a minor role in most of the research on public health history. Sociologists Pekka Sulkunen and Katariina Warpenius have shown that the temperance movement around 1900 embraced competing (or perhaps complementary) logics. On the one hand, the temperance movement propagated general measures such as sales regulations and even prohibition; on the other hand, temperance was regarded as personal development, a duty and an opportunity to overcome the problem by means of individual moral stature. Sulkunen and Warpenius also note that an application of the perspective of New Public Health (NPH; see the introductory chapter in this volume) on the issue of alcohol results in an emphasis on "self-responsibility, as in other areas of new public health discourse".[1]

The public health perspective also tends to be relatively narrow within the field of alcohol research. It might be that public health within alcohol research often is akin to NPH, whereas older – disciplining and controlling – alcohol policies seldom are described in public health terms.[2] An individual-oriented public health perspective also tends to have rather different effects in different alcohol cultures and political contexts and criminologist Ragnar Hauge has argued that (new) public health thinking has weakened alcohol policy measures in the Nordic countries where such measures have sought to minimise damage in the misuser's environment.[3]

Thus, conceptualisations of public health and alcohol consumption occurred as rather separate activities in nineteenth-century public discourse. This was also the century when large and frequently recurring international conferences for the first time served as venues to discuss all sorts of issues of public interest. People and information could travel further and more quickly than before, and the economic, social and cultural development created new possibilities across national borders for various interest groups.[4] The transnational context and the use of an international discourse provided a resource for political struggle and debate. The conferences made demands appear universal, as a fight between good and evil, rather than being about provincial interests.[5]

International cooperation to prevent infectious diseases led to the first international sanitary conference in Paris in 1851. New conferences were held in 1859, 1866 and 1874 – without leading to any substantial agreement on anything.[6] During the same period, the alcohol issue emerged as a field of concern in the international arena. Some international conferences on the topic had been arranged since the first temperance conference in 1846, but the conferences studied here were the first institutionalised and frequently held meetings for researchers, government officials and representatives of non-governmental organisations (NGOs) to gather around a topic often described as one of the most critical issues for Western civilisation at the time.

The organisation behind the conferences, the International Temperance Bureau (ITB) – which in 1923 changed its name to the International Bureau Against Alcoholism (IBAA) and in 1964 to the International Council on Alcohol and Alcoholism (ICAA) – gradually developed from a temperance organisation into a more research-oriented organiser of conferences. The contents of the conferences also reflect this evolution. My primary source materials are the 34 conference proceedings from the years 1885–1992. The proceedings contain formal speeches and other expressions of conference etiquette, in addition to discussion minutes and – what is most important in terms of this study – the participants' papers. The papers covered a wide field of alcohol-related topics, and were also often arenas for competing perspectives and conflicts and when I in this chapter look for connections between the concept of public health and understandings of the alcohol problem, I have been repeatedly forced to give a simplified picture of the rather diversified discussions at the conferences.

The nationalisation of public health (1885–1939)

Individual alcohol problems are frequently referenced at conferences where alcohol misusers are variously described as vicious, criminal or sick, to be remedied by individual corrective admonition, punishment or treatment. However, I am looking for descriptions of how alcohol misuse threatens the whole or important parts of the population and/or society. I am also looking for suggestions to solve these problems.

Threats

The temperance movement that dominated the early conferences shared several presumptions with the public health field, such as the importance of structural preconditions and the view that alcohol was a health risk.[7] The temperance movement was built on an educated middle class who considered working-class alcohol consumption a threat to the social and economic order.[8] Industrialisation made commercially manufactured alcohol cheaper and alcohol misuse more visible in the poorer urban areas, and temperance work consisted in great part of disciplining the working class.[9] Hedonistic drinking habits were in direct opposition to an orderly and entrepreneurial life, and, one could say, in line with Weber's ideas, that the ascetic ideal of the temperance movement enhanced and strengthened "the spirit of capitalism".[10]

In the nineteenth century, the conferences debated forced drinking – *Trinkzwang* – which was still a burden on some occupations (and student life).[11] Thus, working culture could be a threat in the battle against alcohol use. At the same time, the anti-alcohol battle was also thought of as a prerequisite for an efficient working life in the future: "Clear heads and steady hands are needed in all the places of industrial pursuit."[12] Mechanisation of work and Taylorism created a context for definitions of the alcohol problems also in the inter-war period. Conference delegates often condemned unconditionally alcohol in working life.[13]

Not only did the drinking of the male industrial labour force constitute a threat to the economic order, but also women's drinking threatened the new generations of children. Therefore, expectant and breastfeeding women were to be persuaded to abstain from alcohol.[14] Children and the youth were the future, and the increased alcohol consumption in rural Germany in the early twentieth century was therefore alarming because the countryside was "the well of youth from which our tribe shall one day draw its vitality".[15] This patriotism was also manifested in concern for the military, and alcohol was discussed in terms of a potential cause of problems such as lack of discipline, illness and poor performance in the armed forces.[16] Modern warfare needed sober soldiers. According to the renowned race biologist Auguste Forel, the Russians had learnt this costly lesson in the war of 1905 against the sober Japanese.[17]

The undertone of these descriptions was apocalyptic. The predominant problem formulation was future-oriented and occupied itself with such entities as people, culture and nation. To solve the alcohol problem was to secure a better future. The scientific and social advances of the last hundreds of years were now threatened, as the prevalence of mental disturbance increased more rapidly than the size of the population. This was largely due to the consumption of alcohol.[18]

The concept of the nation was strong and demanding; it was through the nation that the people were safeguarded. Care for women, children and youth became important factors in a narrative about the future of the people and the nation. "Save the children and you will save the State!" recited general secretary of the United Kingdom Band of Hope Union, Charles Wakely, in the 1890 conference in Christiania (Oslo). He went on:

> If the children of today are taught to grow up sober and intelligent, the manhood and womanhood of the future will be secure. If, on the other hand, they remain unwarned, and thus become intemperate and sensual, the national shame and degradation will grow with the lapse of years, and the thraldom of drink will restrain as with hand of iron, every effort on behalf of social purity and peace.[19]

The concept of the nation held that force which could take the anti-alcohol battle beyond individual inebriation. The educated middle class of the temperance movement therefore made use of nationalism, as this resulted in wide popular support and confirmed their self-image as the leading force of modern society.[20] For the conference delegates, drunkenness was the cause of "our national disgrace and degradation", and they depicted alcohol in terms of "its baneful effects upon individual and national life".[21] The citizens "should be an asset of the nation, not a liability", which called for a tribute:

> Health, efficiency, wise economy, brotherliness, morality – these are quali-fications which the twentieth century demands of patriotic sons and daughters of the nations in their struggle upward toward the realisation of the ideal state.[22]

The familistic idea of the home as a resource in this fight was also underpinned by a nationalistic subtext. As was argued in the 1909 conference in London, the home was "the seed plot of a nation's continued existence" and "the spring from which proceeds all that is essential to the true patriotism of a people, to the real power of any community, and to the sustained influence of national life and institutions".[23]

The First World War fed on and reproduced these nationalistic frames of understanding, which continued to affect political thinking during the inter-war period.[24] Some pre-war problem formulations, such as the coupling of alcohol and national efficiency or motherhood, were also strengthened by the war.[25] Women's responsibility for the home and for children was a key idea in temperance work. In this context, the home was not only a private sphere but also "an ever widening circle".[26] Women were "the guardians of the race", ultimately responsible for any "influence upon race deterioration".[27]

This thought was expressed most clearly in the discourse on race biology, in which people and nation were thought of as an inseparable unit. This was evident when Nazi Germany's representatives discussed the problem of alcohol at the conference in Helsinki in 1939, only a month before the outbreak of the Second World War. Solutions to the alcohol question were intended to preserve the national community, *die Volksgemeinschaft*.[28] The state constituted a certain way of life, or *Lebensform*.[29] The uniformed German physician Erich Bruns argued that National Socialist ideology redefined the entire relationship between the individual and the collective. Health was no longer an individual concern, but a concern of the nation. In addition, physicians were no longer only serving those who were ill, but would now function as leaders of public health, as *Gesundheitsführer*.[30]

Solutions

One way of describing the conferences under discussion is to see them as part of the growing transnational anti-vice movement. As such, they were also often anti-state – and critics of the state encouraged vice. Nevertheless, the anti-vice movement needed state power to pursue their cause, and during the early twentieth century, advocates more often considered nation states more as part of the solution than the problem.[31] With reference to liberal politician William Gladstone, the 1895 conference therefore viewed that the primary duty of the state "should be so to legislate as to make it easy to do right and difficult to do wrong".[32] Two years later, in Brussels, this idea was formulated as an obligation for the state to act against alcohol misuse in a similar way as it acted against private nuisance or vagrancy. This train of thought could admittedly seem strange in the eyes of a true liberal – as exemplified by *l'école Manchestérienne* – but when something as crucial as the national population was at stake, state intervention seemed the obvious solution.[33]

High state ambitions and high state competence were prerequisites for the structure-oriented and interventionist public health work that dominated before the Second World War. The destructive but logical function of alcohol in industrial society had been discussed ever since the studies by Friedrich Engels on the condition of the English working class and the nature of alcohol as an escapist comforter.[34] Rapid scientific progress and the ubiquitous industrial machines were, for example, identified as the causes of alcohol abuse.[35] The battle against alcohol misuse then came to resemble general social policy, turning into a battle for shorter working hours and improved housing conditions.[36] "The motivation of an individual's sobriety in our time is *social*", and physician Knut Kjellberg consequently listed the suitable social solutions at the Stockholm conference in 1907:

The housing question, long working hours and the more or less exhausting impact that many jobs have on the nervous system, the quality of nourishment and the provision of meals, family life, education at home and school, efforts to provide adult education, cultural recreation [. . .].[37]

During the inter-war period, this social perspective was turned into an almost ideal typical example of structure-oriented public health work and a propaganda piece for the Soviet system. In 1934 the representative of the Soviet Union knew how the alcohol problem would be solved: improve general living conditions; give people more varied leisure time; offer them better housing; create public employment and social services.[38] Most conference delegates, however, had to relate to political systems and problem formulations that focused on alcohol as the crux of the problem and therefore regarded extensive sales restrictions or total prohibition as solutions. When several countries (Russia, Iceland, Norway, Finland and the United States) introduced their own versions of prohibition during or soon after the First World War, the situation looked bright for the radical temperance movement.[39]

The promotion of sales restrictions and prohibition was associated with the identification of alcohol – and thus alcohol producers – as the core problem. This view challenged powerful economic interests and implied that the work towards national sobriety had a clear political dimension. Or, as the Methodist preacher Purley Baker aptly put it at one of the anti-alcohol conferences: "All great moral reforms that seriously affect the monetary interest of a large group of people quickly assume a political aspect."[40]

Structural reforms and identification of pathogenic profiteers are very much in line with classic public health work. The same goes for the description of alcohol misuse as something reminiscent of a contagious plague. Delegates promoted coercion not only as a means of controlling the misusers' bad influence on the environment but also as an opportunity to prevent them procreating.[41] At the turn of the nineteenth and twentieth century, the latter idea was connected to a widespread concern about the degenerating impact of modern society on the population. The anti-alcohol conferences made it clear that the human race was growing weaker because of the sins of one generation.[42]

The answer to this challenge was hygienism. The concept was a loose mix of metaknowledge which could accommodate and legitimate all kinds of demands. Hygienism aimed to improve the quality of the population by means such as improved sanitary conditions, modern housing, spiritual education and racial selection. Hygienism became both an explanatory and legitimating ideology when delegates made a choice between moderation and abstemiousness: "the preaching of moderation in the use of alcohol cannot be the correct aim of the hygienist".[43] It was not only alcohol but also the use of tea and coffee which was not "quite in accordance with the strictest principles of hygiene".[44] Hygienism accommodated both public health objectives of conventional medicine and health ideas of alternative movements. Within the German *gesünder Leben* movement, for example, advocates promoted measures such as natural therapy, physical culture, vegetarianism and nudism.[45] At the conferences, some delegates claimed the vegetarian diet could cure and prevent the misuse of alcohol.[46]

The notion of the people and the nation as a social organism (*l'organisme social*) made the collective into a morally compelling entity that mattered more than an individual's welfare.[47] This way of thinking was most radically reflected in a specific variety of hygienic thought, namely racial hygiene. The eugenic perspective was relatively inquiring and not really put to the test in the pre-war years. A loosely knitted theory of heredity not only lent scientific legitimacy in the battle against drinking, but also more gravity when individual alcohol consumption was linked to the welfare of future generations and national well-being.[48] Several presentations highlighted that alcohol destroyed not only the drinkers themselves but also their offspring: a substandard quality of sorts was expected to be hereditary.[49] In this is way alcohol use ceased to be an individual concern:

> Inasmuch as the interests of the whole, that is, of the human race, must take precedence over those of the individual, an individual's sexual hygiene must subordinate itself to societal sexual hygiene and all the more so as sexual hygiene is first and foremost identical with racial hygiene.[50]

Alcohol would kill the individual and destroy the race – *mort de l'individu et déchéance de la race*.[51] Alcohol would lead to degeneration, and in the end become "a racial illness which is antisocial as it brings down the morals of a nation, encourages impure pleasures and is the enemy of pure enjoyment".[52] This image of a racial war, if not literally then through evolutionary contest, intensified the fateful gravity of the question (see also Paul Weindling's Chapter 2 on eugenics in this volume). At the 1905 conference, Auguste Forel spoke of an Eastern threat – *schwarze Wolken sammeln sich am östlichen Horizont* – and about the white race as being threatened.[53] The races were differently endowed – strong and weak, superior and inferior (*überwertige und minderwertige*) – depending on their different characteristics.[54] However, on top of this was the modern problem of degeneration whereby a race was debilitated by cultural phenomena such as alcoholism, excess and sexual debauchery. The solution was racial hygiene.

The idea of racial hygiene was not, however, accompanied by any obvious solutions to the alcohol problem. Lamarckian eugenics, for instance, contained the idea of investing in social conditions as a response to the problem of degeneration.[55] The first National Conference on Race Betterment, in Michigan in 1914, devoted an entire session to discussion of the alcohol and tobacco problem.[56] There were thus manifest links between the anti-alcohol movement and the eugenic movement, but the anti-alcohol conferences did not at the time debate sterilisation as a response to the alcohol problem. Long periods in institutions could prevent alcohol abusers from having children, but this was deemed an expensive solution.[57] Quite often, eugenic reasoning implied no more than applying "steady common sense with regard to procreation".[58]

In the inter-war period, the aims of turn-of-the-century hygienic movements became government policy, which appeared in many different forms depending on state ideology. Comprehensive public health measures against sanitary problems and unhealthy environments were coupled with measures derived from race biology. As historian Martin Pernick has shown, it is therefore not particularly fruitful to distinguish between inter-war eugenics and public health measures.[59] The collective was a common priority in both areas, and for one of the leading

British public health experts this was also central to the development of civilised societies:

> Each advance in civilization implies increasing communal, supplementary to personal, control and limitation of acts which for the individual may be innocent, but which have been shown by protracted experiment and experience to be inimical to communal well-being.[60]

The war resulted in ideas about national efficiency and about more radical eugenics. Racial hygiene was, however, promoted in many different countries, and not associated with any particular ideology.[61] Inheritance and environment were considered competing and complementary factors, and the usual conclusion was that biological inheritance was the stronger, and that alcohol misusers therefore should be denied parenthood.[62] As internment was considered complicated, ineffectual and costly, and as a marriage ban was seen as similarly ineffective, sterilisation appeared to be the most promising measure. The German Sterilisation Act from 1934 allowed for forced sterilisation in serious cases of alcoholism.[63] But with "the growth of genetic knowledge and with the arousal of a 'Racial Conscience' in the minds of our citizens", many actors hoped people would voluntarily undergo sterilisation, "not as a punishment or a deprivation, but as a privilege, and as a way out of a great difficulty, and as a means of harmonising conflicting individual and racial interests".[64]

One of the few dissenting voices came from the Catholic Church, which argued that sterilisation would be an encroachment on a person's free will and that the solution instead was moral stature.[65] This concept of individual improvement, central to NPH, is also present at the conferences. Some conference papers associated self-control with temperance, and here one must register the ambiguity of the concept itself: while temperance denotes abstinence from alcohol, it may also refer to moderation of sorts. Self-control was therefore both a cause and an effect: it was what one needed to abstain from alcohol and what one lost when drinking.[66]

Ever since the establishment of the temperance movement, personal development and moral suasion were particularly central to the narratives according to which temperance education was an effective measure.[67] This middle-class-based education project aimed not only at sobriety but also sought to discipline the leisure-oriented and politically agitating working class.[68] Temperance education was vividly debated at the pre-war conferences and to a lesser extent at the inter-war conferences.[69] According to Robert Hercod (Executive Director of the organisation behind the conferences between 1907 and 1950), education or propaganda was, however, revitalised in the 1930s "[i]n the totalitarian countries where the State takes upon itself the education of youth outside the school and the home".[70] This was confirmed by the German delegates, who witnessed how the German notion of the state had changed. The fight against alcohol abuse was now more comprehensive and considered the sum of all measures by the authorities who were to guide the people and the nation.[71]

The globalisation of public health (1948–1992)

The transnational temperance movement had made its mark on the pre-war conferences, whereas the inter-war conferences increasingly developed into arenas of national-chauvinist propaganda. The consequences of the Second World War were, however, far more pervasive for the post-war understanding of the alcohol issue. The nations participating in the conferences had once again been thrown into brutal war against each other, and the inter-war nationalism was now greatly challenged. The Holocaust contributed to a general disavowing of the influential eugenics and forced reassessments of once unassailable categories such as people and nation, making it hard to comprehend public health as it had been conceptualised in the early twentieth century.

Potentially even more disruptive for the gatherings that had come to evolve from transnational temperance meetings into scientific conferences was the impact that the atrocities of the immediately preceding years must have had on faith in the presumably ethically neutral science that very much characterised the inter-war discussions. Then there was a humanistic reaction, leading to an anti-authoritarian movement in the post-war period, which in our field of investigations can be associated with a new concept of alcoholism according to which the misuser was regarded as undeservedly ill.[72] In its official historiography, the organisation behind the conferences – the International Council on Alcohol and Alcoholism (ICAA) – consequently emphasised that the post-war conferences were more scientific, a statement associated with this new conceptualisation of alcohol misuse as a disease (alcoholism).[73]

Threats

The role of alcohol in the recently fought war was, of course, a prominent theme in the first post-war conference.[74] Alcohol consumption among key population groups – women, youth and, especially, young women – was also associated with the conditions and consequences of the war.[75] Women's alcohol consumption was modest compared to men's, but it had increased alarmingly in countries like Italy, Germany and Finland.[76] By the end of the post-war period, women's drinking was again considered a problem, as their alcohol consumption was approaching that of men.[77] Increasing youth alcohol consumption was depicted as an "alcohol epidemic among the young", a general increase in consumption that is "particularly steep among young people", something that "has reached endemic proportions to the point of becoming fully institutionalised in our society".[78]

Thus, conference participants identified largely the same problem groups as before the Second World War: soldiers, women and youth. However, the tone was not nearly as apocalyptic. Certainly, the problem was serious and seemingly growing, but it did not imply the imminent downfall of the nation or of civilisation. The same cannot be said, however, of the economic argument found in concern for the workforce. The problem's description from the inter-war years was still valid in the mid-1950s in socialist countries, where alcohol misuse was described as particularly subversive in "a socialist system, which counts with the work of every member of society".[79] In the context of post-war decolonisation, delegates from developing countries also identified alcohol consumption among workers as a threat to economic development.[80]

Even in the West, alcohol constituted a dark spot in the collective self-image of industrialised nations. "Ours is a business civilization", as one of the most influential financiers of the American alcoholism movement, Brinkley Smithers, stated at the 1964 conference in Frankfurt-am-Main, before presenting a text on the importance of curbing alcohol misuse.[81] Throughout the studied period conference delegates depicted alcohol misuse in the workplace as a problem that damaged the national economy.[82]

The openly nationalist discourse withdrew after the Second World War, and with it a more or less articulated logic that equated people and nation and treated threats to them as threats to civilisation. Furthermore, conference delegates discussed the problems associated with alcohol in less concrete terms – perhaps a consequence of the new perspective on alcoholism or because of new scientific ideals. In 1948, we learn that alcoholism cannot be confined to "certain social strata"; the problem had vast implications and thus affected the "whole generation".[83] The idea was not new but it occurred more frequently thereafter, and the use of the concept of public health associated the battle against alcohol problems with established control of contagious diseases. In 1948 a delegate argued that: "as the doctor is rightly in the forefront of the fight against tuberculosis, cancer and the venereal diseases, he ought also to be foremost in the fight against alcoholism, another danger to public health".[84] Compared to the inter-war period, the changes in conceptualisations in the mid-1950s are perhaps not big. A Finnish delegate stated that we "[p]ractically everywhere [. . .] see a growing recognition of alcoholism as a major public health problem" and "a rapidly growing realisation by people of the dangers of small quantities of alcohol in the machine age in which we live".[85]

In the 1950s the problem became anonymised: everybody was the problem; there was talk about "the alcoholization of the world population".[86] Individual misusers were no longer examples of the degeneration of nations and people but, instead, widespread use of alcohol threatened the individual. The post-war period – especially from the 1960s onwards – was therefore characterised by studies that made use of increasingly sophisticated quantitative estimates of alcohol consumption and problems among large population groups (often described as public health problems). From the late 1960s onwards, the term 'public health' also became a political signal calling for action: to describe something as a public or social health problem now served the same function as earlier vivid descriptions of individuals and environments tainted by the misuse of alcohol. The World Health Organization's definition of public health problems – "the most widespread and serious problems" – strengthened such political rhetoric.[87]

In the mid-1970s, a specific causal narrative was established as the total consumption model described the fatal consequences of widespread alcohol consumption. The model was developed in its most sophisticated form mainly in the 1975 WHO publication *Alcohol Control Policies in Public Health Perspective*, and stipulated that a marked increase in average consumption most likely led to an increase in numbers of high consumers.[88] This connection had been discussed at the conferences at least since the early 1960s and remained topical all through the studied period.[89] The total consumption model's significance in legitimising general alcohol restrictions cannot be overestimated, and it certainly inspired large data collections and estimates of total consumption in different countries with different systems of alcohol distribution. These can also be found even before the Second World War, and then mainly from the mid-1950s onwards, but the heyday of alcohol epidemiology would be from the mid-1970s onwards. In 1975, the first separate epidemiological ICAA meeting was also held, from 1987 organised as annual meetings of the Kettil Bruun Society (KBS) for Social and Epidemiological Research on Alcohol.[90]

Solutions

Considering the theoretical/ideological impact of the total consumption model, it is not surprising that many presentations of attractive solutions focused on lowering the total consumption of alcohol. This had certainly been on the conferences' agenda ever since 1885. What was new was the theoretical support for these measures. Alcohol regulation strictly based on the total consumption model was not implemented outside Scandinavia but still ended up in similar means such as alcohol taxes and price controls, techniques that had been in use in various countries at least since the 1700s.[91] Many conference papers also dealt with the importance of accessibility and possibilities to reduce this, for example banning or restricting alcohol advertising, and the development of non-alcoholic alternatives (both drinks and activities).

Concretely, there was thus very little new, and this also applied to the many presentations on preventive education measures that constitute the core of NPH. Although temperance education was considered to have been "debated to death" already in 1907, a remarkable number of conference delegates presented papers on prevention.[92] At the conference in 1964 in Frankfurt-am-Main a delegate reminded participants of the "old wisdom [. . .] that prevention is better than cure".[93]

In the mid-1980s we find an important shift in the motives behind temperance education, when several conference delegates abandoned the negative message that one should renounce alcohol, in favour of a positive message that people's health would benefit from a new lifestyle. This new approach – variously described as health promotion, competence development, lifestyle education or life skills – was holistic and all-encompassing in comparison with earlier notions.[94] When this idea was linked to health as a universal right, quite far-reaching measures could be justified: "besides the right to health which must be protected by special laws, there is also the *duty* of the maintenance of health".[95]

Political scientist Mark Lawrence Schrad has characterised the early conferences as *transnational advocacy networks* – a political resource and an opportunity for the temperance movement to anchor its ideological ambitions in supposedly universal claims. When the temperance movement grew weaker at the conferences between the wars, it came more to resemble *epistemic communities* that, according to Schrad, are only loosely connected to the political process.[96] I believe that Schrad's division is misleading, and have made this case in a previous article.[97] Nevertheless, the conferences did lose their ideological legitimacy during the inter-war period, and this is where the globalised public health model of the post-war years came to create a common framework for the conferences from the 1970s onwards. The new understanding of alcohol problems was, according to a WHO representative at the 1978 conference in Warsaw, "the type of public health approach now being fostered by the World Health Organization".[98] The method, which aimed to solve the most serious health problems, was directly based on measures taken to battle infectious diseases:

> The public health preventive model attempts to interrupt the pathological processes between agent, host and environment or to render the host more resistant, the agent and environment less harmful. So, in the case of alcohol-related problems, preventive measures can be subsumed under the headings of, first, limitation of availability of alcoholic beverages; second, education of the host to limit consumption; and third, introduction of changes in the environment to limit demand.[99]

The ideas were hardly new, and the very same trinity appeared in a conference paper from 1964.[100] Nevertheless, the same old sales restrictions, temperance education and social reform were now associated with the concept of public health. Even though alcohol remained peripheral in the WHO's public health work, references to the organisation strengthened national arguments: "WHO can and must give a lead, both globally and regionally."[101] Everything from availability and pricing to advertising regulations and prevention work was now described as public health work.[102] In the 1990s the conceptual transformation gives a rather pretentious impression. Delegates argued that the public health field was experiencing "a renewed interest in the preventive and health promoting aspects of policies", as well as – with reference to a WHO publication – that "[t]he most widely endorsed descriptions of health promotion now include policy as one of its major components".[103] Everything is public health in this process described as "a major conceptual evolution".[104]

Public health work in accordance with the WHO's work was not necessarily politically neutral, and a focus on "the agent, host and environment" with "changes in the environment to limit demand" could potentially result in radical social reforms.[105] However, the transformation of ideas from sobriety to health promotion is not really fuel for a revolution. Furthermore, opponents argued that a model designed to handle malaria, for instance, was not directly transferable to the alcohol problem. It would require an assimilation of the breeding grounds for mosquitoes with social injustice, and taking a clear political stand:

> It is when we come to consider the environment phase of our three-part public health model that we face the greatest uncertainty. The view that physically

and financially improved living conditions might automatically reduce the pressures that distort people's minds and emotions and make them vulnerable to drug dependence is not borne out by the facts.[106]

Still, this was one of few critiques of social reform-oriented solutions to the alcohol problem.[107] Conference participants did express such ideas throughout the entire period, but rarely framed them as public health measures.[108] Nevertheless, the reluctance explicitly to refer to social reform made the public health model of the late twentieth century somewhat apolitically toothless. Political ambitions have long had an ally in symptom theoretical models focusing social causes on various problems, and public health promoting prevention has been described as a depoliticising of highly political issues.[109] Such criticism was, however, rare at the conferences. There was one paper in 1968 by criminologist Nils Christie and social scientist Kettil Bruun that questioned the medicalisation of the alcohol problem as depoliticising through the fraudulent use of concepts.[110] At the 1985 conference in Calgary, prevention was also criticised in a Marxist analysis advocating the "socialization of the very ways we experience our own needs and desires".[111]

Post-war conceptualisations of public health emphasised individual health and lifestyle choices, indicating an individualisation of society. There was also a reluctance to challenge financial interests. This is why it was difficult to solve the problem of alcohol, if we are to believe one delegate at the 1964 conference: "A major reason for this is the cowardice of politicians and the communications media in doing anything that might antagonize the alcoholic beverage industry and bring economic repercussions."[112] The new perspective on alcohol could certainly be used to promote the interests of the alcohol industry, as exemplified by a review at the 1985 conference where measures taken by the alcohol industry to solve the alcohol problem are listed. Such measures include the recognition of "alcoholism as a treatable illness" and "strengthening and extending the moderation norm", in addition to "responsible decision-making on use, abuse and non-use".[113] Nowhere to be found was the idea that the availability of alcohol should be limited.

Concluding remarks

The framing of the alcohol problem as a public health problem has taken slightly different forms in comparison to how the development of public health in general has been outlined in the introductory chapter in this volume. This might be due to the temperance movement being such a strong social force behind the politicisation of the alcohol issue. By emphasising individual improvement as a core measure, the temperance movement preceded the more comprehensive concept of New Public Health (NPH).

But it might also be due to the alcohol problem being a fundamentally different problem from the sanitary problems and epidemics, which led to demands for collective solutions. Maybe it is this surging contextualisation of what sometimes has been regarded as a contagious disease and sometimes as a chronic disease that has contributed to a loose connection to mainstream public health thinking.

The pre-war conferences were marked by the temperance movement that anchored its moral message on a transnational arena in order to gain legitimacy for its agenda. The movement linked the problem's description to fears of degeneration, and promoted a loosely defined hygienism as the answer to the big questions of the future. Nevertheless, despite vague hopes for producing international conventions, the solutions were reached at the national legislative level and, therefore, the temperance movement was happy to be in the service of the state.

The First World War put an end to hopes of the brave new future beyond national bigotry that many had presaged during *la belle époque*. It also clarified the role of government and the importance of state power in handling foreign powers – both with respect to competing nations and the internationally mobile alcohol industry. This made the inter-war period into a harvest time when the vague ideas about hygienism and social health took concrete form. After the First World War, alcohol restrictions (including total prohibition) were introduced in many countries that previously had not regulated the sale of alcohol in any notable form.

The inter-war nationalist movements, the strong link between people and nation, also led to a focus on the alcohol consumer. Conference delegates identified key groups to target with diverse measures such as information and education, detention and sterilisation. Individual health was a collective problem, and the individual had to submit to the collective represented by the state.

Reactions against the European dictatorships of the 1930s and the Second World War disavowed the state's unlimited authority as a representative of a moral imperative collective. Among post-war reactions we therefore find both nationally transcendent organisations, such as the UN and the European Economic Community (EEC), and an anti-authoritarian humanism manifested in both a thriving youth culture and abolished restrictions on alcohol, as well as a critique of ethically neutral science and a predilection for de-stigmatising notions of disease.

In the absence of the temperance movement's moral universalism and the authoritarian state's mandatory collectivism, the first post-war conferences gave a sprawling and searching impression. Conference delegates eventually formulated new ideas within a framework of post-war public health thinking. According to the new understanding, individual deeds did not threaten people and nation. Instead, aggregated alcohol consumption threatened some kind of abstract public health.[114] Or, as Baldwin has put it, this new democratic public health relied on "the accumulated effect of millions of individual decisions, out of which comes a public good".[115] The total consumption model's connection with the WHO regained the global authority earlier claimed by the temperance movement. The public health discourse of the late twentieth century, supported by the WHO and prevention science, therefore became a strong form of knowledge and a legitimising force in dealing with the alcohol problem (this "epistemic globalisation" is analysed by Matilda Hellman in Chapter 10 of this volume).

Albeit a potential support for severe restrictions on alcohol, public health policy during the late twentieth century has very much been about individualised health promotion. The concept of NPH generalised the problem but individualised the solution, and it is no exaggeration to describe this, as a delegate did at the 1992 conference in Glasgow, as "a major conceptual evolution".[116] This idea of democratic public health did not call for imprisonment or other drastic restrictions, but for joint health awareness for the collective good.[117]

The alcohol problem no longer had a clear locus at the end of the twentieth century. It was no longer people of a different class, sex or age who were to be disciplined in the name of public health. The alcohol problem was everywhere, with everyone, within us. Perhaps this makes the alcohol question unfit for politicisation or for being associated with any radical social reform that could have challenged key voter groups or powerful vested interests. Unsurprisingly, the alcohol industry wholeheartedly endorsed this public health approach that, without threatening alcohol sales, associated individual alcohol dependence as a problem with health awareness as a solution (see also Chapter 10). This understanding breaks with the traditional understanding of public health. Both the problem and the solutions are now thought to be located within the alcohol consumer (host), while the alcohol industry (agent) and the social structures (environment) remain unregulated.

Notes

1 Pekka Sulkunen and Katariina Warpenius, 'Reforming the self and the other: The temperance movement and the duality of modern subjectivity', *Critical Public Health* 10, no. 4 (2000): 423–38, 423.

2 Christoffer Tigerstedt, 'Discipline and public health', in *Broken Spirits: Power and Ideas in Nordic Alcohol Control*, ed. Pekka Sulkunen, Caroline Sutton, Christoffer Tigerstedt and Katariina Warpenius (Helsinki: NAD, 2000), 93–112.

3 Ragnar Hauge, 'The public health perspective and the transformation of Norwegian alcohol policy', *Contemporary Drug Problems* 26, no. 2 (1999): 193–207.

4 Ian Tyrrell, *Reforming the World: The Creation of America's Moral Empire* (Princeton: Princeton University Press, 2010); David T. Courtwright, 'Global anti-vice activism: A postmortem', in *Global Anti-Vice Activism, 1890–1950: Fighting Drinks, Drugs, and 'Immorality'*, ed. Jessica R. Pliley, Robert Kramm and Harald Fischer-Tiné (Cambridge: Cambridge University Press, 2016), 313–24.

5 Mark Lawrence Schrad, *The Political Power of Bad Ideas: Networks, Institutions, and the Global Prohibition Wave* (Oxford: Oxford University Press, 2010).

6 George Rosen, *A History of Public Health* (Baltimore: Johns Hopkins University Press, 2015).

7 Robin Room, 'Alcohol control and public health', *Annual Review of Public Health* 5 (1984): 293–317.

8 Robin Room, 'The liquor question and the formation of consciousness: Nation, ethnicity, and class at the turn of the century', *Contemporary Drug Problems* 12, no. 2 (1985): 165–72.

9 Joseph Gusfield, 'Benevolent repression: Popular culture, social structure and the control of drinking', in *Drinking: Behavior and Belief in Modern History*, ed. Susanna Barrows and Robin Room (Berkeley: University of California Press, 1991), 399–424; Mark Lawrence Schrad, *The Prohibition Option: Transnational Temperance and National Policymaking in Russia, Sweden and the United States* (Madison: University of Wisconsin-Madison, 2007).

10 Sulkunen and Warpenius, 'Reforming the self', 426. See also Michael R. Marrus, 'Social drinking in the Belle Epoque', *Journal of Social History* 7, no. 2 (1974): 115–41; Mack P. Holt, ed., *Alcohol: A Social and Cultural History* (Oxford: Berg, 2006).

11   Carl Rudolf Burckhardt, 'Bitte an die Versammlung, den Trinkzwang bei den Studenten betreffend', in *6me Congrès international contre l'abus des boissons alcooliques à Bruxelles en 1897* (Bruxelles: E. Guyot, 1897) [*CP 1897*]; Dr Bonne, 'Ueber den Trinkzwang beim Broterwerb', in *VIIe Congrès international contre l'abus des boissons alcooliques* (Paris: Au siège social de l'Union française antialcoolique, 1900) [*CP 1899*]. Hereafter *CP* denotes conference proceedings, followed by the year.

12   James H. Kellogg, 'What employers may do to lessen the ravages of strong drinks', in *Bericht des III. internationalen Congresses gegen den Missbrauch geistiger Getränke in Christiania vom 3. bis 5. September 1890* (Christiania: Det Mallingske Bogtrykkeri, 1891) [*CP 1890*], 165.

13   David T. Courtwright and Timothy A. Hickman, 'Modernity and anti-modernity: Drug policy and political culture in the United States and Europe in the nineteenth and twentieth centuries', in *Drugs and Culture: Knowledge, Consumption and Policy*, ed. Geoffrey Hunt, Maitena Milhet and Henri Bergernon (Burlington: Ashgate, 2011), 213–24; Eugene Lyman Fisk, 'The relationship of alcohol to modern health ideals', in *Proceedings of the Fifteenth International Congress Against Alcoholism* (Washington, DC and Westerville, OH, 1921) [*CP 1920*]; William S. Bennet, 'Response', in *CP 1920*; Arthur Newsholme, 'The place of the alcohol question in social hygiene', in *Compte-rendu du XIXe congrès international contre l'alcoolisme* (Bruxelles: Imprimerie Medicale et Scientifique, 1930) [*CP 1928*]; Courtenay C. Weeks, 'Alcohol in relation to professional and industrial efficiency', in *Proceedings of the Twenty-Second International Congress Against Alcoholism* (Helsinki: Raittiuskansan Kirjapaino, 1940–1941) [*CP 1939*].

14   Kate Mitchell, 'Alcohol during pregnancy and the nursing period', in *CP 1890*.

15   J. Gonser, 'Alkoholen på landsbygden', in *Den XI internationella antialkoholkongressen i Stockholm 1907* (Stockholm: Oskar Eklunds Boktryckeri, 1909) [*CP 1907a*], 84.

16   See, e.g., W. J. G. van der Veur, 'Les mesures prises par le ministère de la Guerre, pour combattre l'abus des boissons fortes dans l'armée Néerlandaise', in *Compte-rendu du 4me Congrès international contre l'abus des boissons alcooliques à La Haye du 15–18 Août 1893* ('s-Gravenhage: Smits, 1893) [*CP 1893*]; B. F. Parker, 'Effects of intoxicants in the Spanish–American war', in *CP 1899*; M. G. Popovic, 'Alkohol im Balkankrieg', in *Compte-rendu du XIV congrès international contre l'alcoolisme* (Milan: Bari, 1921) [*CP 1913*].

17   Auguste Forel, 'Alkohol und Geschlechtsleben', in *Xème congrés international contre l'alcoholisme, tenu à Budapest du 11 au 16 septembre 1905* (Budapest: F. Kilián successeur, 1905 [*CP 1905*]. This had been a prominent theme also after the French defeat in the Franco-Prussian war in 1870; see Jean-Charles Sournia, *A History of Alcoholism* (Oxford: Blackwell, 1990).

18   N. S. Davis, 'Is there any causative or etiological relation between the extensive use of alcoholic drinks and the constituted increase of epilepsy, imbecility and insanity, both mental and moral in all the countries of Europe and America?', in *CP 1899*.

19   Charles Wakely, 'The education of children in temperance principles', in *CP 1890*, 126.

20   Sulkunen and Warpenius, 'Reforming the self'.

21   Charles Wakely, 'Primary schools and Bands of Hope as a means of preventing intemperance', in *CP 1893*, 209; J. Martin Skinner, 'Socialism and the drink traffic', in *Bericht über den V. Internationalen Kongress zur Bekämpfung des Missbrauchs geistiger Getränke zu Basel 20.–22. August 1895* (Basel: Schriftstelle des Alkoholgegnerbundes, 1896) [*CP 1895*], 315.

22   Cora Frances Stoddard, 'The relation of juvenile temperance teaching to national progress', in *Proceedings of the Twelfth International Congress on Alcoholism* (London: Paternoster House, 1909) [*CP 1909*], 39.

23   Mr and Mrs Bramwell Booth, 'Alcohol in relation to the home', in *CP 1909*, 125.

24   Arno Mayer, 'Post-war nationalisms 1918–1919', *Past & Present* 34, no. 1 (1966): 114–26.

25 Catherine J. Kudlick, 'Fighting the internal and external enemies: Alcoholism in World War I France', *Contemporary Drug Problems* 12, no. 1 (1985): 129–58; Virginia Berridge, 'The impact of war 1914–1918', *British Journal of Addiction* 85, no. 8 (1990): 1017–22.

26 Laura Pearson, 'The role of the woman-citizen in the fight against alcoholism', in *Compte-rendu du XVIIe congrès international contre l'alcoolisme* (København, 1924) [*CP 1923*], 165.

27 Louise McIlroy, 'Alcohol and womanhood', in *Proceedings of the Twentieth International Congress on Alcoholism* (London: Sainsbury, 1934) [*CP 1934*], 92.

28 Dr Paulstich and Dr Ernst Gabriel, 'Das Problem der Süchtigkeit', in *CP 1939*, 37.

29 Falk Ruttke, 'Erbpflege und Bekämpfung von Alkoholschäden im grossdeutschen Reich', in *CP 1939*, 128.

30 Erich Bruns, 'Ärzte und Alkohol', in *CP 1939*, 171.

31 Jessica R Pliley, Robert Kramm and Harald Fischer-Tiné, 'Introduction: A plea for a 'vicious turn' in global history', in *Global Anti-Vice Activism, 1890–1950: Fighting Drinks, Drugs, and 'Immorality'*, ed. Jessica R. Pliley, Robert Kramm and Harald Fischer-Tiné (Cambridge: Cambridge University Press, 2016), 1–29.

32 J. W. Leigh, 'The tyranny of the liquor traffic', in *CP 1895*, 428.

33 M. l'Abbé Lemmens, 'L'Etat a le droit d'intervenir dans la repression des abus alcooliques', in *CP 1897*, 23.

34 Friedrich Engels, *Die Lage der arbeitenden Klasse in England* (Leipzig: Otto Wigand, 1845).

35 Dr van den Corput, 'L'alcoolisme: Ses causes mésologiques; son extinction physiologique', in *CP 1897*.

36 Otto Lang, 'Alkoholismus und Classenkampf', in *Bericht über den VIII. internationalen Congress gegen den Alkoholismus abgehalten in Wien, 9–14 April 1901* (Leipzig and Wien: F. Deuticke, 1902) [*CP 1901*].

37 Knut Kjellberg, 'Alkoholismen och den sociala frågan', in *CP 1907a*, 179.

38 Ivan Mikhailovich Maisky, 'Alcoholism in the USSR and the measures designed to combat it', in *CP 1934*.

39 Johan Edman, 'Temperance and modernity: Alcohol consumption as a collective problem, 1885–1913', *Journal of Social History* 49, no. 1 (2015): 20–52.

40 Purley A. Baker, 'Political aspects of the prohibition movement in America: Partizan and non-partizan effort', in *CP 1920*, 74.

41 See, e.g., L. D. Mason, 'The pauper inebriate, his legal status, care and control', in *CP 1899*; T. D. Crothers, 'Inebriate asylums in America', in *Bericht über den XI. internationalen congress gegen den alkoholismus: Abgehalten in Stockholm vom 28 Juli–3 August 1907* (Stockholm: Oskar Eklunds Boktryckeri, 1908) [*CP 1907b*]; R. W. Branthwaite, 'Legislation for inebriates', in *CP 1909*.

42 See, e.g., J. J. Ridge, 'Scientific reasons for total abstinence from alcoholic liquors', in *CP 1895*; Dr Lidström, 'Historiens lärdomar i alkoholfrågan', in *CP 1907a*; Taav. Laitinen, 'A contribution to the study of the influence of alcohol on the degeneration of human offspring', in *CP 1909*.

43 Alice Vickery Drysdale, 'Total abstinence and moderation', in *CP 1899*, 603.

44 Ibid., 600.

45 Michael Hau, 'Gender and aesthetic norms in popular hygienic culture in Germany from 1900 to 1914', *Social History of Medicine* 12, no. 2 (1999): 271–92; Florentine Fritzen, Florentine, *Gesünder Leben: Die Lebensreformbewegung im 20. Jahrhundert* (Stuttgart: Steiner, 2006).

46 Jules Grand, 'Du régime végétarien comme moyen préventif et curatif de l'alcoolisme', in *CP 1899*; Dr Larsen, 'Alkoholen som födoämne', in *CP 1907a*.

47 Van den Corput, 'L'alcoolisme', 18.

48 W. F. Bynum, 'Alcoholism and degeneration in 19th century European medicine and psychiatry', *British Journal of Addiction* 79, no. 1 (1984): 59–70; Virginia Berridge,

'Prevention and social hygiene 1900–1914', *British Journal of Addiction* 85, no. 8 (1990): 1005–16; Mariana Valverde, *Diseases of the Will: Alcohol and the Dilemmas of Freedom* (Cambridge: Cambridge University Press, 1998).

49 See, e.g., Mary Clement Leavitt, 'The liquor traffic and native races', in *CP 1890*; Ernst Rüdin, 'Der Alkohol im Lebensprozess der Rasse', in *Bericht über den IX. internationalen Kongress gegen den Alkoholismus* (Jena: Gustav Fischer, 1904) [*CP 1903*]; Karolina Widerström, 'Alkoholen och den sexuella frågan', in *CP 1907a*.

50 Auguste Forel, 'Alkoholen och den sexuella frågan', in *CP 1907a*, 75.

51 Auguste Forel, 'La corruption de la civilization par l'alcoolisme, étudiée au point de vue physiologique et social', in *CP 1897*, 65.

52 Dr Legrain, 'Alkohol och degeneration; rashygien', in *CP 1907a*, 70.

53 Forel, 'Alkohol und Geschlechtsleben', 96.

54 Ibid.

55 Fae Brauer, 'Eroticizing Lamarckian eugenics: The body stripped bare during French sexual neoregulation', in *Art, Sex and Eugenics: Corpus Delecti*, ed, Fae Brauer and Anthea Callen (Aldershot: Ashgate, 2008), 97–138.

56 *Proceedings of the First National Conference on Race Betterment* (Battle Creek, MI: Race Betterment Foundation, 1914).

57 R. W. Branthwaite, 'Alkoholisthemsfrågan', in *CP 1907a*; Curt Wallis, 'Alkoholisthemsfrågan', in *CP 1907a*.

58 Forel, 'Alkoholen och den sexuella frågan', 75.

59 Martin S. Pernick, 'Eugenics and public health in American History', *American Journal of Public Health* 87, no. 11 (1997): 1767–72. On public health as an ever-widening concept and an agenda, see also Martin Gorsky, 'Public health in interwar England and Wales: Did it fail?', *Dynamis* 28 (2008): 175–98.

60 Newsholme, 'Alcohol question in social hygiene', 20.

61 Robert Proctor, *Racial Hygiene: Medicine under the Nazis* (Cambridge, MA: Harvard University Press, 1988); Peter Baldwin, *Contagion and the State in Europe, 1830–1930* (Cambridge: Cambridge University Press, 1999); Nikolay Kamenov, 'A question of social medicine or racial hygiene?', in *Global Anti-Vice Activism, 1890–1950: Fighting Drinks, Drugs, and 'Immorality'*, ed, Jessica R. Pliley, Robert Kramm and Harald Fischer-Tiné (Cambridge: Cambridge University Press, 2016), 124–51.

62 G. H. Carpenter, 'Alcohol, heredity and environment', in *CP 1934*; H. Gachot, 'Alcoolisme et eugenisme', in *CP 1934*.

63 Erich Schröder, 'Neue rassenhygienische Wege zur Bekämpfung des Alkoholismus in Deutschland', in *CP 1934*; Ruttke, 'Erbpflege und Bekämpfung'; Michael Burleigh, 'Psychiatry, German society, and the Nazi "euthanasia" programme', *Social History of Medicine* 7, no.2 (1994): 213–28.

64 J. Bond, 'Discussion', in *CP 1934*, 224.

65 Rev. Hays, 'Alcoholism and a healthy future generation', in *CP 1934*.

66 Ridge, 'Scientific reasons'.

67 Jim Baumohl and Robin Room, 'Inebriety, doctors, and the state: Alcoholism treatment institutions before 1940', *Recent Developments in Alcoholism* 5 (1987): 135–74.

68 Sulkunen and Warpenius, 'Reforming the self'; Harry G. Levine, 'The alcohol problem in America: From temperance to alcoholism', *British Journal of Addiction* 79, no. 4 (1984): 109–19.

69 Edman, 'Temperance and modernity'; Johan Edman, 'Transnational nationalism and idealistic science: The alcohol question between the wars', *Social History of Medicine* 29, no. 3 (2016): 590–610.

70 Robert Hercod, 'Forms of state participation in the fight against alcoholism', in *CP 1939*. A more critical view on the authoritarian states from the same conference is to be found in M. P. van der Meulen, 'The organisation of the leisure time of the labourer and its significance for the struggle against alcohol', in *CP 1939*.

71 Hans Seidel and Ernst Bauer, 'Die Formen der Beteiligung des Staates am Kampf gegen den Alkoholismus. Deutschland', in *CP 1939*, 58.

72 Karl Mann, Derek Hermann and Andreas Heinz, 'One hundred years of alcoholism: The twentieth century', *Alcohol & Alcoholism* 35, no. 1 (2000): 10–15.
73 Edman, 'Temperance and modernity'.
74 See, e.g., Cyril Squires, 'Alcohol and the allied armies', in *Compte rendu du 23e Congrès international contre l'alcoolisme à Lucerne 4 au 9 juillet 1948* (Lausanne: Impremerie du Léman S. A., 1949) [*CP 1948*]; Lt Colonel Jaubert-Jonage, 'L'alcool dans la Résistance français', in *CP 1948*.
75 See, e.g., E. M. Mein, 'The influence of the war on young women', in *CP 1948*; Anna Klara Fischer, 'Der Einfluss des Krieges und der Nachkriegszeit auf die weibliche Jugend in Deutchland', in *CP 1948*.
76 E. Elena Fambri, 'L'alcoolisme et la femme', in *CP 1948*; Dr Riggenbach, 'Der Alkoholismus bei der Frau', in *CP 1948*; J. H. Konttinen, 'The temperance situation in Finland', in *25th International Congress against Alcoholism* (Lausanne: Bureau international contre l'alcoolisme, 1956) [*CP 1956*].
77 See, e.g., Toril Hammer and Per Vaglum, 'Employment, working culture and use of alcohol among women', in *Proceedings of the 35th International Congress on Alcoholism and Drug Dependence* (Oslo: National Directorate for the Prevention of Alcohol and Drug Problems, 1988) [*CP 1988*].
78 W. X. Lehmann, 'The devastating effects of alcohol being noted in teenagers today', in *Proceedings of the 31st International Congress on Alcoholism and Drug Dependence, 23–28 February 1975* (Lausanne: ICAA, 1975) [*CP 1975*], 516; O. Irgens-Jensen, 'Changes in alcohol consumption and frequency of intoxication among Norwegian youth year by year from 1970 to 1978', in *32nd International Congress on Alcoholism and Drug Dependence, Warsaw, 3rd–8th September 1978* (Lausanne : ICAA, 1978) [*CP 1978*], 535; A. M. Ghadirian et al., 'Alcohol and drug use among Montreal high school students', in *Proceedings of the 34th International Congress on Alcoholism and Drug Dependence* (Edmonton: Alberta Alcohol and Drug Abuse Commission, 1985) [*CP 1985*], 22.
79 Jaroslaw Skála, 'On the fight against alcoholism in Czechoslovakia and the part played by health workers', in *CP 1956*, 1.
80 Abdul Jabbar Fahmi, 'The problem of alcoholism in Iraq', in *CP 1956*; Jawaharlal Nehru, 'Message from Prime Minister Jawaharlal Nehru', in *CP 1956*.
81 Brinkley Smithers, 'The problem of alcoholism', in *Selected Papers Presented at the 27th International Congress on Alcohol and Alcoholism* (Lausanne: ICAA, 1965) [*CP 1964*], 55.
82 See, e.g., H. Schaffner, 'Der steigende Alkoholismus in der Welt, ein ethisches, politisches und volkswirschaftliches Problem', in *CP 1956*; Hugh M. Pritchard, 'Economic costs of abuse of and dependency on alcohol in Australia', in *29th International Congress on Alcoholism and Drug Dependence* (London: Butterworth, 1971) [*CP 1970*]; T. Schramm, 'Effective approaches to prevention of drug and alcohol abuse in the workplace', in *CP 1985*.
83 Emile Abderhalden, 'Unsere Verantwortung gegenüber den sozialen Uebeln', in *CP 1948*, 47.
84 H. Müller, 'Le Groupe medical Vaudois de lute antialcoolique de la Société vaudoise de Médecine', in *CP 1948*, 181.
85 Tapio Voionmaa, 'Opening addresses and messages', in *CP 1956*, 2.
86 W. A. Schaffenberg, 'Preventing the alcoholization of the world population', in *CP 1956*.
87 J. Moser, 'Prevention of alcohol-related problems: Developing a broad-spectrum programme', in *CP 1978*, 85. Also I. Khan, 'The responsibility of professionals: The need for cooperation', in *CP 1978*.
88 Kettil Bruun et al., *Alcohol Control Policies in Public Health Perspective* (Helsinki: Finnish Foundation for Alcohol Studies, 1975).
89 See, e.g., H. J. Krauweel, 'Alcohol problems and treatment of alcoholism in the Netherlands', in *Proceedings of the 26th International Congress on Alcohol and*

Alcoholism (Stockholm: Centralförbundet för nykterhetsundervisning, 1963) [*CP 1960*]; Sully Ledermann, 'Can one reduce alcoholism without changing total alcoholic consumption in a population?', in *CP 1964*; Gunnar Nelker, 'Total abstinence – as an attitude and behavior', in *Proceedings of the 30th International Congress on Alcoholism and Drug Dependence* (Lausanne: ICAA, 1972) [*CP 1972*]; A. Haaranen, 'Popular alcohol information in Finland', in *CP 1975*; Keith R. Evans, 'Alcohol policies and political realities', in *CP 1988*; Alex Wodak, 'Reducing alcohol and drug related harm: Past present and future', in *Proceedings of the 36th International Congress on Alcohol and Drug Dependence* (Glasgow: Scottish Council on Alcohol (SCA), 1992) [*CP 1992*].

90 *Kettil Bruun Society* (2017), www.kettilbruun.org.
91 Robin Room, 'Alcohol', in *Oxford Textbook of Public Health*, ed, Roger Detels, Robert Beaglehole, Mary Ann Lansang and Martin Gulliford (Oxford: Oxford University Press, 2009), 5th edn, vol. 3, 1322–33.
92 Curt Wallis, 'Skolan och alkoholfrågan', in *CP 1907a*, 49.
93 Ernst Gabriel, 'The frequency of alcoholism as a phenomenon of cultural pathology', in *CP 1964*, 66.
94 See, e.g., Jan Skirrow, 'Positive approaches to prevention', in *CP 1985*; Svein Larsen, 'Competence development as a preventive strategy', in *CP 1988*; H. Stephen Glenn and C. R. Ming, 'Developing capable people training course', in *CP 1992*. For an early example, see: A. C. Colvin, 'A framework for curriculum construction', in *CP 1970*.
95 Abderhalden, 'Unsere Verantwortung', 47.
96 Schrad, *Political Power of Bad Ideas*.
97 Edman, 'Temperance and modernity'.
98 Moser, 'Prevention of alcohol-related problems', 85.
99 Ibid., 89.
100 Joel Fort, 'Cultural aspects of alcohol (and drug) problems', in *CP 1964*.
101 Marcus Grant, 'The best of both worlds: A retrospective overview of substance abuse prevention', in *CP 1985*, 78. On alcohol's marginal role within WHO's public health work, see Room, 'Alcohol control and public health'.
102 See, e.g., D. V. Hawks, 'The formulation of a national policy on alcohol in Australia', in *CP 1985*; Charas Suwanwela, 'Public health perspective in alcoholism and drug dependence', in *CP 1985*; Arvid J. Johnsen, 'An integrated policy for prevention', in *CP 1988*; Anna Lindh, 'The committee for opinion against alcohol and narcotics', in *CP 1988*.
103 Louis Gliksman, Edward Adlaf, Kenneth Allison and Brenda Newton-Taylor, 'School board drug policies and student drug use: A test of impact', in *CP 1992*, 1211.
104 Ibid.
105 Moser, 'Prevention of alcohol-related problems', 89.
106 H. David Archibald, 'Alcohol and drugs: Government responsibility', in *CP 1970*, 251.
107 See also J. Kaplan, 'Social policy panel', in *CP 1972*.
108 See, e.g., Prof. Dr Horejsi, 'Das wissenschaftliche Studium des Alkoholismus in den slawischen Ländern', in *CP 1948*; Alain Barjot, 'Principes directeurs de l'action des pouvoirs publics en France dans la lutte contre l'alcoolisme', in *CP 1956*; Pat Greathouse, 'The union and the problem drinker', in *28th International Congress on Alcohol and Alcoholism: Washington* (Highland Park, NJ: Hillhouse, 1969) [*CP 1968*]; 'Social policy panel', in *CP 1972*; J. K. Lawton, 'The dilemma facing the preventionist', in *Proceedings of the 33rd International Congress on Alcoholism and Drug Dependence* (Lausanne: ICAA, 1982) [*CP 1982*]; N. N. Ivanets, 'The USSR alcohol policy and the activities of the All-Union Research Center on Medico-Biological Problems of Narcology', in *CP 1988*.
109 E.g., Johan Edman, 'An ambiguous monolith: The Swedish drug issue as a political battleground 1965–1981', *International Journal of Drug Policy* 24, no. 5 (2013):

464–70; Filip Roumeliotis, 'Drug use and affective politics: The political implications of social emotional training', *Contemporary Drug Problems* 43, no. 4 (2016), 331–49.

110 Nils Christie and Kettil Bruun, 'Alcohol problems: The conceptual framework', in *CP 1968*.

111 Udo J. Gedig, 'Prevention as the socialization of experience: Inherent contradiction in prevention', in *CP 1985*, 369.

112 Fort, 'Cultural aspects of alcohol', 29f.

113 Paul F. Gavaghan, 'Social and health issues: The U.S. spirits industry's approach', in *CP 1985*, 465.

114 Tigerstedt, 'Discipline and public health'.

115 Peter Baldwin, 'Can there be a democratic public health?', in *Shifting Boundaries of Public Health: Europe in the Twentieth Century*, ed. Susan Gross Solomon, Lion Murar and Patrick Zylberman (Woodbridge: Boydell & Brewer, 2008), 23–44, 28.

116 Gliksman et al., 'School board drug policies', 1211.

117 Baldwin, 'Democratic public health'.

10 Mainstreaming concepts, discounting variations?

Global policies of alcohol, drugs and tobacco

Matilda Hellman

Introduction

During the twentieth and twenty-first centuries, world polities with a public health ethos have emerged in the areas of alcohol, drugs and tobacco. The road has been staked out with international treaties and cooperation strategies, underpinned by political work by international non-governmental organisations (INGOs) and the World Health Organization (WHO). The developments have looked a bit different in each of the three questions, but a conceptual epistemic mainstreaming has taken place during the past thirty years or so. The discussion in this chapter revolves around two questions: it begins by considering the historical circumstances surrounding the emergence of international collaboration in the three areas. The chapter then discusses certain ideas and concepts that in recent decades have come to mainstream and, in some respect, amalgamate the essence of the three areas as questions of global public health.

As alcohol use is legal and widespread in most parts of the world, the global public health agenda that started to materialize during the second half of the twentieth century has typically applied a grammar of larger epidemiologist, population-based trends and patterns, construed through measures such as the societal burden of non-communicable diseases (NCDs) or disability-adjusted life years (DALYs).[1] However, long before the emergence of such concepts, the nineteenth- and twentieth-century temperance movements had evolved with international alcohol policy collaboration.[2] The population-based health framing of current global health alcohol policies may have alleviated some of the moral valence associated with the historical background.

When it comes to illicit drug policy, the international cooperation developed out of national needs to suppress criminality and work together against the spread of dangerous substances between and within national borders. As drugs have functioned as a "suitable enemy" cooperation has tended to be even more active compared to the international combating of other types of criminality.[3] The international cooperation surrounding illicit drugs has historically concentrated on substance-specific evaluation work and it is partly binding through international juridical agreements. Health-related drug policy objectives may, nevertheless, have been too complicated to grasp, too ideologically invested and too inconsistent in their national variants for arriving at mainstreamed global strategies with a common language. Nevertheless, through connections with other agendas, such as notably the one of HIV/AIDS, the international cooperation has been able to establish a degree of consensus regarding certain general constructs of prevention and reduction of drug-related problems.[4]

In comparison with alcohol and drugs, the global cooperation surrounding tobacco as a matter of public health is of a later date and entails a more archetypical epidemiological narrative of discovery, mobilisation and synchronised attempts for eradication. It grew rapidly as a somewhat clear-cut issue for public health in the latter part of the twentieth century, articulated through an epistemic consensus regarding the evidence on harms caused by smoking for the smoker and their closest environment.[5] The WHO's own account of the history of its Framework Convention on Tobacco Control (WHO FCTC) is formulated as a success story involving a ground-breaking, previously "unused constitutional authority" of the organisation: performances in the "art of negotiation", accounts of "the power of process" and even some "champions" are singled out in the narration of the events.[6]

Concepts and language use, such as the ones in the above-mentioned report on the FCTC, reflect the ways in which alcohol, drugs and tobacco have appeared, and been conceptualised and reproduced as subjects of public health. For example, the normalised cultural position of alcohol use is obvious, given the fact that drug use and smoking have been associated with constructs such as 'epidemics' –"tobacco epidemic",[7] "drug epidemics"[8] – a rhetoric rarely found in documents on alcohol policy.

Seen in a long view, it is of a rather late date that the three questions have been conceptualised as issues related to health. As late as some hundred years ago alcohol, tobacco and opium were primarily items of trade and tools of dominance in the process of European colonial expansion. However, conceptions began to change during the following sixty years.[9] During 1910–1970, alcohol, tobacco and drugs were increasingly conceptualised as different issues.[10] Cigarette smoking became commonplace after the First World War, and a new generation of middle-class youth adopted it as a generational symbol. Consequently, nicotine was separated from concepts such as inebriety and addiction. The same generation also contributed to the failure of alcohol prohibition, which forced key actors to rethink alcohol problems, redefining them from a problem located in the substance to a problem located in the 'alcoholic'.[11] This conceptualisation did not at all fit in the increasingly tighter international prohibition regime for opiates and other drugs, which focused on the drugs themselves as the problem instead of framing them as a social problem or a disease of the will.

However, alcohol, tobacco and drugs have been reintegrated into public health politics since the 1970s.[12] This has occurred simultaneously with ambitions of a global public health agenda, its adherent infrastructure and the political manifest-ation of concepts of public health. As will be shown in this chapter, it can partly be seen as a result of a great global conceptual mainstreaming of diagnostic criteria of dependence and addiction. This is a conceptual public health machinery, executed by epistemic communities in medicine, psychology and pharmacology, with adherent scientific policies of funding and publishing. As a result, drug and alcohol treatment (noticeably though, not tobacco) have been reorganised as a single system in many countries: intoxicants and gambling are treated together in policy strategies; and alcohol, tobacco and drug education in schools is in many parts of the world combined.[13] At the same time, contemporary neuroscientists believe human beings can develop pathological relationships with a seemingly unlimited range of substances and activities.[14]

In what follows, I will present a brief historical backdrop of how each of the three global policy areas arose. In the second part of the chapter, I discuss concepts, worldviews and epistemologies that have associated the three areas with health. In the end, I draw some conclusions regarding the history of ideas relevant for alcohol, drugs and tobacco.

Three global agendas

The rise of a global alcohol agenda

The roots of treating alcohol use as a social question can be traced to the temperance movement, which was internationally organised at the beginning of the twentieth century. The movement for worldwide prohibition was an international arena which began to take an organisational form in 1909, when the International Prohibition Confederation (IPC) was established. In 1919, the IPC was renamed the World Prohibition Federation (WPF). The IPC/WPF – which was a propaganda organisation distributing more than 5 million leaflets, pamphlets and other publications in less than two decades – emphasised that prohibitionists were a moral community, united regardless of race, religion, nationality or politics.[15] It was essentially an Anglo-American organisation in which the Independent Order of Good Templars (IOGT) was a dominant influence.[16] Because of economic difficulties, the Federation failed to compete with the World League against Alcoholism after the Anti-Saloon League of America had established a rival propaganda society in 1919.[17] The World League operated in 185 countries, including European and American colonies. It was most active pushing prohibition in the early 1920s, but the peak of its propaganda activities was in 1927–1930.[18]

At the time, the international temperance movements offered platforms for the dissemination and exchange of ideas associated with societal progress. For instance, the American Women's Christian Temperance Union had a great influence on the manifestation and objectives of the Australian Women's Temperance Movement.[19] The international platforms could also lead to substantial changes in national framings of alcohol control and treatment: the international temperance movement, for instance, influenced Finnish policy makers, who started to look more positively on compulsory treatment towards the late nineteenth century.[20]

The early temperance movement framed alcohol as both a social political and health-related matter. The current global public health frame occurred chiefly through the World Health Organization since its founding in 1948. A recent review of the material from the WHO Expert Committees on alcohol, drugs and tobacco shows that between 1949 and 1963, experts discussed intensively concepts and terminology concerning both alcohol and illicit drugs.[21] The use of alcohol, drugs and tobacco were to be defined as common problems for the world community, through the articulation of a common aetiological understanding.

However, it was difficult to define alcohol and drug use as problems of the human body in a way that would allow for proper public health measures. The experts tried to find a common terminology expressing the phenomenon of 'continuous use despite harmful consequences' (commonly referred to as alcoholism and drug addiction). In the 1950s, the Expert Committee in Drugs Liable to Produce Addiction (ECDLPA) decided that *habit forming* should be replaced with *addiction* in all texts. Different concepts were linked to different control measures, but measures were primarily decided on nationally, outside the frame of the WHO or even outside the public health arena.[22] Between 1964 and 1989 – around the times when ideas of New Public Health (NPH) started to surface and develop[23] – the concept of *dependency* emerged, and allowed for a combination of approaches to different substances. However, after 1990 the WHO singled out tobacco as a policy field largely separated from questions of alcohol and drugs and it started to live a life of its own.

The first alcohol action plan was approved by the WHO's regional office in 1994. The European Charter on Alcohol was approved in 1995 and it has been described as especially important for European countries without a temperance history, such as Portugal. These countries had no sociohistorical reference for dealing with alcohol as a health problem at the level of the population.[24] Developed by the public health community, the WHO's alcohol policy agendas were intended to constitute a fairly indisputable point of reference that would not easily be compromised by trends in national politics. While national policies had previously drawn on both moral and health-related justifications, in the 1980s the public health community explicitly started to concentrate on what was referred to as an evidence-based agenda. This agenda was epistemically speaking heavily intertwined with individualised, medicalised conceptions of control of risk and danger.[25]

In 2010, the international expert community had reached a consensus. At the Sixty-third Session of the World Health Assembly (WHA), it was able to adopt Resolution WHA63.13, which endorsed the global strategy to reduce harmful use of alcohol. The global strategy, which is not legally binding, focuses on ten key areas of policy options and interventions at the national level and four priority areas for global action. The document states that: "WHO and its Member States are dedicated to work together to address the key areas of policy options and interventions, to interact with relevant stakeholders and to ensure that the strategy is implemented both nationally and globally."[26] This document can be viewed as the manifestation of alcohol as a political question on the global health agenda.

Illicit drugs as a global question

Whereas the international cooperation on the alcohol question had a background in the temperance movement, the international drug cooperation had many frontlines in the fight against drug-related crime, in the form of international treaties.

The first international drug control treaty, the International Opium Convention, was signed in The Hague in 1912. The Convention was implemented in five countries in 1915[27] and globally in 1919, when it was incorporated into the Treaty of Versailles. The primary objective was to restrict exports instead of prohibiting or criminalising the use and cultivation of opium, coca and cannabis (added in 1927). A revised International Opium Convention was signed in 1925 and registered in the League of Nations Treaty Series.[28]

The Convention for Limiting the Manufacture and Regulating the Distribution of Narcotic Drugs was a drug control treaty promulgated in Geneva in 1931 and entered into force in 1933. It established two separate detailed groups of drugs, and its scope was broadened considerably in 1948. The Convention was superseded by the 1961 Single Convention on Narcotic Drugs.[29]

The Single Convention on Narcotic Drugs from 1961 (amended by the 1972 Protocol and the Convention on Psychotropic Substances, 1971) states the protection of the health and welfare of humankind as its ultimate goal. The parties of the conventions consider "co-ordinated and universal action" required for restricting use for medical purposes and for making sure there is an opium supply for medical use. The conventions also envisage the use of public health measures to prevent and reduce health and social harm due to "abuse of drugs". The WHO is one of the four treaty bodies in the international drug control conventions; the others are the United Nations Secretary-General, the International Narcotics Control Board (INCB) and the United Nations Commission on Narcotic Drugs (UN CND).

The Single Convention on Narcotic Drugs and the Convention on Psychotropic Substances entrust the WHO with the responsibility of reviewing and assessing substances to determine whether they should be controlled under the conventions. A request for such a review can be initiated by parties to the conventions or by the WHO itself. The review of selected substances is carried out by the WHO Expert Committee on Drug Dependence (ECDD), whose tasks include: carrying out a review of the information available on substances subject to international control or exemption; reassessing the level of control of given substances; and advising the Director-General of the WHO accordingly.[30]

The ECDD, which has had different names at different times, has mostly convened every two years since 1949.[31] It has played a central role in making recommendations to the UN CND on control measures: "In contrast, alcohol and tobacco committees not needing to make scheduling decisions in relation to international conventions have met less frequently often in response to a WHA resolution calling for research on particular area of emerging interest."[32] The frequency of responses may have strengthened the ECDD and slightly compensated for its narrow role, restricted to providing recommendations on the scheduling of drugs.

In comparison to alcohol and tobacco, the global cooperation on drug policy has involved more varied types of substances that need to be classified and standardised according to knowledge of how they affect individuals and societies. The WHO is the only treaty body with a mandate to carry out medical and scientific assessment on substances:

> The advice of the Expert Committee is based on the best available scientific, medical and public health evidence and must comply with the criteria established in the conventions. Specific rules and procedures for the evaluation of substances are published in Guidance on the WHO review of psychoactive substances for international control. The science of substance evaluation has evolved over time and the methods of the Expert Committee are continuously adapted to embrace newly emerging insights.[33]

Through the work of its Expert Committee, the WHO has reviewed more than 400 substances since 1949. Between 1948 and 1999 the number of narcotic drugs under international control increased from 18 to 118, and the number of psychotropic substances from 32 to 111.[34]

The public health community has not been able to agree on global drug policy announcements in the same way as in the fields of alcohol and tobacco. International illicit drug policy bodies have traditionally emerged out of treaties that answer to situations that were not manageable without the involvement of many countries' control systems. It has been more difficult to create a worldwide polity in the area of public health. Not only has the agenda been split between substances, but views on how to approach the problems have also varied greatly.[35] Some countries have promoted a prohibitionist approach (such as Sweden and the US), whereas others (such as Denmark and the Netherlands) have supported a harm-reduction agenda ever since the beginning of the movement.[36]

Mutual understanding has been more common in questions such as dealing with international drug cartels and networks. The latest big advancement was the 2009 Political Declaration and Plan of Action on International Cooperation towards an Integrated and Balanced Strategy to counter the World Drug Problem adopted by the UN CND. The United Nations General Assembly Special Session in New York in 2016 (UNGASS 2016) arranged a special session on 'the world drug problem' with multi-stakeholder roundtable discussion on topics such as demand reduction, supply reduction, human rights, children and regional matters. In comparison with WHO's ECDD, the International Narcotics Control Board (INCB) – an independent, quasi-judicial expert body established by the Single Convention on Narcotic Drugs of 1961 – has been more influential concerning recommendations on control measures.

The WHO has been more successful in formulating a health care-oriented evidence-base to support treatment in member states. In 2009, the WHO published its *Guidelines for the Psychosocially Assisted Pharmacological Treatment of Opioid Dependence*. Compared to the alcohol strategy document, it is more heterogeneous in its worldview, acknowledging the many different drug abuses and problems. Still, it is more clinically oriented and targeted at 'health systems' – a generalised term used to cover national models for treatment supply. The readership targeted consists of policy makers and administrators, a global policy and practitioner community in health care administration. The recommendations in the guidelines are based on systematic reviews of the available literature and on consultations with a range of experts from different regions of the world. The word 'evidence' appears 179 times in the 134-page document, and 'recommend' appears 171 times. Scientific reviews are accounted for in an appendix concerning information mostly gathered from randomised controlled trials (RCTs).

In the field of drugs, the international arena was long occupied primarily by meetings of and around the official international drug control system. However, as Robin Room explains, while many countries remain conservative and supportive of the drug control system, it is out of tune with progressive public opinion, and independent expert opinion has become increasingly sceptical.[37] Under such circumstances, international sets of meetings and societies have emerged and developed a critical stance. These meetings include the annual International Conference on the Reduction of Drug Related Harm, which has been organised by the International Harm Reduction Association (IHRA) since 1990. In addition, drug user movements run by active and former drug users have started to become increasingly organised in international arenas.[38]

A smoke-free world: Tobacco as a global question

In the 1960s, new evidence on the relationship between tobacco and health hazards gained public attention in the USA and in Europe. In 1962, a report from the British Royal College of Physicians was the first to document a causal relationship between smoking and cancer. In their study on Finnish and Norwegian tobacco policy developments, Matilda Hellman et al. point out three stages of mainstreaming the tobacco policy agenda since the 1950s. The first period entailed an ontology of harm to the smoker, and harm reduction was an articulated goal. In the second stage, as of the 1970s, harm to others became an important driver in the promotion of smoke-free environments. In the third period, as of the 1990s, the focus shifted onto the problems of addiction and dependency, which entailed technical solutions and biological explanations for controlling physical cravings.[39] Similar developments have also occurred elsewhere, which is partially attributable to the strong role of the medical profession in the anti-smoking agenda. In the collective memory of the global health policy community, the process was perceived as rather unique: a success story in public health mobilisation setting the example also for other lifestyle-related fields.[40]

The tobacco question entered WHO cooperation rather late, towards the end of the twentieth century. When Norwegian physician Gro Harlem Brundtland became Director-General of the WHO in 1998, its Tobacco Free Initiative (TFI) raised the profile of tobacco control. The WHO initiated a process of developing a framework that permitted member states to adopt a comprehensive tobacco control policy, which included transnational tobacco control measures.[41] While the ECDD had deferred tobacco for further consideration in 1996, by 1999, new evidence of greater liability for abuse brought tobacco into focus again.[42] The WHA adopted the WHO Framework Convention on Tobacco Control (FCTC) in 2003 and put it into effect in 2005. The convention became the first international treaty negotiated under the auspices of the WHO.

The WHO's political strategies involved the creation and validation of a collective reality to be reflected and implemented in regional and national policies. Suzanne Taylor et al. characterise the period 1990–2013 as a movement towards a more sustainable and combined approach to substance abuse.[43] This was reflected in the creation of the WHO's Division of Mental Health and the Prevention of Substance Abuse's Programme on Substance Abuse (PSA). This period was marked by the development of global tobacco control strategies.

The tobacco question represents a unique global mainstreaming of views on a problem and its subsequent policies. Consensus and conformity upheld the mandate and kept it together. Civil society engagement was important for the development of framework conventions – –in particular, industry forces that were actively working against them.[44] This institutional agenda provided a framework for activities, goals and policies.[45] The mainstreaming and the isomorphism of tobacco policy and control can be seen as extremely functional and with a strong focus on problem-solving. Tobacco policy is a good example of a broadly shared view on a problem whose agenda led to a rather rapid breakthrough. The Framework Convention has subsequently served as an aspirational success story for other substance control agendas (alcohol policies, in particular).[46]

Mainstreaming concepts and ideas

The framing of alcohol, drugs and tobacco as public health problems has been related to broader social developments underpinned by rationales based on science and technology. These have relied on specific worldviews, concepts and discourses, some of which follow general developments in public health discourses, whereas others have been specific to questions of substance use. In the later part of the twentieth century, collective welfare solutions in Western countries were beginning to cover broader areas of concern whereby public health measures, policies and discourses were also formulated. This framework enabled the institutionalisation of alcohol, drug and tobacco policies.

Alcohol, drug and tobacco policies would, partly through the expanding global polity of public health, develop into a somewhat more consensual psychological and medical polity. This community sought to establish large-scale, systematic and mechanical methods for identifying problems and developing solutions. For alcohol, drug and tobacco abuse to be included in the agenda of public health problems, they have been required to involve normative, ontological and epistemological conceptions of human functioning and societal prosperity in relation to the value of health.[47] The concept of health – an embodied and modifiable status – has brought the problems aetiology closer together and enabled the focus to shift away from, e.g., disagreements regarding export and import of different substances, or from the moral responsibility to abstain from alcohol.

The WHO Expert Committees on alcohol, drugs and tobacco were active in formulating concepts and definitions in an attempt to unify the world behind the universal problems of humans and human societies. Sometimes terminology was revised several times, e.g., when the somewhat opaque term *habit-forming* was replaced by *addiction*. However, *addiction* quickly proved to be unsatisfactory in links to control measures, after which it was replaced by *dependence* and a focus on *dependence-producing drugs*.[48]

The WHO Expert Committee first suggested replacing *addiction* and *habituation* by *dependence* in 1962, after which it would include dependency concepts in its International Classification of Diseases (ICD, updated since 1949). In retrospect, it can be seen as an early contribution to a larger project of combining different substances on the health agenda. The ICD serves as a problem-defining tool and a manifestation of a joint global terminology.[49] The WHO emphasises the ICD's role in identifying health trends and interpreting statistics on a global level; in short, in allowing the world "to compare and share health information using a common language".[50]

The ICD involved an understanding of the syndrome of *dependency* as definable, countable and counteractable in populations – a notion that resonated well with the rise of governance ideas of NPH.[51] This was a rather long conceptual step from the international crime control ambitions of the Opium Convention or the morally invested social ideals of the temperance movements.

Terms such as *dependency* and *addiction* highlight similarities between illicit and licit substances, and created an opportunity for a seemingly universal global approach to a variety of problematic behaviours. This holds true at least in the areas of research and treatment, but the psy conceptions of dependency and addiction would entangle with and spread to popular discourse.[52] On a super-ficial level, *dependency* seems to offer a possibility to steer away from social, political and cultural complexity by concentrating on a diagnosable, health-related syndrome. This was a manageable construct familiar from the WHO's global endeavours for communicable diseases. For example, alcohol as a *dependence-producing drug* cuts across the public health spectrum, from a diagnosable physical/mental problem in the individual to the measurement of the prevalence of the problem in any given population. These goals and measures are shared by policies related to illnesses such as malaria, HIV/AIDS or hepatitis. For the global health community seeking consensus, the 'dependency' diagnostic tool involved important connotations. It associated severe substance use with a problem conception that was seemingly more clean-cut, technical and morally detached compared to the frail balance between the freedom of consumers to drink alcohol and health protection through limited alcohol availability.

Drawing on Law's concept of collateral realities,[53] Suzanne Fraser et al. scrutinise the literature that influenced and formed the basis of the dependency concept, which would turn out important for the construction of a commonality between alcohol, drug and tobacco policies.[54] Clinical knowledge and the need for addiction treatment have depended on such a conception of the problems. The *dependence syndrome*, as introduced by the WHO, can also be seen to have marked a globally accepted definition for a phenomenon embracing compulsive acts or thoughts beyond those directly related to drugs.[55] It illustrates an emerging contemporary interest in linking addiction to a spectrum of other behaviours.[56] Important for this conceptual trend has been that "[t]he 'dependent person' is a pre-constituted subject whose diseased condition improves or worsens according to the impact of external social processes."[57]

In all areas of epidemiology, international measurement synchronisation and diagnostic criteria constitute mainstreaming forces. They define problems and lay the ground for how the prevalence and solutions are formulated. Concepts of addiction and dependency have been propelled and underpinned by transnational discourses by epistemic communities and organisations. The construction of dependence allows for expertise to reign over a broad spectrum of behaviours. At the same time, the repertoire of solutions is sealed within the concept's epistemologies and the professions executing and reproducing their rationales.[58] Its connotation thus inherently creates ambivalence. While it formulates a core shared by a variety of problems – excessive alcohol use, gambling, eating or any other behaviour thinkable – it excludes, by definition, non-diagnosable and fuzzy problem variants and their surrounding realities. These variants and realities are bound to prevail on a larger scale than the ones that fit the criteria of 'dependency'.

While the forthcoming ICD-11 has retained *dependence*, the American Psychiatric Association (APA) has replaced dependency in its *Diagnostic and Statistical Manual of Mental Disorders* (DSM-5) of 2013 with 'Substance-Related and Addictive Disorders'. Both ideas fit agendas underpinned by medical, epidemiological and psychiatric expertise. At the same time, the large neuro-biological-ontological endeavour, commonly referred to as the brain disease model of addiction (BDMA), has pushed this project further by looking for supportive evidence in line with the diagnostic constructs. Its proponents claim the moral extra bonus of avoiding stigmatisation by sticking to physical expressions and excluding individual self-interpretations of the problems.[59] At the same time, the brain disease model is largely intertwined with systems of psy science in order to manifest itself in practice. The BDMA is an epistemic project of which knowledge on socio-political and ethical consequences is urgently needed.

The concept of the world as one single place in which problems of dependency and addiction appear and are dealt with is embedded in an international normative regime operating with common concepts, words and ideas.[60] The norms of this global culture will inevitably reflect the interests of the elites who champion them. In the case of global addiction policies during the past forty years or so, the elite has primarily consisted of experts in pharmacology, medicine and epidemiology. The epistemic globalisation of conceptions and standards is an ongoing rationalisation in which dependence, addiction and substance use disorders are only a small part of the picture. More contemplative literature on concepts in the area seems to be mushrooming, and the problems with implementing concepts in different cultures are being acknowledged.[61]

Discourse on threats and enemies

An inherent discursive objective of the global health policy documents on alcohol, drugs and tobacco is to gather the global community behind a worldview that calls for national action, political processual collaboration and joint action. Such ideas materialise through arguments that highlight the urgency of the project by emphasising threats to humankind and its societies. Health risks and threats typically involve notions of the problems' scale and their fatal consequences. For example, the Framework document 1997 programme for substance abuse is committed to address "the substantial health, social and economic costs related to the use of psychoactive substances, which have become a major global health concern, affecting millions of people throughout the world".[62] The guidelines for the psychosocially assisted pharmacological treatment of opioid dependence state that:

> UNODC estimates that there are 25 million problem drug users in world, of whom 15.6 are problem opioid users and 11.1 problem heroin users (approximately 0.3% of the global population). ... The cost of this epidemic is counted in the millions of lives lost each year and the billions of dollars spent.[63]

Typically, the widespread nature of the problem is emphasised by tying in questions that overlap and attribute to the problems. In the global alcohol strategy from 2010, the harmful use of alcohol is estimated to cause 2.5 million deaths every year, and alcohol use is named as the third leading risk factor for poor health globally:

> The harmful use of alcohol is one of the four most common modifiable and preventable risk factors for major noncommunicable diseases (NCDs). There is also emerging evidence that the harmful use of alcohol contributes to the health burden caused by communicable diseases such as, for example, tuberculosis and HIV/AIDS.[64]

The alcohol strategy also involves another typical element of current global health rationales, namely, a focus on world inequalities. While reducing health inequalities on a global scale has been an embedded objective of the WHO from the start, globalisation has further sharpened this focus.[65] According to Andrew McMichael and Robert Beaglehole, due to globalisation, "[c]ontemporary public health must encompass the interrelated tasks of reducing social and health inequalities and achieving health-sustaining environments."[66] The expansion of the scope involves a general mainstreaming of the concept of globalisation (referring to 'the way in which the world is collectively going'), as well as acknowledging that a global perspective nevertheless involves different realities (e.g., poorer and richer countries, good and less favourable circumstances for implementing and upholding good health).

According to the 2010 alcohol strategy:

> Reducing the harmful use of alcohol by effective policy measures and by providing a relevant infrastructure to successfully implement those measures

is much more than a public health issue. Indeed, it is a *development issue*, since the level of risk associated with the harmful use of alcohol in developing countries is much higher than that in high income countries where people are increasingly protected by comprehensive laws and interventions – and by mechanisms to ensure that these are implemented.[67] (my emphasis)

The statement above portrays alcohol as more than merely a public health issue; it is represented as a structural problem that goes beyond the health scope. In the world health polity, a responsibility for low-income countries has developed into an ethical premise. There is not enough room (political mandate and economical resources) to involve the structural dimensions relating to poverty and equality that were already raised by the temperance movement in the nineteenth century. In the twenty-first century world health polity, structural problems are often arti-culated through a linear narrative of countries' different extent of resources and of evidence-based policy implementation. Political and ideological explanatory factors and themes related to, e.g., labour, gender equality or systemic social margin-alisation might be overlooked. The international cooperation under the temperance umbrella may have been a better platform to spread and integrate such ideas.

As mentioned above, modern global health policy agendas had perceived inequality as a central theme already before the emergence of current globalisation forces. Partly due to the increasing AIDS/HIV awareness, the Ottawa Charter for Health Promotion of 1986 expanded definition(s) of public health and strived for a broader cross-sectional social perspective. While the initiative enabled a more contextual framing of public health issues, it has later on been seen as too wide a scope for the WHO, an organisation with specialised epistemic views and limited resources.[68] The period between 1964 and 1989 has been characterised as the era when New Public Health ideas were emerging and consolidated – of which the Ottawa Charter is an important manifestation. During this period, the WHO Expert Committees on alcohol, drugs and tobacco also introduced and established the concept of *dependence*. The Ottawa Charter did not entail new social framings for questions regarding alcohol and drugs, which both had different contextual and conceptual backgrounds compared to epidemiology and public health. However, its zeitgeist perhaps constituted a welcome reminder of the complex overall picture of the problems' nature as well as social dimensions that went beyond aspects of health.

In 1984, an advisory group for European WHO member states outlined Health for All targets for the European region. One set of the targets promoted "a social model of health" through a package of five lifestyle and health targets that addressed healthy public policy, social support systems, knowledge and moti-vation, positive health behaviour, and health-damaging behaviour. While the advisory group still addressed individual behaviour, it focused on the interactions between individuals and their environments, as well as the political instruments needed for addressing health determinants. In line with the growing epistemic movement on social contextualisation of the 1970s and 1980s, the advisory group sought to expand the territory of health into other policy arenas, and emphasised the complex political and social processes necessary for achieving changes in health.[69]

The Ottawa Charter thus initiated an attempt at redefining and repositioning institutions, epistemic communities and actors at the 'health' end of the disease–health spectrum. By abandoning an individualistic conception of lifestyles and instead highlighting social environments and public policy, health promotion sought to shift the focus from the modification of individual risk factors or risk behaviours to the "context and meaning" of health actions and health-supporting determinants. In its Health for All strategy, the WHO framed health as a core value of development policy. Furthermore, it defined the goal of health policy as "providing all people with the opportunity to lead a socially and economically productive life". Governments were seen as accountable not just for the health services they provided, but also for the health of their populations.[70]

In the 1980s, the scope of the political project for world health was actively aiming to expand, demanding greater national governmental involvement. The initial global project began resembling a national political programme. Lifestyles were understood as collective behaviours deeply rooted in structural contexts; but how were these shifting conceptions to be translated into policies of alcohol, drugs and tobacco, particularly as the concept of *dependence* was rising? As the complexity and extent of public health policies were being acknowledged, it was also acknowledged that many issues were difficult to address to a satisfactory degree through a global agenda.[71]

Since the Ottawa Charter, the world has witnessed a globalisation which could not have been foreseen at the time.[72] Solidarity between low- and high-income countries has become an even more central goal of the WHO, although perhaps less structurally defined in comparison with the 1980s. This solidarity is, indeed, one of the most frequently raised 'geographical' variations acknowledged in WHO documents on alcohol, drug and tobacco policies. It enunciates a solidarity among the world polity, calling for collaboration in order to deal with world inequality. The potential partners and promoters of the global agenda are state governments, INGOs and the private sector.[73]

While the inequality theme has received more space, the enemy has become more pronounced: the global alcohol and tobacco industry, as well as producers and sellers of drugs who recruit consumers in low-consumption or traditionally abstinent geographies.[74] Globalised health challenges along with global scopes and agendas for dealing with them have led to a more severe polarisation between public health and industry interests, one which resembles a new left–right constellation.[75]

The health versus industry constellation involves tremendous competition among global and national stakeholders to legitimise their own standpoint in order to get people's beliefs to conform to their own agendas.[76] One of the most aggressive intrusions of the global alcohol industry in politics is the brewing multinational SABMiller and the industry-funded International Center for Alcohol Policies (ICAP) formulation of official National Alcohol Policy draft documents for Lesotho, Malawi, Uganda and Botswana.[77] The industry is a very real, yet no doubt a gathering and convenient, enemy in the worldview of the global epistemic order of alcohol and tobacco policies. A strong global industry entails various problems, from scientists with funding from vested interests to industry intrusions into policy-making.[78] Global public health and global industries are entwined with each other's modus operandi.

The world health polity has not only brought more and more issues into its purview; globalisation has also increased the odds of finding an elite ally for any given movement. The global NGO networks in questions regarding alcohol, drugs and tobacco are involved in influencing and implementing agendas and frame conventions of the WHO or the UN, aiming for these to become, partly or fully, integrated in policy and praxis. Transnational NGOs have been referred to as "the citizen sector" and agents of accountability.[79] O'Gorman and colleagues have reviewed and mapped over 200 EU-based drug policy advocacy organisations, showing that NGOs and large-scale civil society organisations (CSOs) have great capacity to access and engage in governance spaces at national, EU and UN levels.[80]

Conclusions

In this chapter, I have outlined the background for the appearance of alcohol, drugs and tobacco on the world polity's health agenda. The nineteenth-century temperance movement was the first to engage in international cooperation regarding the social aspect of alcohol. The international cooperation concerning drugs, for its part, has mostly focused on aspects of criminality and on categorising substances, partly due to a lack of political consensus. Finally, in current times, tobacco has rapidly risen as a clear-cut question of public health.

The chapter has also suggested some mainstreaming forces that have enabled seeing alcohol, drug and tobacco policies as involving similar core problems as well as mainstreaming forces that have emphasised them as global problems, hence to be addressed in a world polity. The word 'dependency' and the idea of this phenomenon (also in terms of addiction and substance use disorders in the DSM) have supported both of these mainstreaming objectives.

The worldview that materialises in the account of this global health policy sphere on alcohol, drugs and tobacco largely disregards regional and cultural variations. The emphasised structural and geographical variations are those between high- and low-income countries, which reflects a solidarity project. This chapter suggests that this project became more articulated due to the rise of interest in societal and contextual framings of problems – e.g., through the Ottawa Charter in the 1980s, or other global health challenges such as AIDS/HIV. The focus on balancing out resources between low- and high-income countries by spreading good practices reflects a moral project that sometimes resembles a welfare state idea in the aims to overcome inequalities between people. To some extent, it involves a positivist view on low-income countries as simply being in the earlier stages of implementing the 'right' kind of evidence-based interventions. Another important element of this ontology is shared notions of enemies and threats regarding ill health and criminality, and a demoralised global industry.

Drawing on a strong evidence-based movement (EBM) and disciplines such as medicine, pharmacology, public health and epidemiology, the global epistocracy in these areas of public health have entangled roles of political activists and researchers. This epistemic project is morally invested. In its *raison d'être*, EBM pursues a moral imperative in producing interventional efficacy and therefore better health, a largely uncontested moral good. At the core of this project lies the ontological idea of a controllable reality (within the individual body, or the evidence-based policy task) – i.e., an external reality that might influence health status but is seldom formulated within cultural and societal frameworks. How this is reproduced in the mainstream of addiction science is an urgent research task.

What has unfolded in this chapter is the narrative of a simultaneously inclusive and exclusive agenda. On the one hand, the problems are seen as stemming from similar disorders and circumstances. On the other hand, the narrative is highly dominated by somewhat synchronised ontologies of the psy, medical and biological disciplines. Some major ethical concerns for the enormous projects covered in this study reflect attempts to homogenise or to see heterogeneities. In the future, the question of the scientific community's different roles in relation to science production and policy needs to be scrutinised and discussed more thoroughly.

Notes

1 Robert Beaglehole et al., 'Priority actions for the non-communicable disease crisis', *The Lancet* 377, no. 9775 (2011): 1438–447; David H. Jernigan et al., 'Towards a global alcohol policy: Alcohol, public health and the role of WHO', *Bulletin of the World Health Organization* 78, no. 4 (2000): 491–9.
2 See also Chapter 9 by Johan Edman in this volume.
3 Niels Christie and Kettil Bruun, *Den goda fienden* (Kristianstad: Rabén & Sjögren, 1985).
4 Alex Wodak, 'Harm reduction is now the mainstream global drug policy', *Addiction* 104, no. 3 (2009): 343–5.
5 Matilda Hellman, Pekka Hakkarainen and Gunnae Sæbø, 'Underpinnings of tobacco policy: An epistemic governance perspective', in *Concepts of Addictive Substances and Behaviours across Time and Place*, ed. Matilda Hellman et al. (Oxford: Oxford University Press, 2016), 151–67.
6 *World Health Organization History of the World Health Organization Framework Convention on Tobacco Control* (Geneva: World Health Organization, 2009).
7 World Health Organization and Research for International Tobacco Control, *WHO Report on the Global Tobacco Epidemic* (Geneva: World Health Organization, 2008).
8 Dale D. Chitwood, Sheigla Murphy and Marsha Rosenbaum, 'Reflections on the meaning of drug epidemics', *Journal of Drug Issues* 39, no. 1 (2009): 29–39.
9 Robin Room, 'A century of societal responses to alcohol, tobacco and drugs', Archer Tongue Memorial Lecture, 50th International ICAA Conference on Dependencies, Stockholm, Sweden, 10–15 June 2007.
10 Ibid.
11 Niels Christie and Kettil Bruun, 'Alcohol problems: The conceptual framework', in *Proceedings of the 28th International Congress on Alcohol and Alcoholism*, vol. 2, ed. M. Keller and T. Coffey (Highland Park NJ: Hillhouse, 1969), 65–73; Ron Roizen, *The American Discovery of Alcoholism, 1933–1939* (Berkeley: University of California Press, 1991).

12 Room, 'A century'.
13 Tamiko Ysa, Joan Colom, Adrià Albareda, Anna Ramon and Lidia Segura, *Governance of Addictions: European Public Policies* (Oxford: Oxford University Press, 2014).
14 Suzanne Fraser, David Moore and Helen Keane, *Habits: Remaking Addiction* (Basingstoke: Palgrave Macmillan, 2014); WHO, *Neuroscience of Psychoactive Substance Use and Dependence* (Geneva: World Health Organization, 2004).
15 David M. Fahey, 'Temperance internationalism: Guy Hayler and the World Prohibition Federation', *Social History of Alcohol and Drugs* 21, no. 2 (2005): 247–75.
16 Jack S. Blocker, David M. Fahey and Ian R. Tyrrell, *Alcohol and Temperance in Modern History: An International Encyclopedia, vol. 1* (Santa Barbara, CA: ABC-CLIO, 2003), 396.
17 Ibid., 692; Fahey, 'Temperance internationalism', 247.
18 Blocker et al, *Alcohol and Temperance*.
19 Ian Tyrrell, 'International aspects of the Women's Temperance Movement in Australia: The influence of the American WCTU, 1882–1914', *Journal of Religious History* 12, no. 3 (1983): 284–304; Ian Tyrrell, *Woman's World/Woman's Empire: The Woman's Christian Temperance Union in International Perspective, 1880–1930* (Chapel Hill: University of North Carolina Press, 1991).
20 Jukka-Pekka Takala, 'Ideas and organizations: Notes on the Finnish Alcoholics Act of 1936', *Contemporary Drug Problems* 13, no. 3 (1986): 527–54.
21 Suzanne Taylor, Virginia Beridge and Alex Mold, 'WHO expert committees and key concepts for drugs, alcohol, and tobacco, 1949–2013', in *Concepts of Addictive Substances and Behaviours across Time and Place*, ed. Matilda Hellman et al. (Oxford: Oxford University Press, 2016), 57–85.
22 Taylor et al., 'WHO expert committees', 57–85, 61.
23 See Chapter 1 in this volume.
24 Blocker et al., *Alcohol and Temperance*, 488.
25 Cf. Ellen K. Silbergeld, 'Risk assessment: The perspective and experience of US environmentalists', *Environmental Health Perspectives* 101, no. 2 (1993): 100–104, 100; Ulrich Beck, *Risk Society: Towards a New Modernity* (London: Sage, 1992); Wee-Kiat Lim, 'Understanding risk governance: Introducing sociological neoinstitutionalism and Foucauldian governmentality for further theorizing', *International Journal of Disaster Risk Science* 2, no. 3 (2011): 11–20.
26 World Health Organization, *Global Strategy to Reduce the Harmful Use of Alcohol, 2010*, www.who.int/substance_abuse/alcstratenglishfinal.pdf (accessed 7 Aug 2017).
27 The five countries were the United States, Netherlands, China, Honduras and Norway.
28 It introduced a statistical control system to be supervised by a Permanent Central Opium Board, a body of the League of Nations. See *League of Nations Treaty Series, vol. 8*, available at https://treaties.un.org/Pages/showDetails.aspx?objid=08000002800 46862&clang=_en (accessed 10 Oct 2017).
29 See United Nations Treaty collection.
30 World Health Organization, *International Classification of Diseases (ICD)*, www.who.int/classifications/icd/factsheet/en/ (accessed 7 Aug 2017).
31 It sometimes met more often, but between 2006 and 2012 it did not convene at all.
32 Taylor et al., 'WHO expert committees', 61.
33 WHO, *ICD*.
34 Ibid.
35 Floyd LaMond Tullis, *Unintended Consequences: Illegal Drugs and Drug Policies in Nine Countries* (Boulder: Lynne Rienner, 1995); Hans-Jorg. J. Albrecht and Anton van Kalmthout, eds, *Drug Policies in Western Europe* (Freiburg: Max-Planck-Institut für ausländisches und internationales Strafrecht, 1989).
36 Leif Lenke and Börje Olsson, 'Swedish drug policy in the twenty-first century: A policy model going astray', *Annals of the American Academy of Political and Social Science* 582, no. 1 (2002): 64–79; Tim Boekhout van Solinge, *Dealing with Drugs in Europe:*

An Investigation of European Drug Control Experiences: France, the Netherlands and Sweden. (The Hague: BJu Legal Publishers, 2004).

37 Room, 'A century'.
38 Bagga Bjerge et al., 'Exploring user groups as stakeholders in drug policy processes in four European countries', in *Concepts of Addictive Substances and Behaviours across Time and Place*, ed. Matilda Hellman et al. (Oxford: Oxford University Press, 2016), 108–29; Jørgen Anker et al., 'Drug users and spaces for legitimate action', in *Empowerment and Self-Organisations* [sic] *of Drug Users: Experiences and Lessons Learnt*, ed. Georg Bröring and Eberhard Schatz (Amsterdam: Foundation Regenboog AMOC, 2008), 17–40; Thomas Babor, *Drug Policy and the Public Good* (Oxford: Oxford University Press, 2010).
39 Hellman et al., 'Underpinnings of tobacco policy'.
40 Eric A. Feldman and Ronald Bayer, 'The triumph and tragedy of tobacco control: A tale of nine nations', *Annual Review of Law and Social Science* 7, no. 79 (2011): 79–100.
41 Taylor et al., 'WHO expert committees'.
42 World Health Organization, *Expert Committee on Drug Dependence: Thirty-First Report* (Geneva: WHO, 1999); see also Taylor et al., 'WHO expert committees'.
43 Taylor et al., 'WHO expert committees'.
44 Hadii M. Mamudu and Stanton A. Glantz, 'Civil society and the negotiation of the Framework Convention on Tobacco Control', *Global Public Health* 4 (2009): 150–68; Derek Yach and Douglas Bettcher, 'Globalisation of tobacco industry influence and new global responses', *Tobacco Control* 9 (2000): 206–16; Heide Weishaar et al., 'Global health governance and the commercial sector: A documentary analysis of tobacco company strategies to influence the WHO Framework Convention on Tobacco Control', *PLoS Medicine* 9, no.6 (2012), e1001249.
45 Deborah Barrett and Charles Kurzman, 'Globalizing social movement theory: The case of eugenics', *Theory and Society* 33, no. 5 (2004): 487–527; Ronald L. Jepperson, 'The development and application of sociological neoinstitutionalism', in *New Directions in Contemporary Sociological Theory*, ed. Joseph Berger and Morris Zelditch Jr (Lanham, MD: Rowman & Littlefield, 2002), 229–66.
46 See, e.g., Robin Room, Laura Schmidt, Jurgen Rehm and Pia Mäkelä, 'International regulation of alcohol', *BMJ* 337, no. 7681 (2008): 1248.
47 See John Coggon, *What Makes Health Public? A Critical Evaluation of Moral, Legal and Political Claims in Public Health* (Cambridge: Cambridge University Press, 2012), 49.
48 Taylor et al., 'WHO expert committees'.
49 See Robin Room, 'Alcohol and drug disorders in the International Classification of Diseases: A shifting kaleidoscope', *Drug and Alcohol Review* 17, no. 3 (1998): 305–17.
50 WHO, *ICD*.
51 See Chapter 1 in this volume.
52 Matilda Hellman, *Construing and Defining the Out of Control: Addiction in the Media* (Helsinki: University of Helsinki, 2010).
53 John Law, 'Collateral realities', in *The Politics of Knowledge*, ed. Fernando Dominguez Rubio and Patrick Baert (London: Routledge, 2011), 156–78.
54 Fraser et al., *Habits: Remaking Addiction*.
55 See also Taylor et al., 'WHO expert committees'; Isaac Marks, 'Behavioural (non-chemical) addictions', *British Journal of Addiction* 85, no. 11 (1990): 1389–94.
56 Fraser et al., *Habits: Remaking Addiction*, 198–9.
57 Ibid., 142–3.
58 Ibid., 137.
59 Nora D. Volkow and Ting-Lai Li, 'Drug addiction: the neurobiology of behaviour gone awry', *Nature Reviews Neuroscience* 5, no. 12 (2004): 963–70; Nick Heather, 'Q: Is

addiction a brain disease or a moral failing? A: Neither', *Neuroethics* 10, no. 1 (2017): 115–24.
60 See e.g. Deborah Barrett and Charles Kurzman, 'Globalizing social movement theory: The case of eugenics', *Theory and Society* 33, no. 5 (2004): 487–527.
61 Taylor et al., 'WHO expert committees'; Robin Room, Matilda Hellman and Kerstin Stenius, 'Addiction: The dance between concepts and terms', *International Journal on Alcohol and Drug Research* 4, no. 1 (2015): 27–35; Robin Room, 'Taking account of cultural and societal influences on substance use diagnoses and criteria', *Addiction* 101, no. 1 (2006): 31–9.
62 World Health Organization, *Strategy Framework and Work Plan 1997*, http://apps.who.int/iris/bitstream/10665/63317/1/WHO_MSA_PSA_97.2.pdf (accessed 8 Aug 2017).
63 World Health Organization, *Guidelines for the Psychosocially Assisted Pharmacological Treatment of Opioid Dependence* (Geneva: WHO, 2009), www.who.int/substance_abuse/publications/opioid_dependence_guidelines.pdf (accessed 8 Aug 2017).
64 WHO, *Global Strategy*.
65 Laurie Garrett, *Betrayal of Trust: The Collapse of Global Public Health* (Oxford: Oxford University Press, 2003); Don Nutbeam, 'What would the Ottawa Charter look like if it were written today?', *Critical Public Health* 18, no. 4 (2008): 435–41.
66 Andrew J. McMichael and Robert Beaglehole, 'The changing global context of public health', *The Lancet* 356, no. 9228 (2000): 495–9, 495.
67 WHO, *Global Strategy*.
68 Alfred Uhl, 'How to camouflage ethical questions in addiction research', in *Drugs in Society: European Perspectives*, ed. Jane Fountain and Dirk Korf (Oxford: Radcliffe, 2007), 116–30.
69 Ilona Kickbusch, 'The contribution of the World Health Organization to a new public health and health promotion', *American Journal of Public Health* 93, no 3 (2003): 383–8.
70 Ibid., 383.
71 Ibid.
72 See Nutbeam, 'Ottawa Charter'.
73 WHO, *Global Strategy*.
74 David Michaels, *Doubt Is Their Product: How Industry's Assault on Science Threatens Your Health* (Oxford: Oxford University Press, 2008); Peter Anderson et al., *The New Governance of Addictive Substances and Behaviours* (Oxford: Oxford University Press, 2016); Øystein Bakke and Dag Endal, 'Vested interests in addiction research and policy. Alcohol policies out of context: Drinks industry supplanting government role in alcohol policies in sub-Saharan Africa', *Addiction* 105, no. 1 (2010): 22–8; David Jernigan, 'The global alcohol industry: An overview', *Addiction* 104, no. 1 (2009): 6–12.
75 Fiona Ross, 'Beyond left and right: The new partisan politics of welfare', *Governance* 13, no. 2 (2000): 155–83.
76 Anderson et al., *New Governance*.
77 Bakke and Endal, 'Vested interests'.
78 Thomas Babor, 'Alcohol research and the alcoholic beverage industry: Issues, concerns and conflicts of interest', *Addiction* 104, s1 (2009): 34–47; Benjamin Hawkins, Chris Holden and Jim McCambridge, 'Alcohol industry influence on UK alcohol policy: A new research agenda for public health', *Critical Public Health* 22, no. 3 (2012): 297–305.
79 Anderson et al., *New Governance*, 197.
80 Aileen O'Gorman, Eoghan Quigley, Frank Zobel and Kerri Moore, 'Peer, professional, and public: An analysis of the drugs policy advocacy community in Europe', *International Journal of Drug Policy* 25, no. 5 (2014): 1001–8.

11 Science, politics and public health

The North Karelia Project 1972–1997

Johannes Kananen

The governance of public health is intimately connected to the production of scientific knowledge. Therefore, it is interesting to observe the linkages between various knowledge production regimes and associated forms of knowledge in the conceptual history of public health. This chapter focuses on connections between forms of medical knowledge, epidemiology and conceptualisations of public health.

In the nineteenth century, several schools of medical thought coexisted, including homeopathy (established by Samuel Hahnemann, 1755–1843) and hydropathy (established by Vincent Priessnitz, 1799–1851).[1] By the early twentieth century, allopathic medicine, however, had established a hegemonic position in the Western world. In the US, the Flexner Report of 1910 – commissioned by the American Medical Association's (AMA) Council of Medical Education and supported by the Carnegie Foundation – was crucial in this struggle for hegemony. It succeeded in establishing uniformity in the previously pluralistic scene of medical higher education.[2] After the concentration of resources on a single school of thought, US medical schools emerged as important centres of medical knowledge production.

Allopathic medicine typically operates under the following conditions:

- *Distinction between normal and pathological conditions* of the human being. The role of medicine is thought to be to identify pathologies through diagnosis and the re-establishment of normality through evidence-based interventions, such as surgery, or by prescribing chemical drugs.
- *Separation between physical and psychological aspects* of the human being. Allopathic medicine accepts only limited interaction between psychological and physical aspects. An example of an accepted interaction is the placebo effect of drugs.
- *Reductionism.* The various aspects and characteristics of the human being may be reduced to biological and material phenomena and processes. Concepts such as 'the gene' and 'the brain' are important in this respect. Normative questions are ruled outside the sphere of knowledge.[3]

While allopathic medicine was established as a hegemonic form of knowledge related to the individual body, there was an epidemiological turn in public health science whereby knowledge production had begun to focus on chronic, non-communicable diseases (NCDs) such as cardiovascular diseases and its causes, instead of contagious diseases such as cholera.[4]

The Finnish North Karelia Project of community control constitutes an interesting case in the evolving relationship between public health and medicine. The project shows how medical knowledge has been important for Nordic (and international) conceptualisations of public health – and vice versa: how the pursuit of public health has been important for the establishment of a particular form of medical knowledge.

Heralded by the World Health Organization (WHO) as a prime example of efforts to prevent non-chronic illness, the North Karelia Project became an international success story. Lasting for about a quarter of a decade, the project took place between the 1970s and the 1990s and involved public health experts mobilising an Eastern Finnish region in an effort to reduce incidents of cardiovascular disease.

On the web pages of the Finnish National Institute for Health and Welfare, an official describes the project in the following way:

> There has been a very wide international interest in the groundbreaking results and experiences of the North Karelia Project. They have been used not only in scientific cooperation but also in the health programmes of various countries and especially the WHO.[5]

In existing literature, besides being presented as an international success story, the North Karelia Project is often portrayed as progressing in a linear way from its beginning until the point in time when results are evaluated. The longer the project progressed, the more mortality rates associated with heart disease decreased in North Karelia.[6] Breaking with this conventional understanding, this chapter will place the North Karelia Project in a context of generating new meanings for the concept of public health. I show how such new meanings were generated in four phases particularly during the first decade of the project's operation. Each new phase changed the project and its relation to society. Hence, I argue that the project underwent a metamorphosis during the time it was active, rather than progressing in a linear fashion towards a predestined goal.[7] The four phases developed here are:

1. an initial phase of formulating a medical scientific understanding of the causes of cardiovascular disease;
2. acquiring administrative authority for public health experts;
3. establishing a social and ideological movement at the local level; and
4. identifying the real needs of the people.[8]

The chapter ends with some reflections on the subjects and objects of knowledge in public health at a more general level.

The Finnish 1972 Act on Public Health

Chapter 5 by Minna Harjula in this volume indicates the centrality of the concept of *kansanterveys* (public health; literally, 'people's health') in the history of the Finnish welfare state from the 1970s onwards. I argue that the North Karelia Project of community control had a fundamental role in generating new meanings for this concept from the 1970s and 1980s onwards.

The Public Health Act of 1972 was important for the North Karelia Project as it established an administrative structure, which was used in the infrastructure of the project. The opening paragraph of the Public Health Act used *kansanterveys* as a rather all-encompassing and collectivist concept:

> Public health work means health care targeted at the individual and their surroundings, individual hospital care and associated activities, the purpose of which is to maintain and enhance the well-being of the population.[9]

The Act generated a certain kind of meaning for public health work (*kansanterveystyö* in Finnish). It tells us how public health is to be achieved in practice. The Act defined health care as action aimed at affecting the population as a whole. This is a collectivist understanding of public health in terms of health care measures seen as existing not primarily for the individual citizen, but for managing the population as a whole. Hence, we might interpret an individual person's visit to a health clinic as an expression of the government's effort to direct the health behaviour of the population, rather than as an expression of the individual's choice to care for her or his health. In other words, the Public Health Act perceived individuals as being part of a whole, rather than as a group of individuals with separate identities.

The Public Health Act of 1972 establishes a bureaucratic structure for *kansanterveystyö*, i.e., the pursuit of public health in Finland. The Act defines the duties and responsibilities of various authorities at the central and local level. Paragraph 2 states that "the highest leadership, government and monitoring of public health work belongs to the Board of Medicine [*lääkintöhallitus*]", which is assigned the responsibility of producing five-year plans for the organisation of public health work. The Board of Medicine was to report directly to the Finnish government.

Under the Board of Medicine were the various Regional Boards (*lääninhallitus*) that assumed responsibility for public health work at the regional level. The local municipalities were assigned the responsibility of executing the various tasks associated with public health promotion at the local level.

Although the administrative structure described in the 1972 Act was hierarchical, local municipalities had some autonomy as they could levy their own taxes and manage their own budgets. Citizens could also run for office and vote in municipal elections. The municipal council decided on the financing and implementing of policy at the local level – not only concerning health and social care, but also regarding education, culture, sport and recreation.

The Public Health Act stated that each municipality (some of which were rather small, with only a few thousand inhabitants) should have a health care centre (*terveyskeskus*) in order to implement the tasks assigned in the law.

The North Karelia Project of community control

Phase I: Creating a medical scientific discourse

As a consequence of the Public Health Act of 1972, public health science and public administration continued to merge. The government used public health science to justify the policy reform. The new administrative structure was to improve the health of the population by putting scientific knowledge into practice. Uniform intervention at the individual level was supposed to produce beneficial results for the entire population.

The Public Health Act provided fertile soil for the subsequent North Karelia Project, which sought to tackle mortality rates and cardiovascular disease (CVD), particularly in Eastern Finland. Previous studies had established that both mortality rates and the occurrence of cardiovascular disease were higher than average in Eastern Finland, and in North Karelia in particular. Public health science had also established the risk factors of cardiovascular disease: smoking, cholesterol levels and blood pressure. Furthermore, public health science had established that certain eating habits were associated with high blood pressure and high cholesterol levels. For instance, eating greasy food containing unsaturated fats would raise the level of cholesterol in the blood, and thus increase the risk of cardiovascular disease, and, ultimately, untimely death.[10]

In the first phase of the North Karelia Project, experts demonstrated areas of knowledge that led to an understanding of the causes of chronic illness and of ways to prevent such disease. This understanding drew on previously established epidemiological knowledge about the causes of cardiovascular disease and the connections between high incidents of cardiovascular disease and mortality.

Previous research presented the project's experts with a rationale concerning mortality: smoking and eating the wrong types of food increased mortality rates of the general population. The obvious solution was to try to influence the health behaviour of men (initially) in order to reduce the risk factors of cardiovascular disease and thus mortality rates. Nordic and Western societies in general were going through a phase of social engineering and rational administrative planning in the 1970s, so it was not surprising that soon after the establishment of the Public Health Act in 1972, a community intervention project was initiated in Northern Karelia.

In 1972, prominent representatives of the North Karelia region signed a petition demanding action in order to reduce mortality rates and incidents of cardiovascular disease. This petition was important for raising the public and political awareness needed for launching a large-scale campaign aimed at community control. It was also an important discursive act that consolidated the particular construction of mortality and cardiovascular disease outlined by public health research (Figure 11.1).[11] The discursive act constructed not only a health problem but also a social problem in a particular region, and a population group – namely, men.

In this initial phase of the project, the construction of cardiovascular disease was still a neutral scientific analysis of the causes of cardiovascular disease (notwithstanding an unintended bias regarding gender and class).

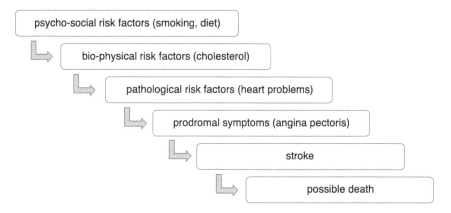

Figure 11.1 The biomedical construction of cardiovascular disease

Phase II: The establishment of administrative authority

The petition signed by the North Karelian politicians was successful, and soon the North Karelia Project of community control was initiated. Its aim was "to reduce mortality rates and incidents of disease in the entire population of North Karelia, especially concerning cardiovascular disease".[12]

Pursuing this aim, the project sought to; 1) reduce the known risks of coronary heart disease (smoking, high cholesterol, high blood pressure); and 2) establish early recognition and diagnosis of incidents of coronary heart disease, and thus effective care and rehabilitation. In practice, the project sought to increase awareness of the causes of cardiovascular disease, and indicate healthy lifestyles for the people living in the North Karelia region. The project was set up quite professionally and efficiently, with a clear organisational structure. The official status of the project was emphasised several times:

> When the National Board of Medicine in 1972 assigned the North Karelia Project the status of an official public health development programme, the local responsibility of coordinating the programme was transferred from the county council to the regional board of social and health administration.[13]

> The status of the project as an official testing and development programme of public health strengthened the participation of the health care centres in organising services and planning activities in accordance with the project's aims.[14]

Along with involving local administrations in the project, the construction of cardiovascular disease gained a double legitimation: the construction was not only scientifically but also politically and administratively legitimate. In addition to its official status, the project also made use of publicity, as one of its major objectives was to educate people about health and how it could be maintained. The experts involved in the project thought it important for the messages delivered to the general public to be simple and frequently repeated so they could be comprehended.[15]

The fact that the project used publicity in order to promote its aims indicates that those responsible for the project consciously wanted to influence not only the behaviour of people but also how they thought about themselves and their health. However, at this stage, the project was merely giving practical advice, and people could decide for themselves how to change their own behaviour:

> Communicative activities were designed in order to support the project's other interventions in order to produce lasting behavioural changes. The project's communications gave practical advice so that following such advice people themselves could start behaving in a healthier manner.[16]

Considering that during its first five operative years the project generated 1,509 articles in local newspapers, organised 251 public events and published half a million leaflets, one gets the impression that publicity was a very important aspect indeed. The people of North Karelia were strongly convinced to follow the advice generated by experts.

At the same time, the North Karelia Project appears to have been somewhat hostile to alternative constructions of cardiovascular disease:

> By increasing general communicative activities and health knowledge it was possible to prevent and to clear up many sensational pieces of news, rumours, witchcraft, etc. related to the prevention of cardiovascular disease.[17]

The project's experts, who saw themselves as representatives of public health science, sought to establish their own conception of cardiovascular disease as hegemonic. The project was obviously facing existing, traditional ways of looking at health, and it had to replace these existing forms of reasoning in order to establish its own construction of cardiovascular disease.[18] In other words, in the second phase of the project, the neutral undertone started to change. By dismissing old conceptions as 'rumours' and 'witchcraft' – i.e., unscientific by definition and therefore untrue – the project's experts tried to depoliticise their own form of knowledge.[19] Paradoxically, the political decision to grant the project official status contributed to this depoliticising.

Phase III: Creating a social and ideological movement

The project report of 1983 seems to have been conscious of an asymmetrical power relationship between experts and laymen. Instead of trying to establish symmetry, the project utilised the asymmetry in order to promote its aims. In addition to noting that 87 per cent of the North Karelian population was aware of the project in 1973,[20] the report stated that:

The sign of the North Karelia Project was made into a collective symbol. On different occasions it was reminded that it was about a popular appeal and a movement originating in the local community. The researchers clarified the background of the problem and demonstrated ways in which the population themselves could affect the matter. The aim was to establish a kind of social obligation to participate in the organised activities of the North Karelia Project.[21]

In sum, the project engaged in an interaction with its audience, further indicating that the aim was to affect the collective psyche, including unconscious or deep-seated motives and beliefs of the population. The project report describes how the researchers framed their work as neutral, and that the people themselves could decide how to react to the information presented. However, the information presented was no longer neutral: participating in project activities was presented as a social obligation. Thus, in the third phase of the project, the tension between authority and autonomy became fundamental.

Another example of this interaction was the way the project intervened in public transportation. The project distributed stickers prohibiting smoking inside buses. The stickers read: "Smoking not allowed – we are a part of the North Karelia Project."[22] The stickers conveyed the implicit message that North Karelia was the target of community control, and therefore passengers on buses should not smoke. By not smoking, people showed their (moral) commitment to the collective effort of decreasing mortality rates in North Karelia. The spirit of this kind of communication was that even death could be combated by determinate and rational collective decision-making.

In an article in the *American Journal of Public Health* those responsible for the project explained that this particular aspect of the project was a conscious effort to associate its goals with feelings of local patriotism:

> There was a conscious effort by the Project to associate the goals of the project with the pride and provincial identity of the population. People were urged to participate and to make changes not only for themselves, but for 'North Karelia'. For instance, signs reading 'Do not smoke here – we are in the North Karelia Project' were everywhere and fostered a kind of local patriotism.[23]

In 1974, the project started to cooperate with a local sausage producer (*Makkaratehdas Oy Halonen*) in the development of a new sausage, labelled 'Karelia' (*Karjala*). "Management of a local sausage factory was particularly interested in cardiovascular disease prevention after two managers suffered heart attacks."[24]

Karjala contained only 6 per cent fat, whereas other sausages on the market contained 18–20 per cent. This discursive act was also important for the project as it succeeded in connecting the positive sentiments associated with the name of the region with a sausage containing significantly less fat than others. This was in line with the aims of the project. As in the case of the no smoking signs, the goal was to associate the project's aims with feelings of provincial identity.

In addition to feelings of patriotism and fear of death, the managers presented traditional gender roles when promoting the project. They noted that in rural Finland most women occupied the traditional role of homemaker, and that adding more vegetables to the family diet might require the homemaker to change long-standing patterns.[25] Invoking traditional gender roles, the project assumed that women had a major responsibility in shaping the eating habits and in calming cigarette-craving husbands:[26]

> women were shown how potatoes and other roots can replace meat fat in soups, while still producing acceptable appearance and consistency. Guidance and feedback was presented by the course leaders as the new skills were practiced. The rest of the families were invited in the evening to enjoy the meal with them, creating good opportunities for natural reinforcement. [. . .] Wives of smokers were informed about how to deal with nervousness on the part of a recent ex-smoker and how to be patient and reinforcing as their husband learned to live without cigarettes.[27]

In sum, the third phase of the North Karelia Project was essentially about the mobilisation of the local community. In order to change people's behaviour and combat cardiovascular disease, the project engaged with the local community beyond simple education and training. The aim was to win the hearts and minds of the local population by appealing to their various identities – as Finns, Karelians and housewives – and to anticipate and suppress possible counter-arguments:

> In communicating new ideas, Project staff arranged for their messages to be disseminated from many different sources – deliberately seeking a mix which would maximize perceived credibility. Explicit endorsements were obtained from prestigious institutions such as the World Health Organization. In addition, opinion leaders from both formal and informal groups were involved. These individuals were targets of especially intense persuasive communication from respected medical and other experts. [. . .] The content of the messages was carefully constructed to anticipate and suppress counter-arguments. . . . messages . . . pointed out that one of the most famous distance runners from Finland, H. Kolemainen, was a vegetarian.[28]

Phase IV: Identifying the real needs of the people

In its fourth phase, the project expands on the previous phases. This phase occurred when the project was complete and its results evaluated.[29] Central to the fourth phase was a distinction between the real needs of the population and those experienced by the lay people themselves:

> It was central to direct the measures in such a way that they would result in the best possible outcome for the entire community. The population's real needs, as estimated by epidemiological knowledge, were defined as foundation of

the measures, instead of the needs experienced by the health care centres or those patients seeking advice from those centres.[30]

The fourth phase completes the metamorphosis of the project during its formative period between 1972 and 1983. The project almost abandons the ideal of neutrality as the experts take on the responsibility of identifying people's real needs.

Two features characterise the fourth phase of the North Karelia Project. First, it builds on the previous three phases. The medical discourse on cardiovascular disease (i), the administrative structure (ii) and the ideological movement (iii) were all needed in order to successfully identify the real needs of the people (iv).

Second, the fourth phase was qualitatively different from the first three phases. It established a hierarchical power relationship between experts and lay people. In this phase, the experts judged the *experience* of people inferior to their knowledge. In other words, whatever people may say about their own health is always less important than what the scientist or the expert says.

In retrospect, in 1983, those responsible for the North Karelia Project could state that "the programme had the desired implications for changing the health behaviour of the population" and that mortality rates associated with cardiovascular disease had decreased. They also noted the national benefits the project had produced and the international attention it had received.[31]

From the project's own perspective, its initial period in 1972–1977 was successful. The project constructed a notion of health that it sought to consolidate by appropriate communicative action. It also defined what improvement in health at the collective level might mean. It carried out an intervention accordingly and established a distinction between real and perceived health needs.

The organisers of the North Karelia Project concluded that the simple distribution of information about healthy lifestyles was not enough, but that intervention aiming at health promotion should seek ways to change the population's health behaviour:

> We are products of our environment, but we can change our environment through concerted action. Thus, we may be held collectively responsible for public health, and we must learn to use our political system more effectively to create a favorable environment for all segments of society if we hope to limit the current burden of illness. Efforts to persuade those whose options are limited and whose values are distorted by economic and social problems to accept responsibility for their own health may be futile. Yet many public health activists seeking basic social or economic change are acutely aware of the difficulty of winning popular support for their views and recommendations.[32]

This quotation takes up the issue of self-reflexivity. The authors talk about 'we', but they do not reflect upon their own role as part of this 'we'. Do they see themselves as part of the collective responsible for public health? Are they acting on behalf of "those whose options are limited and whose values are distorted"?

Or do they see themselves as public health experts who possess the knowledge about healthy life? Are these roles compatible with each other?

The experts in the North Karelia Project were also aware of the fact that part of the authority of medical experts comes from the management of anxiety and the fear of death. The project presented the risk of death and hazardous life-styles and the managers were aware that this might cause anxiety among the population. However, they did not detect such anxiety.[33]

In conclusion, the managers thought that the project was fairly successful. In 1982 they felt that the project was "a promising case study rather than a critical test of the effects of health promotion" and that further studies were needed.[34]

McAlister et al. also made an interesting remark concerning cultural differences and health promotion. They think that Finns are more likely to trust public authorities than people in the US, for instance:

> There are critical differences between the Finnish and North American cultures that probably make health promotion easier to implement in Finland. United States citizens do not uniformly perceive governmental agencies as credible sources of information, whereas Finns are generally more willing to accept public recommendations and to cooperate with community health workers. Thus, public health interests in Finland find it easier to regulate promotion and marketing of products such as tobacco and cigarettes. ... Cultural acceptance of the notion that health is a public responsibility in Finland facilitates perception of the wisdom of shifting investments toward the prevention of disease.[35]

Other medical experts contested at least some of the truth claims made by those responsible for the North Karelia Project. In the *American Journal of Public Health* Edward H. Wagner (MD, MPH) noted that cardiovascular disease mortality rates and risk factor prevalence had been declining in many parts of the developed world during the time of the project. He raised the question: "can we justify intervening on an improving patient?"[36] Wagner was raising here the question of whether community level intervention was necessary at all if incidents of cardiovascular disease were declining in any case. He did not, however, question the overall rationale of the North Karelia Project.

Wagner also highlighted some of the controversies of targeting an entire community of people. He said that cardiovascular disease was conceptualised as a community problem related to the life-style of the region rather than to that of a particular group of people. He also noted this was a radically different approach compared to most of the major clinical trials of cardiovascular disease prevention, which typically focus on what he termed "individual high-risk subjects". According to Wagner, "community-oriented interventions require broad political support and public financing and may be viewed by some as impinging on individual freedom".[37]

In the same issue of the *American Journal of Public Health*, Donald M. Klos and Irwin M. Rosenstock contested the truth claims made by the North Karelia Project. They noted that there was no evidence that dietary advice given by the project was received, understood or followed.[38] They also noted that it was possible that, by observing a reduction of risk factors of cardiovascular disease, the North Karelia Project had in fact merely observed a trend that had started already before the project – rather than observing effects caused by it.[39] This observation challenged the interventionist strategy and its effects on the local community.

The impact of the North Karelia Project

The North Karelia Project is significant for the conceptual history of Finnish public health in two ways. First, it contributed to establishing distinct forms of knowledge that were associated with the Finnish (and possibly also Scandinavian and English) use of *kansanterveys*. Actors important for the history of public health operated within the structures created by this project.

Second, it is also a significant event in the dynamic and ongoing construction of the archetypical forms of knowledge associated with *kansanterveys*. To give a few examples, still in 2017 the WHO promoted the North Karelia Project by highlighting it as one of the first two settings for the first real community intervention programme, whose goal was "to bring about social and health oriented behavioural changes". According to the WHO, "the population risk factor levels have greatly reduced", and mortality rates decreased between 1970 and 1995 in North Karelia.[40]

One of the most crucial background assumptions of the North Karelia Project (in line with the background assumptions of allopathic medicine outlined above) was a clear distinction between physical and mental health. Coronary heart disease and mortality were only discussed as matters of physical health. Of course, psychosocial risk factors (e.g. eating habits) were seen as important, but such factors were important because the wrong physical food items entered the physical body (if one reconstructs the logic to some extent). The project thus did not, for instance, consider the option that a person might be depressed and therefore eat the wrong kind of food. Such a consideration might have led to a completely different intervention.[41]

Psychological factors were indeed central to an interpretation of the causes of cardiovascular disease that became popular in the US. In the 1950s, American cardiologists identified a masculine behaviour pattern, which they labelled 'Type A man'. This pattern of behaviour was associated with competitiveness, and with an inclination to work to deadlines and a struggle to achieve more and more in less and less time. An interpretation which traced the causes of heart attack and cardiovascular disease to 'Type A man' became popular in the US. The Type A hypothesis was, however, declared scientifically invalid in the 1980s.[42]

What is crucial for the form of knowledge that the North Karelia Project represents is the construction of cardiovascular disease referred to earlier in Figure 11.1. This construction gave rise to an authoritative narrative that served as a framework for individual life-stories in order to create uniformity where there was complexity. Presentations such as the one by the WHO referred to above reinforce and reproduce the construction of cardiovascular disease and, consequently, the form of knowledge associated with the North Karelia Project.[43]

Furthermore, such presentations consolidate the particular forms of knowledge in question as fundamental parts of a collective understanding of (and language around) public health (internationally) and *kansanterveys/folkhälsa* in the Finnish and Scandinavian contexts.

In the Finnish context, the North Karelia Project was important for the evolution of public health science (subsequently labelled *kansanterveystiede*). The Finnish-language textbook on *kansanterveystiede*, published in 1994, consolidated the construction of cardiovascular disease by stating that half of all people living in 'rich countries' die of cardiovascular disease, and that 600,000 Finns (more than 10 per cent of the population at the time) suffer from cardiovascular disease.[44] The textbook thus presents CVD as the prime example of *kansanterveysongelma* (a public health problem). Furthermore, it devotes six pages to a description of the North Karelia Project, stating for instance that at the beginning of the 1970s "the entire Finnish society was struck by the serious public health problem of cardiovascular disease" and that North Karelia was hit particularly hard. However, the project produced valuable experiences for the WHO and the rest of the world. The book also noted that the project was awarded the WHO's health education award in 1991.[45]

An important condition for the North Karelia Project, and hence for the subsequent Finnish conceptualisation of *kansanterveys*, was the tight connection between biomedicine, the medical profession and public health administration. In practice, the Public Health Act of 1972 helped the North Karelia Project mobilise a large group of publicly employed professional physicians for the work of preventing cardiovascular disease. Public health and biomedicine entered into a kind of symbiosis where public health was dependent on professional physicians for the implementation of goals, and professional physicians were able to consolidate their dominant form of knowledge (allopathic medicine) with the support of public administration and public funding.

Again, the contrast with the US is striking. In the US, the medical profession and public health administration have traditionally been separate from each other, at least in comparison with the Nordic countries and Finland. They have not merged in the same way as they did in Finland after the North Karelia Project.[46]

Subject and object of knowledge, subjectivation and objectivation of people

In sum, one of the most important results of the North Karelia Project was the establishment of forms of knowledge, i.e. rules concerning how knowledge should be expressed and organised systematically. In doing so, the project's representatives participated in a process where the object of knowledge was constructed.

There is a sense in which the object of knowledge in public health science (and other sciences as well) is linguistically constructed. And according to the prevailing forms of knowledge this object is at the most merely an aspect of the human being: the human being and the human body (and even aspects of the physical body); the human being as a member of a community; the psyche of the human being, etc.

When this kind of knowledge is connected with public administration, the result is a distinct process of subjectivation.[47] Once the object of knowledge is created (as in the case of the North Karelia Project, for instance), people start to adjust their behaviour in accordance with these objects and the way they are represented in public (scientific and political) discourse. Cardiovascular disease (or coronary heart disease) is only one of countless diagnoses in medical science, each of which has its own logic but each of which roughly corresponds to the form of knowledge associated with the construction of cardiovascular disease. Medical diagnoses, for example of cardiovascular diseases, capture people's imagination because they get mixed with the fear of death every human being is prone to.

This is thus one aspect of the object the medical sciences, public health sciences and the discourse around *folkhälsa* has created: human beings may be controlled, and positions of authority among human beings may be established by management of the fear of death (or, conversely, the hope of prolonged life).[48]

Another aspect of this object is that psychological and physical aspects of the human being are strictly distinguished from each other. This distinction, of course, originates in the Cartesian distinction of mind and body (subject and object), but it developed when the disciplines of medicine and psychology evolved into different branches of science. The analysis above shows that the whole discourse around the concept of *kansanterveys* – at least in 1970s' Finland – centred on the assumption that the physical and psychological aspects of the human being are distinct from each other.[49]

A third aspect of the object established by medical science (and the politics of public health) is the effort to establish normality where there is pathology. In terms of the object of knowledge (the human being), what is important is that the human being is made attentive towards cultural images and expectations concerning normality, and that such expectations are presented as desirable so that they create uniformity where there is plurality.

Such efforts work in the following way: in the case of cardiovascular disease, for instance, certain symptoms are defined as fulfilling the criteria of a diagnosis of coronary heart disease. This diagnosis indicates a pathological state which must be normalised.[50] Normalisation may occur, for instance, by a change in eating habits. And, at least in Finland in the 1970s and 1980s, this change in eating habits occurred for the sake of the local community and the entire national community. Thinking about the object established by this sort of activity, one comes to think of the human being as lacking a distinct personal identity – or the capacity to establish such an identity. And this is important because, true or not, the process whereby people constructed their identities was governed in accordance with this constructed object.

At the same time, despite the various constructions of the object of knowledge and despite the ways in which this object is used for governance, and in order to establish hierarchies, the human being has remained somewhat of a mystery. We still do not seem to know very much about the human being as a whole, in all its complexity. This may be because we have thus far not been able to observe ourselves in relation to others.

Notes

1 For a survey of different medical schools of thought, including numbers of associated medical schools in the US, see Elianne Riska, *Power, Politics and Health: Forces Shaping American Medicine* (Helsinki: Finnish Society of Sciences and Letters, 1985), 19.

2 Ibid., 32; Paul Starr, *The Social Transformation of American Medicine: The rise of a sovereign profession and the making of a vast industry* (New York: Basic Books, 1982), 118.

3 This list is not exhaustive, and is intended only to provide a general picture of allopathic medicine (sometimes also referred to as biomedicine or scientific medicine). The background assumptions of hegemonic forms of knowledge, despite being subject to historical change, are seldom discussed or questioned – precisely because they are hegemonic and equated with 'science'. The foundations and grounds for generally accepted knowledge claims in allopathic medicine have evolved throughout history and constitute an interesting subject for study from the perspective of conceptual history. Generally speaking, allopathic medicine rests on a naturalist philosophy regarding the way it looks at the human being. On naturalism, see e.g. Willard Van Orman Quine, *Theories and Things* (Cambridge, MA: Harvard University Press, 1981).

4 Allan M. Brandt and Martha Gardner, 'Antagonism and accommodation: Interpreting the relationship between public health and medicine in the United States during the 20th century', *American Journal of Public Health* 90, no. 5 (2000): 707–15, 711.

5 Terveyden ja hyvinvoinnin laitos [Institute for Health and Welfare], 'Pohjois-Karjala projekti muutti terveysnäkymiä Suomessa ja maailmalla' [The North Karelia Project transformed health outlooks in Finland and worldwide] (Helsinki: THL, 2017), www. thl.fi/fi/-/pohjois-karjala-projekti-muutti-terveysnakymia-suomessa-ja-maailmalla (accessed 28 Aug 2017).

6 See e.g. Pekka Puska, 'Why did North Karelia-Finland work? Is it transferrable [*sic*]?', *Global Heart* 11, no. 4 (2016): 387–91; Pekka Puska, E. Vartiainen, T. Laatikainen and P. Jousilahti, eds, *The North Karelia Project: From North Karelia to National Action* (Helsinki: National Institute for Health and Welfare, 2009); Pekka Puska, 'Successful prevention of non-communicable diseases: 25 year experiences with North Karelia Project in Finland', *Public Health Medicine* 4, no. 1 (2002): 5–7. For sociological analyses of the project, see Mikko Jauho, 'Contesting lifestyle risk and gendering coronary candidacy: Lay epidemiology of heart disease in Finland in the 1970s', *Sociology of Health and Illness*, doi: 10.1111/1467-9566.12542 [e-pub ahead of print]; Mikko Jauho, '"Give people work, and the blood pressure will sink": Lay engagement with cardiovascular risk factors in North Karelia in the 1970s', *Health, Risk and Society* 18, s1–2, 21–37.

7 The idea of linear progression is contradicted by the fact that the North Karelia Project was a victim of its own success. It was extended many times, and the Finnish National Archives contain newspaper articles associated with the project collected between 1971 and 1997. In other words, it was not initially planned as a project that would last for more than 25 years.

8 I would like to acknowledge the helpful suggestion by Ulla-Britta Broman-Kananen when developing the interpretation about these four phases.

9 Parliament of Finland, Public Health Act 66/1972, §1 (my translation).

10 See also HE 98/1971. *Hallituksen esitys Eduskunnalle kansanterveystyöstä ja sen voimaanpanosta annettaviksi laeiksi* [Government bill for Parliament about Public Health Work and the Laws concerning its Implementation] (Helsinki: Government of Finland, 1972), 1.

11 Figure 11.1 is adapted from Pekka Puska et al., *Pohjois-Karjala-projekti: Pohjois-Karjalan läänissä vuosina 1971-1977 toteutetun yhteisötason sydän- ja verisuonitautien torjuntaohjelman kuvaus ja keskeiset tulokset* (Helsinki: Lääkintöhallitus, 1983), 27.

The report does not mention possible death as the cause of stroke, but instead speaks of a rehabilitation process. I think, however, that death as a possible outcome is an important element of the construction of cardiovascular disease. More specifically, the construction gains its potential power from the (conscious or unconscious) fear of death people may have.

12   Puska et al., *Pohjois-Karjala-projekti*, 17.

13   Ibid., 36.

14   Ibid., 38.

15   Alfred McAlister, Pekka Puska, Jukka T. Salonen, Jarkko Tuomilehto and Kaj Koskela, 'Theory and action for health promotion: Illustrations from the North Karelia Project', *American Journal of Public Health* 72, no. 1 (1982): 43–50, 44.

16   Puska et al., *Pohjois-Karjala-projekti*, 42.

17   Ibid.

18   Marja-Liisa Honkasalo's research illuminates traditional ways of understanding heart disease in North Karelia, as well as experiences of disease and illness at the local level. See e.g. Marja-Liisa Honkasalo, *Reikä sydämessä: Sairaus Pohjois-karjalaisessa maisemassa* (Tampere: Vastapaino, 2008).

19   Also see Chapter 7 by Sophy Bergenheim in this volume, where she presents a similar attempt at depoliticising racial hygiene/hereditary hygiene in the 1940s.

20   Puska et al., *Pohjois-Karjala-projekti*, 57.

21   Ibid., 20.

22   Ibid., 90.

23   McAlister et al., 'Theory and action', 46.

24   Ibid., 47.

25   Ibid., 46.

26   See also Elianne Riska, 'Sukupuoli [Gender]', in *Sosiaaliepidemiologia: Väestön terveyserot ja terveyteen vaikuttavat sosiaaliset tekijät*, ed. Mikko Laaksonen and Karri Silventoinen (Helsinki: Gaudeamus, 2011), 60–72, 64. For an analysis of gender and coronary heart disease, see Elianne Riska, *Masculinity and Men's Health: Coronary Heart Disease in Medical and Public Discourse* (Lanham, MD: Rowman & Littlefield, 2004).

27   McAlister et al, 'Theory and action', 46.

28   Ibid., 45.

29   As noted earlier, the project was to be extended after its first evaluation in the early 1980s.

30   Puska et al., *Pohjois-Karjala-projekti*, 21.

31   Ibid., 239–41. The report states, however, that the decreases in mortality were not necessarily due to the North Karelia Project.

32   McAlister et al., 'Theory and action', 45.

33   Ibid.

34   Ibid., 49.

35   Ibid.

36   Edward H. Wagner, 'The North Karelia Project: What it tells us about the prevention of cardiovascular disease', *American Journal of Public Health* 72, no. 1 (1982): 51–3, 52.

37   Ibid.

38   Donald M. Klos and Irwin M. Rosenstock, 'Some lessons from the North Karelia Project', *American Journal of Public Health* 72, no. 1 (1982): 53–4, 54.

39   Ibid.

40   WHO, 'Chronic diseases and health promotion', www.who.int/chp/about/integrated_ cd/en/index2.html (accessed 28 Aug 2017).

41   The assumption of a strict distinction between physical and mental health was contested in 1979 by medical sociologist Aaron Antonovsky in his book *Health, Stress and Coping* (San Francisco: Jossey-Bass, 1979), where he challenged the medical scientific way of focusing on pathologies, and instead introduced the concept of 'salutogenesis'.

Antonovsky was more interested in what makes people stay healthy rather than risk factors of disease. He operated with a more holistic understanding of health compared to the assumptions of the North Karelia Project and compared to the characteristics of allopathic medicine listed at the beginning of this chapter.

42 Elianne Riska, 'Gender and medicalization and biomedicalisation theories', in *Biomedicalisation: Technoscience, Health, and Illness in the US*, ed. Adele E. Clarke, Laura Mamo, Jennifer Ruth Fosket, Jennifer R. Fishman and Janet K. Shim (Durham, NC: Duke University Press, 2010), 147–72, 157–8.

43 In 2017 the English-language Wikipedia page for North Karelia stated that "North Karelia is renowned among public health officials." It referred, obviously, to the North Karelia Project. Wikipedia, 'North Karelia', https://en.wikipedia.org/wiki/North_Karelia (accessed 28 Aug 2017).

44 Aulikki Nissinen, Jussi Kauhanen and Markku Myllykangas, *Kansanterveystiede* (Helsinki: WSOY, 1994), 223.

45 Ibid., 333, 337.

46 Brandt and Gardner, 'Antagonism and accommodation'.

47 On subjectivation, see also Michel Foucault, *The Order of Things: Archaeology of the Human Sciences* (London: Routledge, 2001) and Nikolas Rose, *The Politics of Life Itself: Biomedicine, Power, and Subjectivity in the Twenty-First Century* (Princeton: Princeton University Press, 2006).

48 See also Chapter 12 by Helena Tolvhed and Outi Hakola in this volume.

49 Nikolas Rose has shown how notions of the relationship between mind and body are changing as scientific knowledge changes. Most recently, the phenomenon termed 'biomedicalisation' by some scholars has reshaped our understanding of the relationship between mind and body. See Rose, *Politics of Life Itself*.

50 As noted in the characterisation of allopathic medicine at the beginning of the chapter.

12 The individualisation of health in late modernity

Helena Tolvhed and Outi Hakola

Introduction

The maintenance of a healthy population has been a major goal for social and welfare policies in the Nordic countries. During the twentieth century, the health status of the individual was not considered a strictly private concern, but part of the general collective capital, and medical expertise and research had important roles in constructing notions of societal development.[1] In the late twentieth century, however, the emphasis on consumption and individual expression was followed by an individualisation of health. The prevention of illness has increasingly come to be understood as the responsibility of each individual citizen rather than that of the state, and lifestyle management has replaced traditional structural and economic explanations of public health concerns.[2] However, this emphasis on illness prevention and individual responsibility for one's own health is not entirely new for the post-1970 society; as Karin Johannisson has pointed out, the Swedish welfare state presupposed and relied on the efforts of individuals to improve their own health, and was built to support and facilitate these efforts.[3] The individualisation of health is a general development in the Western world, but in the Nordic countries it has fundamentally changed the logic of the welfare state at an ideological level. During the last decades, the state-run Swedish and Finnish public health regimes, which had close ties to the national sports movements, have been supplemented and partly replaced by a commercial health and fitness industry whose agenda is largely set by private operators. This industry includes a booming market for health and training magazines, as well as internet forums, taking over the role as primary advisor and regulator on health maintenance. This development means that health is increasingly managed without the government's involvement.

In this chapter, we study new norms and discourses in health management, and the meanings related to it, through Swedish health and fitness magazines and periodicals and Finnish tabloid health journalism. Central to the methodology is the comparison of representations and the ways in which the reader is addressed. When analysing and scrutinising representations and values related to health, we give special attention to gender issues, since men and women have faced rather different expectations. Late modernity introduced new gender ideals in the form of the physically active and well-trained female, as well as the appearance-oriented man. For women, this stands in stark contrast to a history where modern sports during the nineteenth and well into the twentieth century were often considered incompatible with conceptions of respectable femininity. Women were warned of the physically and mentally harmful and masculinising effects of sport and strenuous physical activities.[4] In today's field of health and fitness, however, women no doubt occupy a central position as subjects/consumers. Hence, gender needs to be taken into account when analysing how the media constructs, normalises and challenges different understandings of health.

An interest in health and diet is far from new. Likewise, prescriptions of body management and diet and its association with moral life have existed for a long time. What is new, we suggest, is the extent to which this is part of popular and commercial culture in a neoliberal economy targeting the individual consumer. We will illustrate how health journalism in Sweden and Finland reflects Western processes of individualisation, commercialisation, feminisation and de-politicisation of health. The impact of this is underlined by the growth of the health and training magazine market (including supplements in tabloids), and later on social media (from the 1980s onwards), with more and more niches and titles on the market.[5] Our analysis of the individualisation of health is framed by the concept of 'healthism', which is discussed in relation to changes in power relations and citizenship.

'Healthism' and bio-politics in late modernity

Robert Crawford has identified an ideology of 'healthism' – where health and a fit body are lifestyle markers and metaphors for morality and a good life in late modern society. Subjects are constructed as autonomous agents responsible for their own wellbeing, without considering social and economic determinants. Health has, according to Crawford, become a "super value", implicating not only the absence of sickness but also happiness, sense of self, ability to function and productivity.[6]

The concept of healthism can be connected to Michel Foucault's theoretical concept of bio-politics, a regulating regime where human life is managed through knowledge and power, and the related processes of subjectivity.[7] Foucault argued that the character of bio-politics changed during the twentieth century, from the disciplinary regimes of families, hospitals, schools and factories towards more sophisticated techniques of governing. In late modern consumer culture, power primarily works through stimulation and internalised self-monitoring, influencing the way people think, feel and perceive.[8]

Late modern governance, hence, works not through the imposing of constraints but through shaping a citizen capable of exercising regulated freedom – conceptualised as 'free choice'. Here, subjects actively participate in the process of governance. In the new modes of regulating health, individuals are addressed on the assumption that they *want to be healthy*, not least due to the synonymous use of healthiness and happiness, and enjoined to seek out the ways of living most likely to promote their own health. Experts instruct us on how to be healthy, advertisers picture the appropriate actions and fulfilments, and entrepreneurs develop a market for health.[9]

The concept of 'free choice' has been central in the rise of neoliberalism since the mid-1970s.[10] An underlying assumption within the 'healthist paradigm' is that illness is (largely) preventable and that individuals have a choice in matters of health.[11] Whereas the 'healthy' body is perceived as a reflection of self-control and a 'healthy' inner world of the subject, the 'unhealthy' body is read as a moral and aesthetic personal failure.[12] The body is constructed as a project, in need of constant maintenance and open to reconstruction and improvement – it is forever unfinished.[13] With the increasing demand for self-management, critical voices in public debate have noted a growing 'health stress' and body fixation, and question a development where an employee's health becomes a concern for employers and a means to compete in today's "flexible labour market".[14]

Self-management and individualisation of training have been connected to a more general individualisation of Western culture.[15] Since the 1970s, alternatives to the traditional sport movements have emerged: jogging/running and exercising in gyms have transformed from rather marginal phenomena into being part of everyday culture.[16] Late modern physical culture is individualist and social interaction, even in gym classes, is often limited.[17] New forms of exercise, body treatments, diets and wellbeing strategies appear constantly, and health coaches and personal trainers are growing professions. This expanding market includes health media – magazines, newspapers and online media – that circulate the latest ideas of diet and exercise, news of health-related studies and changing trends in well-being. The number of niches seems to keep growing constantly: for different kinds of diets and 'healthy eating', yoga, triathlons or weight-training, running for women over 40 and so on. Athletes and various celebrities publish books and talk on television shows about their healthy living and give their best exercise tips.

Offering advice on how to live, eat and exercise, the health media are useful sources in order to capture a broader discourse on health. In its own way, the health media participates in Foucauldian bio-politics and rationalisation of social power by addressing citizens who are supposed to use the available information for their own best interests.[18] In this chapter, we approach the changing social values and politics of health and healthism as cultural processes where the media is regarded as a co-creator of reality and of human identities.[19] We will start our analysis from Swedish health magazines, and continue with Finnish tabloids before turning to a discussion on gender and health.

The Swedish *Journal of Health* 1960–2010

Tidskrift för Hälsa (*Journal of Health*, 1940–present) is the oldest extant Swedish periodical specifically dealing with the subject of health.[20] It was the only magazine on the Swedish market directed at the general public focusing on the subject of healthy living until the introduction of *iForm* in 1987.[21] The analysis here is based on the volumes from the years 1960, 1970, 1980, 1990, 2000 and 2010.

In the volumes of 1960 and 1970, *Tidskrift för Hälsa* takes a firm position on threats to the individual's health as well as to society as a whole. Health was to be achieved through natural living and diet, and the magazine favoured bio-dynamic and organic farming, eating raw vegetables and wholegrain food, animal protection, alternative medicine, hiking and gymnastics. Articles and editorials argue against environmental toxins and chemicals, artificial sweeteners, sugar, fluoride, nuclear power, processed food, war, tobacco, alcohol and world famine.[22] The covers show pictures of natural scenery, photos of children or health movement profiles. The indigenous people's way of life, and at times also the Vikings and 'Eastern wisdom', is idealised and used for critiquing modern society's materialism, shallowness and environmental degradation. Industrial meat and egg production is regarded as both morally wrong and wasteful of resources.[23] Critique of the consequences of the global market economy is also voiced; for example, an article from 1970 demonstrates the headline "Everything we don't need is available to buy",[24] and an editorial against nuclear power critiques "short-sighted economic interests".[25]

Hence, in 1960 and 1970, readers were addressed as a kind of vanguard group of the 'health conscious', urged to take action and lead the way for a general reform and betterment of the Swedish population. Concepts such as 'people' (*folk*), 'public/people's health' (*folkhälsa*) or 'the health standard' (*hälsonivå*) of the population are commonly referred to in the articles. Editorials recommend readers to arrange marches and other activities for the general public, and sports activities in order to make youth interested in health promotion.[26] Hence, a message of the responsibility for one's own individual health was clear, but the ultimate cause and goal was wider: a national – and by extension global – reform of the people.

In the journal's 1980 editions, the cover photographs have changed completely, with the majority now showing only food. The covers hence reflect a shift towards consumer advice, and away from social and political commentary and critique; articles commenting on society, economy and environment have now almost disappeared.[27] *Journal of Health* had adopted a narrower focus on healthy eating, presenting the nutritional value of different foods as well as the occurrence and dangers of food additives and preservatives. Articles on how to cure various forms of disease with the right diet are frequent. The cover pages exhibit short quotes with an urging and direct reader address: "End your bad habits", "How to treat stomach pains", "How to handle you back", "How to get better sleep", "The best diet from morning to evening". From a previous broad definition of health, embedded in a social and political context, the journal's focus had moved towards the management of individual health.

Journal of Health 1990 (now called just *Health*) featured another noticeable change: a strong focus on weight-loss, and the use of smiling, posing and slim female models for most of the cover photos (face or full/part body), making it look similar to general women's magazines. The first issue shows a jumping model holding the waistband of her trousers, which are obviously too big for her. The main headline reads "The ten best ways to slim down".[28] Other examples of main headlines on the covers of this volume are "Become slim without dieting", "Great shape after 40" and "Lose weight without dieting". Calories and 'slim food' are also in focus in the recipes section – it seems that slim now equals healthy. Like in 1980, health is constructed as a de-contextualised and de-politicised phenomenon; the content is oriented towards prescribing ways for the individual care of one's own body. The trimmed (female) body has now emerged as the prime manifestation of health. Health is now understood as an individual responsibility as well as a feminised field.[29]

The use of female – slim, smiling and usually white – models on the cover photos persists in the magazine's volumes of 2000 and 2010. The focus is on healthy food, but also on alternative medicine and therapies, together with mental balance and stress relief methods such as meditation. Alternative medicine and 'mainstream' medicine are presented as complementary, and there is no mentioning of any conflict between the two fields. The content is more explicitly feminised, with sections advising on nail, skin and hair care. Like in the 1960 and 1970 volumes, the magazine recommends natural and ecological products and food without additives, but there are no longer any references to global political and economic conditions or structures impacting on health. Weight loss and weight maintenance are represented as central aspects of health, and exercise has become a more important theme.

The urging way of addressing the reader and the imperative to change one's behaviour is continuously present in *Journal of Health* during the studied time period. However, from 1980 onwards, the focus shifts from changing the world to perspectives on how to take care of one's own body and avoid hazards to personal health. The organic view of human beings as part of a world society and the ecosystem is replaced by exclusive attention to the individual body. This implies disconnecting from social and political contexts; these no longer appear relevant to the conceptualisation of health. The shift is also underlined by the fact that we are dealing with a commercially viable genre, with new magazines starting up during the 1980s, 1990s and 2000s. In *Journal of Health*'s volumes from 1960 and 1970, the reader is urged to see maintaining their own fitness and health as a duty of citizenship, one which would benefit both the nation and humanity. The focus shifts from social citizenship with obligations deriving from membership of a collective body to an individualistic discourse emphasising personal gains and making informed consumer choices.[30] As Wendy Brown has formulated in discussing the 'post-political' state: "The model neo-liberal citizen is one who strategizes for her/himself among various social, political and economic options, not one who strives with others to alter or organize these options."[31]

Finnish tabloids 2010–2016

In the 1980s and 1990s, ideas of individualism and the rise of neo-liberalism slowly emerged in Finland as well. State documents and reports that had previously emphasised the nation's role in active social politics began addressing individuals as subjects involved in a constant process of developing themselves, similarly to self-help literature.[32] At the same time, health-inspired rhetoric appeared in Finnish magazines in the 1980s and, in the 1990s, consumerism increased its importance. Earlier values of community and shared responsibility were at least partially replaced when the discussion moved towards personal choices in the fields of health, diet and exercise.[33] Yet, even in contemporary Finnish popular media, state or community responsibility and individual responsibility continue to coexist. Pertti Suhonen, for example, argues that health as a value has increasing importance in Finnish culture and society. This is reflected not only in people's beliefs, but also in the increasing amount of official health education, health marketing and health communication.[34]

In the following, health journalism in contemporary Finnish tabloids *Ilta-Sanomat* and *Iltalehti* is analysed through "wellbeing and health" articles published between 2010 and 2016. The focus is on health discussions involving mortality. Mortality rate[35] and life expectancy[36] are ways to compare the state of health between nations, and they may be regarded as proxies for quality of life, social equality and peace. Thus, when a newspaper article dealing with health chooses to emphasise the quantifiable mortality rate, national success is related to personal health, and personal health becomes a social concern as well. This practice exemplifies what Nikolas Rose and Carlos Novas refer to as 'biological citizenship'. Late modern citizens are made aware of and evaluated according to their biological conditions, including both medical conditions and vitality, such as health and exercise.[37] Thus, the citizens' responsibility is to actively shape their lives through acts of choice.

An individual's health and wellbeing is not just about having or giving the right kind of information; it is also about emotions, experiences and a sense of self. Health-related articles in *Ilta-Sanomat* and *Iltalehti* indeed emphasise the importance of choice, underlined by addressing the reader directly as 'you' – your health, your actions. They also address the readers through two main types of discourse. The first, and more common one, is threat: the articles provide information on unhealthy habits such as smoking or immobility. This approach invokes the reader to feel guilty about their lifestyle choices by emphasising negative effects.[38] For example, in a story about the dangers of being overweight, *Ilta-Sanomat* proclaims "The harsh truth: all extra weight shortens life-span", and continues to list negative consequences such as diabetes, cancers, heart problems, etc.[39]

The other strategy to address readers relies on hope: the articles provide information on how some habits make you healthy, and encourage the reader to continue, or in some cases to acquire, these habits. For example, *Ilta-Sanomat* greets its audiences with: "Good news! A couple of hours of weekly exercise is enough to increase life expectancy."[40] This hopeful strategy assumes the reader actively seeks to increase their own wellness, health and quality of life. Sometimes articles are also open to different kinds of interpretation – the readers can think of the same story as educational or as showing a way to a good and happy life.

In tabloid journalism, threats and hopes alike are backed by information, expert commentary and scientific facts. The difference to openly commercial magazines can be explained by different understandings of journalism – magazines publish stories, whereas tabloids define their articles as 'news'. Thus, sources are of importance. Ulla Järvi has identified three styles of argumentation in Finnish health communication: scientific argumentation built on research; economic reasoning regarding the costs of unhealthy lifestyles to society; and human argumentation based on our consciousness of mortality.[41] The Finnish tabloids utilise these health communication strategies, in particular the scientific approach (many health stories refer to scientific research, statistics or the expertise of doctors or researchers). The economic communication strategy is the rarest form, although sometimes health care costs are presented as the amount of taxpayers' money spent on health care, and especially on health issues that could have been minimised by different lifestyle choices or preventive practices.[42] The third argumentation type, human interest, is reflected in stories based on personal experience, such as testimonials about how 'I' lost weight or quit smoking. The human argumentation utilises people's fear of dying, pain, sickness and loss of autonomy by playing with threats and hope in an intimate fashion. Human argumentation also plays with beauty ideals that add to questions of vitality and wellbeing. For example, when discussing the dangers of sunbathing, *Ilta-Sanomat* reminds its readers about the paradoxes of mixed beauty ideals – beautiful tanned skin leads to undesired wrinkles in older age.[43] Here, fitness and beauty support the mortality strategy to create an image of desirable life.

Analysing the articles that use mortality as a narrative strategy, two major issues become apparent. First of all, in these articles, health is understood in a wide sense. It is related to lifestyles, whereas illnesses are framed as consequences of undesired individual choices. The wellness section of the tabloids, unsurprisingly, deals with nutrition, weight issues and exercise, and addictive habits such as drinking alcohol or coffee, using drugs or smoking. Yet, the stories also include other issues. Wellbeing can be achieved by owning a dog, getting married, being social and active, or by winning a Nobel Prize. Individual choices have indeed become part of healthism. The most varied aspects of life can be understood in terms of health. The self-management of one's health and wellness is represented as a condition for high quality of long life. In a sense, the articles convert social norms into personal desires – setting the cultural agenda and shaping human subjectivity in a context of a consumer society.

Secondly, mortality is used in the context of calculative measures. The articles sometimes count the years certain habits either give or take from one's life. Finnish tabloids, for instance, have observed how childhood obesity threatens increasing life expectancies in Western countries,[44] how four lifestyle changes give ten more years to over-65-year-olds,[45] and how a firm handshake increases the lifespan.[46] Also, several articles include tests in a spirit of participatory health communication: with the help of questionnaires or activities, readers can calculate their own life expectancy and test the sustainability of their lifestyle choices. These articles suggest that the success of health management can be measured in terms of an increase in life expectancy and the length of a potentially productive working career.

Although the information about life expectancy can be useful for 'shopping' between lifestyles, this argumentation style is also related to public health. Alan

Petersen and Deborah Lupton have argued that, already since the nineteenth century, public health projects have relied upon "'scientific' and 'rational' methods of monitoring, measuring and regulating the population".[47] This bio-political strategy focuses more on risk groups than individuals, and uses biostatistics, such as life expectancy statistics, to create an idea of factual or objective information.[48] Similarly, Finnish tabloids do not represent health issues as intertwined or individual choices as part of a complex entity. Instead, the presented issues encourage individual choices and actions; and the same logic places the responsibility on the individual instead of on 'the population' or 'the public', who are framed as bearing the consequences of individual choices.

By constructing health as something that can be measured, it becomes associated with productivity. The quantification of health creates a narrative of a 'good life' by establishing the increase in life expectancy as an ultimate goal. An extended lifespan becomes equated with being an active and successful individual. The underlying messages are clear: in order to have a good life and in order to be a happy and responsible citizen, one should take care of one's health. This new form of healthy and responsible citizenship requires diligence, self-control and hard work.

Feminisation of the health and fitness media

Historically, new gender ideals in late modernity – the physically active and well-trained woman and the appearance-oriented man – are closely aligned with diet and exercise practices. Gender permeates forms of exercise practices, as well as media representations of body and health.[49] Women have often been expected to be more conscious of health and fitness in comparison to men, due to the special role of care-giver and mother, where women are seen as responsible for providing health care and education as well as a sound home environment. For example, Finnish health and fitness magazines such as *Kauneus & Terveys*, *Kunto Plus* and *Voi hyvin* define their target audiences as (middle-class) women by claiming to write for 'active women' who take care of their fitness, beauty, health and wellbeing.[50]

Lund Kirkegaard has identified career-orientated middle-class women as a core group for the fitness industry since the 1980s, with Jane Fonda's rise as an exercise icon. The gym offers a variety of different classes, and does not demand as much coordination with others as sports usually do. Hence, it could more easily fit into the busy everyday life of work and family.[51] Regarded against a history where muscles and physical strength have often been perceived as unfeminine and unwanted for the female body, the rise of the fit female body ideal could be seen as emancipatory, as symbolising activity and power. But feminist researchers have questioned the emancipatory potential, pointing out the limiting and harmful bodily norms of the fit and toned ideal.[52]

In a study of the Swedish health magazine *iForm* from 1987, 1997 and 2007, Helena Tolvhed identifies an individualist discourse becoming more prominent during the time period. Traditional sports and play are replaced by more 'rational' and time-effective forms of exercise that cut out the social elements present in sport and maximise physical exercise. The very definition of health becomes narrower; areas such as sex and relationships have disappeared from the magazine in 2007, as have more general educational articles on the body. Instead, the focus on diet and exercise has increased.[53] The female models that are used to represent 'health' are conventionally beautiful, smiling, white and predominately thin, rather than obviously muscular. This, Tolvhed concludes, limits the destabilising potential of the 'fit' woman in *iForm*. Her arms might be more 'toned', but today's mediatised representation of the 'fit' and 'healthy' woman still conforms to a narrow and largely stereotypical ideal of femininity.

Through the advice given on how to eat, how to exercise and how to lose weight, the body is constructed as inherently flawed, constantly in need of work. The way to avoid becoming unfit and unattractive is to partake in and to become more knowledgeable about exercise and healthy eating – this is the road to success and happiness.[54] The responsibility for success as well as failure is the individual woman's own, and no attention is paid to the impact of limiting power structures, for example related to gender or class. The visual representation of physical health in health magazines and tabloids is obviously "closely aligned with the cultural conventions of beauty", as Christy Newman has put it.[55]

Finnish tabloids also contribute to a feminisation of healthism with their imagery. In general, tabloids aim to address all genders, and most health articles do not differentiate between genders – except in cases where the article deals with gendered phenomena such as motherhood or increased health problems within the male population. Yet, the visualisation of the stories reveals some degree of feminisation. The photos used in the health-related articles can be divided into four categories: photos of women and/or men; unidentified genders; close-ups of hands or feet; and pictures without people in them. The least popular option is pictures of just men, which are used in connection to stories about athletics and work life. The third category includes pictures without any people, and these stories often deal with nutritional information; stories about medicines and vaccinations; and occasional stories about climate issues, gambling, prisoners, or city and work lives.

The second most popular category does not differentiate clearly between genders. These pictures either include both men and women (stories about sex life, divorce and getting old) or the gender is unclear in the picture (pictures of hands, feet, etc.) when the story concerns overeating, work life or handshaking issues. The most popular category includes women. Here, a distinction between 'unattractive' and 'attractive' women is visible. Unattractive women are overweight, messy and poorly dressed, whereas attractive women are white, slim, well-dressed and well-groomed. The first category illustrates health risks related to overeating and smoking, whereas conventionally beautiful female models represent issues such as exercising, sunbathing and stories about wellbeing and motherhood, as well as stories about how being nice and happy increases life expectancy. These categories reveal how men are connected to working life or athletics, whereas women's health issues are more concentrated on their body image and body management.

Consumer culture encourages self-reflection, with the media and advertising providing pictures of (mainly young and female) bodies that show consumers what they can, and should, become. It represents happy, healthy and beautiful people as role models for consumers to aspire towards.[56] In a gendered, healthist culture, the success of women, in particular, is increasingly assessed in terms of health, fitness and wellbeing instead of other areas of life. There is a noticeable overlap between the meanings of health and beauty that works in both directions; health is understood as equalling a slim, toned body, and looking good becomes equal to being healthy.

Conclusions

The post-war welfare states relied on an authoritarian expert community and the assumption that there was a right way to act. In contrast, the late modern health market is inhabited by different kinds of 'experts', such as dieticians, personal trainers, health or life coaches – not only scientists and doctors; and there is no official authority present to sort out the flurry of advice, treatments and methods. The journalist or magazine generally does not have a consistent perspective, but functions in accordance with the principles of free market and identification rather than traditional medical authority. Instead of a critical reviewer, the health media journalist is a mediator and supplier of research findings and advice from different 'experts', leaving the reader 'free to choose'. Being healthy has become a private concern and responsibility, albeit one that is simultaneously constructed as a prerequisite in order to be an acceptable member of the socio-cultural community. On a normative or ideological level, which has here been examined through health media, the social support system seems to have been taken out of the equation. The creation and maintenance of health is, instead, to be achieved through consumption and making the right choices in diet and exercise. In the increasing mediatisation of health management, health has become something that can be filtered, understood, controlled, shared and communicated through media practices.[57]

In a time period of "retreat from welfare interventionism and of reaffirmation of the importance of 'markets' as regulators of economic activity", the concept of rights begins to appear limited and untenable.[58] Yet, the new modes of regulating health, building on self-management and the discourse of freedom of choice, tend to assume that everyone has the same access, ability and skills to understand and relate to the complex and at times paradoxical health messages available. As discussed above, this also limits the emancipatory potential of the 'fit' and 'healthy' woman. While a physically active lifestyle and 'toned' muscles are historically new elements as far as ideal femininity goes, the (female) body is still constructed as being in need of work and change, and in accordance with narrow conceptualisations of female beauty.

The health media contains a broad and multifaceted range of news and advice on health, weight-loss and exercise. The advice offered sometimes seems paradoxical; but, within a neoliberal paradigm, where consumers choose 'freely' between different options, it actually makes complete sense. Rather than subjects defined or supported by the state, citizens are constructed as rational, active and responsible consumers and opportunists who participate in the national project through competitive and free markets. These subject-citizens consume health services and create their own wellbeing. Similarly, any problems related to health or wellbeing appears to be caused by an inability to control one's own life.[59] The health and fitness media capitalises on this idea of choice by offering information about different services, products and diet advice. This is a definition of freedom that hides the fact that not everyone has the same opportunities – because of variations in place of residence, different bodily abilities/medical conditions, educational or social and financial circumstances – to access the products and services that are being marketed.

Notes

1   Annika Berg, *Den gränslösa hälsan. Signe och Axel Höjer, folkhälsan och expertisen* (Uppsala: Uppsala universitet, 2009); Yvonne Hirdman, *Att lägga livet tillrätta. Studier i svensk folkhemspolitik* (Stockholm: Carlsson, 1989); Helena Hörnfeldt, *Prima barn, helt u.a. Normalisering och utvecklingstänkande i svensk barnhälsovård 1923–2007* (Göteborg: Makadam, 2009); Karin Johannisson, *Kroppens tunna skal. Sex essäer om kropp, historia och kultur* (Stockholm: Norstedt, 1997); Ulf Olsson, *Drömmen om den hälsosamma medborgaren* (Stockholm: Carlsson, 1999); Eva Palmblad and Bengt Erik Eriksson, *Kropp och politik. Hälsoupplysning som samhällsspegel från 30- till 90-tal* (Stockholm, Carlsson, 1995).

2   Allan M. Brandt and Paul Rozin, eds, *Morality and Health* (New York: Routledge, 1997), 65–70; Olsson, *Drömmen om den hälsosamma*; Palmblad and Eriksson, *Kropp och politik*; Dorothy Porter, 'The social contract of health in the twentieth and twenty-first centuries: Individuals, corporations, and the state', in *Shifting Boundaries of Public Health: Europe in the Twentieth Century*, ed. Susan Gross Solomon et al. (Woodbridge: Boydell & Brewer, 2008), 45–60, 46–7; Arttu Saarinen, Suvi Salmenniemi and Harri Keränen, 'Hyvinvointivaltiosta hyvinvoivaan valtioon. Hyvinvointi ja kansalaisuus suomalaisessa poliittisessa diskurssissa', *Yhteiskuntapolitiikka* 79, no. 6 (2014): 605–18.

3   Karin Johannisson, 'The people's health: Public health policies in Sweden', in *The History of Public Health and the Modern State*, ed. Dorothy Porter (Amsterdam: Rodopi, 1994), 165–82, 178, 179.

4   Susan K. Cahn, *Coming on Strong: Gender and Sexuality in Twentieth-Century Women's Sport* (Cambridge, MA: Harvard University Press, 1995); Jennifer Hargreaves, *Sporting Females: Critical Issues in the History and Sociology of Women's Sports* (London: Routledge, 1994); Helena Tolvhed, *På damsidan. Femininitet, motstånd och makt i svensk idrott 1920–1990* (Göteborg: Makadam, 2015).

5   Such as *Voi hyvin* (1982–), *iForm* (1987–), *Hälsorevyn* (1987–1990), *KuntoPlus* (1988–), *B&K Sports Magazine* (1989–, today *Body*), *Hyvä Terveys* (1993–), *Sport* (2002–), *Topphälsa* (2004–), *Body* (2005–), *Fit* (2008–), *LCHF-magasinet* (2010–), *Fitness Magazine* (2001–, today *Women's Health Sverige*), *Hälsa & Fitness* (2011–), *Apu Terveys* (2014–), *ET terveys* (2014–). The magazine market has grown overall, but health and training magazines have wide circulation. In Finland, for example, *Hyvä Terveys* had the third highest circulation of all magazines in 2016 (behind *Aku Ankka* and *ET-lehti*). Kansallinen Mediatutkimus (KMT), 'KMT 2016 lukijamäärät ja koko-naistavoittavuus', MediaAuditFinland, http://mediaauditfinland.fi/wp-content/uploads/2017/03/KMT-2016-lukijamaarat.pdf (accessed 21 Mar 2017).

6   Robert Crawford, 'Healthism and the medicalization of everyday life', *International Journal of Health Services* 10, no. 3 (1980): 365–88; Alan Peterson and Deborah

Lupton, *The New Public Health: Health and Self in the Age of Risk* (London: Sage, 1996).

7 See also Chapter 1 in this volume.

8 Michel Foucault, *Discipline and Punish: The Birth of the Prison* (New York: Pantheon, 1977); Michel Foucault, 'Body/Power', in Michel Foucault: *Power/Knowledge*, ed. Colin Gordon (New York: Pantheon, 1980).

9 Nikolas Rose, *Powers of Freedom: Reframing Political Thought* (Cambridge: Cambridge University Press, 1999), 86–7.

10 Neo-liberalism was born in Anglo-American cultures, but the ideology has influenced Nordic welfare societies as well. The change towards neo-liberal values might have been slower, but similar debates about 'bureaucratic' state systems and 'efficient' competition models have been introduced to Nordic political spheres since the late twentieth century. See, for example, Jason Read, 'A genealogy of homo-economicus: Neoliberalism and the production of subjectivity', *Foucault Studies*, no. 6 (2009): 25–36; Saarinen et al. 'Hyvinvointivaltiosta'.

11 Nikolas Rose, 'Government and control', *British Journal of Criminology* 40, no. 2 (2000): 321–39, 337.

12 Erika Björklund, *Constituting the Healthy Employee? Governing Gendered Subjects in Workplace Health Promotion* (Umeå: Umeå universitet, 2008); Shari L. Dworkin and Faye Linda Wachs, *Body Panic: Gender, Health, and the Selling of Fitness* (New York: New York University Press, 2009); Kathleen LeBesco, 'Neoliberalism, public health, and the moral perils of fatness', *Critical Public Health* 21, no. 2 (2011): 153–64; Petersen and Lupton, *New Public Health*, 68–9; Helena Sandberg, *Medier & fetma. En analys av vikt* (Lund: Sociologiska institutionen, 2004).

13 Chris Shilling, *The Body and Social Theory* (London: Sage, 1993), 4–8, 199–200.

14 Carl Cederström and André Spicer, *The Wellness Syndrome* (Cambridge: Polity, 2015).

15 Jesper Andreasson and Thomas Johansson, *Fitnessrevolutionen. Kropp, hälsa och gymkulturens globalisering* (Stockholm: Carlssons, 2015), 59; Dworkin and Wachs, *Body Panic*, 1–3, 10; Christina Hedblom, *The Body Is Made to Move: Gym and Fitness Culture in Sweden* (Stockholm: Acta Universitatis Stockholmiensis, 2009).

16 The gym and fitness industry has been expanding steadily, mainly in the Western world but also in countries such as Brazil, Japan and China. Andreasson and Johansson, *Fitnessrevolutionen*; M. J. Stern, 'The fitness movement and the fitness center industry, 1960–2000', *Business and Economic History On-line* 6, no. 1 (2008).

17 Kasper Lund Kirkegaard, *Fitnesskultur.dk – fitness-sektorens historie, de aktive udøvere og breddeidrættens kommercialisering* (Odense: Syddansk universitet, 2011), 182, 206–9.

18 Foucault (*Discipline and Punish*) emphasises the role of knowledge in body governance: borders of society and humanity are formed, defended and renegotiated in practices of knowledge and power.

19 Norman Fairclough, *Media Discourse* (London: Edward Arnold, 1995); Sara Mills, *Discourse* (London: Routledge, 2004); Diane Negra and Yvonne Tasker, 'Gender and recessionary culture', in *Gendering the Recession: Media and Culture in an Age of Austerity*, ed. Diane Negra and Yvonne Tasker (Durham, NC: Duke University Press, 2014), 1–30, 1–2.

20 The title of the magazine has changed over the years: 1940–1944: *Solvikingen*; 1944–1953: *Waerlands månads-magasin: tidskrift för hälsa*; 1953–1978: *Tidskrift för hälsa*; 1978–present: *Hälsa*.

21 The journal *Hälsovännen* existed from 1886 to 1961, but was more orientated towards medicine and sanitation.

22 See, e.g., 'Vad har DU med miljövård att göra?', *Tidskrift för hälsa*, no. 1 (1970): 28–31.

23 Johan Börtz, 'Vetenskapliga höns', *Tidskrift för hälsa*, no. 3 (1960): 9; Tidskrift för hälsa no. 5 (1960): 7.

24 Alf Ahlberg, 'Allt det vi inte behöver finns att köpa', *Tidskrift för hälsa*, no. 1 (1970): 16–17.
25 Richard Jobson: 'Krigsförklaring mot fredlig atomkraft', *Tidskrift för hälsa*, no. 4 (1970): 11.
26 Lennart Warodell, '1960: Ett hälsofrämjande år', *Tidskrift för hälsa*, no. 1 (1960): 21.
27 With the exception of an article on the upcoming vote on nuclear power in March 1980, where the no-alternative was advocated as the better choice for health and future, *Tidskrift för hälsa*, no. 3 (1980): 14–17.
28 *Tidskrift för hälsa*, no. 1 (1990).
29 A similar point has been made by Kardemark in a study of Swedish health journals at two points in time: 1910–1913 and 2009. Wilhelm Kardemark, *När livet tar rätt form. Om människosyn i svenska hälsotidskrifter 1910–13 och 2009* (Göteborg: Göteborgs universitet, 2013).
30 Karin Johannisson, 'Den undflyende hälsan: hälsostrategier i Sverige under 1900-talet', in *I väntan på framtiden. Rapport från forskarseminariet i Umeå januari* (Stockholm: Försäkringskasseförbundet, 2000), 38–49; Charlotte Macdonald, *Strong, Beautiful and Modern: National Fitness in Britain, New Zealand, Australia and Canada, 1935–1960* (Vancouver: University of British Columbia Press, 2013); Porter, 'Social contract of health'; Malin Österlind and Jan Wright, 'If sport's the solution then what's the problem? The social significance of sport in the moral governing of "good" and "healthy" citizens in Sweden, 1922–1998', *Sport, Education and Society* 19, no. 8 (2014): 973–90, 986.
31 Wendy Brown, *Edgework: Critical Essays on Knowledge and Politics* (Princeton, NJ: Princeton University Press, 2005).
32 Saarinen et al., 'Hyvinvointivaltiosta', 615.
33 Jallinoja and Suihko have studied the values related to nutrition discussions in *Sotilaskoti*, a Finnish magazine published by a voluntary service to provide free-time spaces, or military homes, for soldiers. This magazine, obviously, differs from some other commercial health magazines, but provides some information about the Finnish magazines. Piia Jallinoja and Johanna Suihko, 'Munkkiperinteestä pizzaelämykseen: Terveys ja ruoka sotilaskoti-lehdessä 1967–2007', *Tiedotustutkimus* 30, no. 4 (2007): 41–3.
34 Pertti Suhonen, 'Suomalaisten eriytyvät ja muuttuvat arvot', in *Uskonto, arvot ja instituutiot. Suomalaiset World Values -tutkimuksissa 1981–2005*, ed. Sami Borg et al. (Tampere: Yhteiskuntatieteellinen tietoarkisto, 2007), 26–46, 40.
35 The mortality rate is a measure of the number of deaths in a particular population and is typically expressed in units of deaths per 1,000 persons per year. Because the rate is scaled to the size of the population and often used in relation to a specific cause of death, rates become comparable.
36 Life expectancy is a statistical measure of how long a person might live based on the year of their birth.
37 Nikolas Rose and Carlos Novas, 'Biological citizenship', in *Global Assemblages: Technology, Politics, and Ethics as Anthropological Problems*, ed. Aihwa Ong and Stephen J. Collier (Oxford: Blackwell, 2004), 439–63.
38 See also, Katariina Kyrölä, *The Weight of Images: Affect, Body Image and Fat in the Media* (Farnham: Ashgate, 2014), 31–92.
39 'Karu totuus: Kaikki liikakilot lyhentävät elinikää. Katso pienimmän riskin painoindeksi!', *Ilta-Sanomat* 19 May 2016.
40 'Hyviä uutisia! Pari tuntia liikuntaa viikossa riittää jo pidentämään elinikää', *Ilta-Sanomat* 14 Apr 2015.
41 Ulla Järvi, '"Suomalaistutkijat tekivät mullistavan havainnon". Analyysi vuoden 2004 terveysaiheisista tiedotteista', *Tiedotustutkimus* 30, no. 4 (2007): 53–60.
42 This approach, which often invokes or utilises feelings of guilt and blame, is a visible trait in some of the health journalism in Finland. For example, STT, the Finnish News

Agency, announced how the overweight issues costs 300 million euros a year to Finnish health care. STT 8 Jul 2010.

43 'Nuorten suomalaisnaisten syöpätilastossa hyppäys. Uudenmaan ja Etelä-Suomen ilmiö', *Ilta-Sanomat* 20 Apr 2016.
44 'Lapsuuden lihavuus lyhentää elämää', *Iltalehti* 23 Feb 2010.
45 'Yli 65-vuotias: Nämä 4 asiaa tuovat sinulle 10 vuotta lisää elinaikaa', *Ilta-Sanomat* 27 July 2014.
46 'Luja kädenpuristus pidentää elinikää', *Iltalehti* 22 Sep 2010.
47 Petersen and Lupton, *New Public Health*, 27. See also Chapter 11 by Johannes Kananen in this volume.
48 Petersen and Lupton, *New Public Health*, 27–60.
49 Dworkin and Wachs, *Body Panic*.
50 The press material from 2017 as written in the marketing pages of Finnish magazine platform Aikakausmedia, 'Jäsenluettelo', www.aikakauslehdet.fi/jasenet/?lista=lehdet (accessed 21 Mar 2017).
51 Kirkegaard, *Fitnesskultur.dk*, 27, 40–41, 186, 194–5.
52 Dworkin and Wachs, *Body Panic*; Angela McRobbie, *The Aftermath of Feminism: Gender, Culture and Social Change* (London: Sage, 2009); Jennifer Smith Maguire, *Fit for Consumption: Sociology and the Business of Fitness* (Abingdon: Routledge, 2007).
53 Helena Tolvhed, 'Hälsosam femininitet och postfeministiska subjekt. En undersökning av hälso- och träningsmagasinet iForm 1987, 1997 och 2007', *Tidskrift för genusvetenskap* 37, no. 3 (2016): 77–94.
54 Kerry R. McGannon and John C. Spence, 'Exploring news media representations of women's exercise and subjectivity through critical discourse analysis', *Qualitative Research in Sport, Exercise and Health* 4, no. 1 (2012): 32–50, 36, 46; Tolvhed, 'Hälsosam femininitet'.
55 Christy Newman, 'Reader letters to women's health magazines: Inscribing the "will to health"', *Feminist Media Studies* 7, no. 2 (2007): 155–70, 163.
56 Annemarie Jutel and Stephen Buetow, 'A picture of health? Unmasking the role of appearance in health', *Perspectives in Biology and Medicine* 50, no. 3 (2007): 421–34; Chris Shilling, *The Body and Social Theory* (London: Sage, 2003).
57 The concept of 'mediatisation' addresses the changing logic of media that influences everyday practices, experiences and communication of (health) issues. Andreas Hepp, 'Differentiation: Mediatization and cultural change', in *Mediatization: Concept, Changes, Consequences*, ed. Knut Lundby (New York: Lang, 2009), 139–58; Stig Hjarvard, *The Mediatization of Culture and Society* (London, New York: Routledge, 2013); Friedrich Krotz, 'Mediatization: A concept with which to grasp media and societal change', in *Mediatization: Concept, Changes, Consequences*, ed. Knut Lundby (New York: Lang, 2009), 21–40.
58 Peterson and Lupton, *New Public Health*, xiii, xiv.
59 Brown, *Edgework*; Saarinen et al., 'Hyvinvointivaltiosta', 604, 612–14.

13 Editors' notes

Transitions in the conceptual history of public health

Johannes Kananen, Sophy Bergenheim and Merle Wessel

They say you should not judge a book by its cover. In this volume, we have suggested that you also should not judge a concept by the way it appears in language.

Concepts and the words for expressing them can be deceiving. They might share the same spelling, but nevertheless carry different, unwritten meanings – even in the same language, time period and geographical area. This, of course, easily leads to confusion and misinterpretation. Even more confusion ensues when the same word or term has been in use for decades (such as 'public health' or the Germanic varieties of 'people's health') or for centuries (such as 'people' or 'race').

The chapters in this anthology have analysed various historical and contemporary health-related concepts and their discourses. On the one hand, the chapters have made a valuable contribution to dispelling conceptual confusion. On the other, they demonstrate that the work should not end here, but that further key concepts should be stripped of their seemingly self-evident disguise.

Some of the recurring key concepts in this volume include 'people', 'race' and 'citizen', which are intertwined with notions of 'nation' and 'state'. At first glance, 'people' and 'citizenship' may seem like universal and inclusive categories, as they refer to a community and collective. However, they also mask various gate-keeping criteria – who is included and who is not – which vary according to time and place. Nowadays, citizenship is primarily associated with a formal belonging to a nation state. However, throughout the twentieth century, various formal and informal characteristics, traits and criteria have been attributed to the concept. In other words, it has not been a fixed, but a flexible and negotiable category. (Chapters 4, 5 and 8.)

Similarly, 'people' has not been a neutral and all-inclusive concept; rather, it is to be regarded as a political and historical concept. For example, 'people' has also been understood as the working class or lower classes; alternatively, the working class and lower classes have been understood as a specific part of the people or race (Chapters 3, 5, 6, 7 and 9).[1] Left-wing movements have used the concept for empowering the working class and distinguishing it from the bourgeoisie and the elite. Respectively, the 'people' or the working class and lower classes have been a source of particular concern for the middle and upper classes: a group that should be educated and/or controlled by the social or medical elite.

The latter notions have been intertwined with an objective to protect the 'nation' and the 'race' from social and health characteristics associated with the lower classes (such as alcoholism, tuberculosis, STDs, criminality, prostitution, etc.). In addition to the diseases being health- or even life-threatening, in the nineteenth and early twentieth century, these characteristics were seen as posing social, moral, economic, and defence/military threats. In addition to class-based perspectives, this conception of protection also had a gendered aspect. The future of the nation or race was seen as resting on the shoulders of women and children whereby various attempts at controlling or educating (often working-class or lower-class) women were seen as vital and legitimate. (Chapters 2, 3, 5, 6, 7 and 9.)

Social, moral and health characteristics were thus intertwined, as was their heredity. Nineteenth- and early twentieth-century racial hygiene and racial biology were scientific and social ideas based on this understanding. They are often characterised as striving to improve the race or population, but another important viewpoint is protection. Actors favouring and promoting racial hygienic policies, measures and legislation strived to protect the collective (the nation or the people or population) from social, moral and physical degeneration and social unrest by inhibiting or discouraging undesired traits from being passed on to future generations. Racial hygiene was closely linked with family policy, population policy, social policy and social medicine. As noted in the introductory chapter, racial hygiene should not be perceived merely as an apparatus of coercive control and exclusion; it should also be seen as an attempt to include excluded people in the community or collective, on condition that they consent and conform to racial hygienic measures and criteria. (Chapters 2, 3, 5, 6, 7 and 9.) However, not everyone was enchanted by the narrative of protection, and voices condemning racial hygienic ideas and practices as a threat to individual and civic rights were also raised (Chapter 4).

Racial hygiene was a complex and multifaceted phenomenon that took many forms. It was, for instance, a part of a Social Democratic model for social progress ('welfare eugenics', as labelled by Albert Spektorowski and Elisabet Mizrachi[2]) in Sweden and Norway (Chapter 6). In Finland, the pronatalist population policy and public health ideas promoted by actors from the political centre-right included marked racial hygienic features (Chapter 7). The most notorious form of racial hygiene is, of course, Nazi Germany (Chapter 2). These examples illustrate how the idea was attributed to different social and political entities.

Likewise, the idea of racial hygiene should not be attributed to a strictly delimited time period. In the early twentieth century, racial hygiene ideas and public health ideas shared many features; for some actors, they even meant largely the same thing. After the Second World War, countries and actors changed their vocabulary at varying pace. Some held on to 'hygiene' concepts (Chapter 7), some adopted concepts such as 'population policy' (Chapters 5 and 7), some favoured 'people's health' with varying meanings throughout the twentieth century (Chapter 6). A change in vocabulary did not, however, necessarily reflect a change in ideas and policies; but legislation and practices with racial hygienic features continued to exist in the Nordic countries until the 1960s and 1970s.

Furthermore, eugenics has been an important idea in Eastern and Southern Europe, as well as in China, Japan, India and Latin America. China's one-child policy (1978–2002) is an example of post-war eugenics whereby the main aim was to limit population growth. Japan implemented the Eugenic Protection Law in 1948, which allowed the sterilisation of individuals with a genetic disposition to crime, other mild genetic disabilities (like albinism or colour-blindness), as well as those who were mentally ill, for example with manic-depression or schizophrenia. In 2002, India started a programme to sterilise predominantly (lower-caste) women to limit the population size. The women are rewarded with land, money or loans if they agree to be sterilised.

Central questions posed in this book have been: whose health? and what is 'health'? There has been a distinction between the health of the collective and the health of individuals. The various conceptions of the collective whose health has been of concern can be illuminated through the discussion regarding 'people', 'race', 'population', 'nation', etc. In addition, the collective has been broadened to encompass the population of the entire world or to transgress national borders (Chapters 6, 9 and 10). The individual, for its part, may carry (unwritten) assumptions of gender, class, ethnicity, physical condition, age and so forth.

The chapters in this volume have demonstrated various historical and contemporary struggles in defining 'health'. These have manifested themselves, for example, as rivalry (and collaboration) in defining (public) health problems, producing health- and medicine-related knowledge, and setting health policy agendas (their targets, scope, objectives, etc.). From a Foucauldian perspective, this book has, in other words, analysed how actors have strived to contribute to the 'regime of truth'[3] of health. They have sought to create and influence a conceptual, symbolic and discursive framework for health: health ideals and, respectively, health problems. The regime of truth determines what is deemed politically and socially important, accurate information and knowledge, proper treatment, desired development and so forth.

In addition to medical experts and policy makers (Chapters 2, 3, 5, 6, 7, 8, 9 and 11), participants in this struggle or interaction around the regime of truth of health include, among others: national and transnational temperance movements (Chapters 9 and 10); other non-governmental actors involved in health policy (Chapter 7); and cultural figures, journalists and the media (Chapters 4 and 12). The contributions of these actors have resulted in different interpretations of 'health' – for example, health understood as little to no prevalence of specific illnesses, or as abstinence, or as able-bodiedness, fitness and attractiveness.

Reinhart Koselleck has coined the terms 'space of experience' and 'horizon of expectation'.[4] They illustrate a perspective where the past is approached as a past present, with its own past and future. The space of experience refers to the past of the past: experiences that have led to present of the past and have sculpted the perceived reality of that present. The future, by definition, is unknown – but not limitless. The space of experience delimits the expectations of what the future can or will bring; in other words, the horizon of expectation.

In a Koselleckian vein, all themes discussed in this book can be seen as attempts to influence the future in one way or another – as a tension between experience and expectation. As noted earlier, the focus has been on health: of the collective, individuals, future generations, the present generation. It has all been about trying to have a positive influence on the future of health. Whose health, through which measures and according to what criteria, for their part, have been determined by past events, the reality of the present and the resulting expectations for the future.

The people, the state and modern science

The Second World War was followed by a political, economic and social transition period. It was the starting point of the Cold War and the domination of two different political systems – capitalism and socialism. It changed the face of nationalism in most countries. This had effects on conceptualisations of public health concepts, as we have shown in the book. Global ideas were added to concepts of national public health with the development of the World Health Organization (WHO). The individual and the global perspective started to prevail over the collective and national one, respectively. International cooperation had existed before, but what was new about the WHO was its ambition to eradicate diseases such as smallpox and tuberculosis. Public health was no longer only a concern of individual states and their citizens; it was also of concern across nations. The Western world started to transport its public health values to non-Western countries in organised form, and supported developing countries in health crises. At the same time, there was an 'epidemiological' turn in public health whereby the focus in many countries shifted from infectious to chronic diseases. Epidemiological knowledge began to focus on individual risk factors, and public health experts developed ideas of preventing chronic disease.

The concept of 'people's health' (*folkhälsa* in Swedish) and its various post-war uses in the different Nordic languages illustrates some of the ambiguities associated with the Nordic welfare state model. At the same time, such ambiguities reveal important differences between Nordic uses of the concept in comparison with other geographical areas.

Similar to the concept of 'universalism', another key concept of the Nordic welfare state, 'people's health', has been an ambiguous concept. When Nordic governments have established and expanded publicly provided health care services during the 'golden era' of welfare state development (the decades after the Second World War), they have promoted 'people's health'. However, the same governments have also promoted 'people's health' through paternalism, control of individual behaviour, compulsion and normalisation.

Directing individual behaviour from above was motivated after the Second World War – for instance in the case of Axel Höjer in Sweden – by a balance between rights and obligations. The government (at central and local levels) granted universal access to publicly provided health care. In return, the government could expect certain behaviours from citizens, including efforts to live healthy lives. (Chapter 6.)

In the Nordic countries, both medical science and the medical profession were integral parts of public administration. Consequently, public health and biomedicine were closely connected. The situation was different in the US, for instance, where the two fields have traditionally been separate in various ways. American public health has often been involved in a struggle for prestige and power, competing with a respected medical profession operating outside the state apparatus.[5] In the US, the states or the federal government did not offer public health insurance or public health care services like the Nordic governments did after the Second World War.[6]

In comparison with the US, it is interesting to note that the Nordic medical profession has been, in part, an extension of public health – organised by public authorities and fulfilling goals and policies established by public health officials. This is a fundamental difference, reflecting different conceptualisations and different understandings of the relationship between individual and society – in addition to the more obvious differences in political preferences. Comparative welfare state research has demonstrated what this difference implied at the collective level in terms of social equality.

Restriction of alcohol consumption in the name of public health

Another example of the comparatively wide field of meanings associated with Nordic usages of the concept of 'people's health' is the central role of alcohol policy in efforts to promote public health. Ideas about how to govern and regulate alcohol consumption have been central to Nordic conceptualisations of public health (Chapters 9 and 10). Again, key actors derived central ideas from scientific evidence. This evidence demonstrated the harmful effects of alcohol on the individual human body, the association between social problems and alcohol consumption, and the distribution of consumption at the level of the population.

Confronted with this evidence, Nordic policy makers proceeded by regulating the price and availability of alcohol as part of efforts to reduce total consumption. Experts had shown that the distribution of alcohol consumption among the population followed the clock-shaped Gauss curve. Most people consumed an average (or close to average) amount of alcohol, while a minority consumed extremely high and extremely low (or zero) amounts of alcohol. Furthermore, statistics showed that alcohol consumption levels per head were comparatively high among Nordic populations. Therefore, alcohol-related problems were thought to affect the Nordic populations in a particularly severe manner.

Hence, Nordic policy makers – especially in Finland and Sweden – focused on comparatively strong regulations on sales and the price of alcohol. The legitimation of such measures was often derived from usages of the concept of 'people's health'. Rhetoric could include, for instance, statements of the harmful effects of high alcohol consumption on 'people's health' – trying to create an atmosphere where regulations were ultimately beneficial for all members of society, including moderate consumers. The Nordic countries were the only countries where the total consumption model had a central role in conceptualisations of public health

(Chapter 9). In most other countries, the model remained at a level of abstract reasoning without practical implications such as sales and price regulations.

Joining the European Union created a challenge for Swedish and Finnish conceptualisations of public health in the 1990s. The EU looked sceptically on sales monopolies, regardless of good intentions associated with 'people's health'. Thus, the Finnish and Swedish governments had to negotiate special deals in order to maintain state monopolies and price regulations of alcohol in the EU. The European four freedoms (freedom of movement of goods, labour, capital and services) are in stark contrast with Nordic notions of regulating the sales and price of alcohol.

Contemporary drivers of change

Since the 1980s and 1990s there have been at least four important drivers of conceptual change. These include cultural individualisation, cultural globalisation, economic globalisation and changes in knowledge production.[7] Each of these processes challenges past meanings of 'people's health' and forces key actors wishing to affect social development to create new meanings of the concept.

Cultural individualisation has involved increased efforts by individuals to determine the content of their lives and the weakening of traditions, undermining traditional Nordic conceptualisations of collectivistic citizenship. This process has forced actors wishing to promote public health to rethink ideas about governing the population. In the 2010s, in the age of social media and smartphones, it would be inconceivable to start a community control project in the fashion of the Finnish North Karelia Project in the 1970s (Chapter 11). People would no longer respond to such a project in the way they did thirty or forty years ago. Compared to that period, people behave in a more unpredictable way,[8] and mechanisms of governance are bound to change.

After the collapse of the Soviet Union and with the increasing influence and dominance of Western ideas, the Nordic countries have been confronted with ideas of individual rights in new ways. The international discourse on human rights and social rights looks at the issue of rights from the individual's perspective. The individual is granted rights to achieve and receive various things in addition to freedom from oppression and discrimination.

Such ideas are quite different compared to the traditional ideas associated with the Nordic welfare state.[9] While citizenship rights, including social rights, were comparatively comprehensive in the post-war Nordic countries, these rights were established with respect to various groups and segments of society – workers, parents, mothers, children and pensioners, for instance. The perspective was that of society as opposed to the US, for instance, where the Constitution specifies individual rights. From the perspective of the human rights discourse, such a rationale created little room for individual choice.

The idea of individual rights forces Nordic actors to rethink ideas of 'people's health'. Should future public services be designed from the perspective of the individual or from the perspective of the population? Would this imply a rolling back of past public welfare state institutions?

At the same time, cultural globalisation has challenged the very notion of population.[10] As noted in the contributions to this volume, in addition to various notions of class, the notion of an ethnically unified people has been another central feature of Nordic conceptualisations of public health.[11] 'People's health' has (among other things) implied the health of the (ethnically unified) people. The global mobility of people has resulted in increasing migration to the Nordic countries, which have responded in different ways. Sweden, Norway and Denmark have welcomed more immigrants per native population compared to Finland, for instance. At the same time, it has become increasingly difficult to maintain ideas about an ethnically unified population as lifestyles and subcultures have begun to diverge under the influence of individualisation and multiculturalisation.

This challenge to earlier notions of *folk* has led to a strong counter-reaction. In the Nordic countries, like elsewhere in Europe, populist right-wing parties have channelled public anxiety in the face of social change.[12] Such a channelling has occurred through wishes to maintain old notions of *folk* by restricting the number of immigrants and refugees. Right-wing populist parties have appealed to and encouraged xenophobia, hatred and racism.

As traditional parties relying on the left–right division and an opposition between workers and employers have failed to renew their rhetoric, populist parties have been successful in channelling destructive forces of social change in an atmosphere of increasing hatred where groups of non-immigrants exploited by the labour market are turning against immigrant groups. Such developments have led to demands to restrict public health care services to non-immigrant population groups.

Puzzled by this great social question of our era but unable to find solutions, Nordic governments have continued to reform societies according to neoliberal ideals. In the 1980s, economic globalisation introduced neo-classical economic ideas in the Nordic countries.[13] The idea that market forces – the laws of supply and demand – should allocate resources in society was rapidly adopted by key Nordic policy makers, and especially by organised business and their think tanks. Similar to ideas about individual human rights, most neo-liberal ideas were in stark contrast with the ideas associated with the traditional Nordic welfare state where the state had acquired a special role in social planning, social engineering, and allocation and redistribution of resources. While publicly adhering to such classical welfare state ideals, including redistribution of resources, Nordic governments have, since the 1990s: deregulated markets; privatised public services; tightened the eligibility criteria of welfare benefits; introduced sanctions in social assistance; and participated in the international financialisation of the economy.[14]

In the area of public health, the potential influence of neoliberalism lies in the idea that the provision of health care and pharmaceuticals could be organised along the lines of private enterprises trying to generate returns for privately invested capital. Gradually, Nordic governments have begun to widen the reach of the market mechanism in the provision of health care, allowing private companies to increase market shares in an area previously dominated by public provision. Welfare state professionals, including the medical profession, previously organised by the state and public authorities, have to increasing extent been able to choose between public and private employers. Socioeconomic inequalities in access to health and social care services have tended to persist, however.[15]

Neoliberalism creates a context for public health reminiscent of the period before public health care provision when health care services and the distribution of pharmaceuticals were organised and provided by private actors and enterprises. The main problem of this development is that multinational corporations are driven by the profit motive, and their interests are hard to combine with a pursuit of social justice and equality at the national and local level.

In practice, the most recent widening of the market mechanism has started with a differentiation between purchaser and provider in welfare services. Private service producers have the opportunity to act as producers of public health and social care services as public authorities have outsourced service production in accordance with tendering processes. At the same time, outsourcing and public private partnerships have increasingly become subject to European competition law.

The emerging molecular gaze

Yet another important driver of conceptual change in the Nordic countries stems from the development of the so-called life sciences (i.e. biology and its various subdisciplines such as molecular biology and neuroscience).[16] Scholars have termed this shift the emergence of the molecular gaze, comparable to the emergence of the clinical gaze in the eighteenth and nineteenth centuries along with modern medical science.[17] Since this transformation, the life sciences have broadened their focus to include the molecular level instead of mainly focusing on the level of tissues and organs. The shift in focus has had, and continues to have, enormous implications for the meanings of key concepts, including life, disease and, indeed – public health.[18]

The combination of new knowledge production with the ideas of neoliberalism and economic globalisation has brought forth new kinds of rationales and objectives. Capital investors have discovered that the great promises associated with technoscience and new biomedical knowledge can be coupled with the development of new products to be distributed and sold in health care markets. The human body, with its cells and genes, becomes raw material in this process of generating profits for private investors.[19]

Nordic governments have embraced this new development, signalling a willingness to break with past understandings of public health. For the governments, the business potential of this new development appears tempting. They see the search for techno-scientific innovations and the development of new health care products and services as desirable and potentially beneficial for the economy and for the creation of new jobs.[20] Therefore, Nordic governments want to participate in the international race for new techno-scientific innovations in the area of bioscience. For this purpose, scientific research needs to be cutting-edge, which requires sufficiently large research facilities with enough resources.[21]

From another direction, Nordic governments seek to attract private investors as part of an effort to secure funding for the development of new products for private health care markets. Efforts to widen the scope for markets in health care can also be viewed from this perspective: bigger markets attract bigger investors.

Thus, a completely new understanding of the role of the Nordic state is emerging: whereas before, the link between state and science was fundamental for the organisation of society, more recently, the state is acquiring a new role by trying to tighten the links between science and private markets. In a sense, states are also becoming actors in a global market. Before, the state sought to apply the knowledge produced by the life sciences in the name of public health. More recently, the governments try to compete with other states in a race for international capital and job creation through capital investment in multinational corporations. This is a major shift in the political imaginary.

Given past efforts to promote 'people's health', the Nordic countries have a strong tradition in focusing on the health of the population. This tradition puts these countries in a special position regarding the latest development in the life sciences that have started to value large data sets (or Big Data). Such Big Data have existed for decades (or even centuries) in the Nordic countries, in the form of personal identification numbers and data on health and social security clients. Personal screening of mothers and women has been part of traditional efforts to promote public health. As a result of such screenings, large data sets exist containing biomedical information that can be linked to individual persons and, hence, combined with other public registers of information.[22]

Following the development of life sciences, the Nordic countries have established biobanks – i.e. collections of samples of human tissue or blood which can be used for research at the molecular level. In the Nordic countries, such samples could be connected to existing public registries with all their information.[23]

Constructing the object of knowledge

Generating meanings of public health concepts is part of the activity that may be understood as the construction of the object of the knowledge that our modern societies heavily rely on. A central condition for modern science has been a distinction between the subject and object of research – i.e., a distinction between the one who carries out the research and the object of knowledge.[24]

Modern researchers have been able to accumulate knowledge because they have been able successfully to delimit and delineate the object of knowledge. From our perspective, the act of delineating the object of knowledge is linguistic. In other words, it occurs through conventions, rules concerning scientific discipline, and definitions of what counts as knowledge and what the scientific method is about.[25] 'The human mind' as discussed by psychology does not, in other words, necessarily exist outside the discursive space created by the scholars participating in maintaining the praxis commonly labelled as 'psychology'.[26]

In this process of establishing or constructing the object of knowledge through linguistic acts, theory and practice have been deeply intertwined. The various contributions to this volume shed light on the processes and linguistic acts whereby the objects of scientific knowledge have been constructed from the point of view of public health. We might say that the object of knowledge in public health and the (bio)medical sciences is – like in all humanities and social sciences – the human being and life itself.[27] While countless efforts have been made to increase scientific knowledge in the humanities and social sciences, the object of knowledge – the human being as a whole and life itself – has remained rather unknown. The delimited objects only include aspects of the human being, never the human being in all its complexity. Conceptualisations of public health certainly have had enormous consequences for how we live our lives as human beings and how we understand ourselves, our bodies and our minds and our identities.[28] Yet, the contributions to this volume, alongside other contributions in the field of sociology of health, indicate that such consequences often occur rather indirectly, unintendedly and sometimes even accidentally.

The objects of our knowledge are linguistically constructed in a process of social and public interaction of authorised scientists, and scientific and public debate consequently tends to focus on words rather than concepts and phenomena behind words and concepts. From what is happening we can, however, judge that the object of our knowledge is changing, and so is our collective understanding of ourselves. These changes create new meanings for key concepts we use to grasp and shape our social reality and our personal lives.

Advances in life sciences imply that future physical conditions of the human being may be affected in the present – through applications of knowledge about genes, for instance. The risk of having a disease in the future may be controlled in the present. Stem cell research contains the promise of engineering embryos, for instance in order to improve future quality of life. Thus, there is a sense in which we are able to imagine future physical conditions and manipulate our bodies in accordance with this image. Nikolas Rose regards this as 'an emergent form of life'.

In this type of future-orientated intervention, the object of knowledge is no longer clearly distinct from the knowledge-producing subject. If we are able to imagine ourselves in the future, and manipulate our physical bodies (or that of an embryo) in accordance with that image, the distinction between the perceiving subject and an external world of objects (including the physical body) becomes blurred. Cartesian duality is being transgressed by a science that once held this duality as constitutive for knowledge production. The time has come to discover ourselves in relation to the objects we study.

Notes

1   See also Ilkka Liikanen, 'Kansa', in *Käsitteet liikkeessä: Suomen poliittisen kulttuurin käsitehistoria*, ed. Matti Hyvärinen, Jussi Kurunmäki, Kari Palonen, Tuija Pulkkinen and Henrik Stenius (Tampere: Vastapaino, 2003), 257–309.
2   Alberto Spektorowski and Elisabet Mizrachi, 'Eugenics and the welfare state in Sweden: The politics of social margins and the idea of a productive society', *Journal of Contemporary History* 39, no. 3 (2004): 333–52.

3   Michel Foucault, 'Truth and power', in *Power/Knowledge: Selected Interviews and Other Writings 1972–1977* by Michel Foucault, ed. Colin Gordon (New York: Harvester, 1980), 109–33.
4   Reinhart Koselleck, *Futures Past: On the Semantics of Historical Time* (New York: Columbia University Press, 2004).
5   Allan M. Brandt and Martha Gardner, 'Antagonism and accommodation: Interpreting the relationship between public health and medicine in the United States during the 20th century', *American Journal of Public Health* 90, no. 5 (2000): 707–15. On the relationship between public health and medicine in Sweden, see Annika Berg, *Den gränslösa hälsan: Signe och Axel Höjer, folkhälsan och expertisen* (Uppsala: Uppsala University Press, 2009).
6   Countries like Germany and the UK have general and inclusive access to health care. Germany implemented the first health insurance for workers in 1884, and the UK founded the National Health Service (NHS) in 1948 to provide all residents with health care services.
7   See also Adele E. Clarke, Laura Mamo, Jennifer Ruth Fosket, Jennifer R. Fishman and Janet K. Shim, eds, *Biomedicalization: Technoscience, Health, and Illness in the US* (Durham, NC: Duke University Press, 2010).
8   If the idea of individualisation is true, see e.g. Ulrich Beck, Anthony Giddens and Scott Lash, *Reflexive Modernisation: Politics, Tradition and Aesthetics in the Modern Social Order* (Cambridge: Polity, 1994).
9   This observation was originally made by Johan Strang.
10   For discussion of globalisation and cosmopolitanism, see Ulrich Beck and Edgar Grande, *Cosmopolitan Europe* (Cambridge: Polity, 2004) and David Held, *Cosmopolitanism: Ideals and Realities* (Cambridge: Polity, 2010).
11   At the same time, there have been efforts to transcend national boundaries in public health work, for instance by Axel Höjer in Sweden and by the WHO.
12   Ann-Cathrine Jungar and Anders Ravik Jupskås, 'Populist radical right parties in the Nordic region: A new and distinct party family?', *Scandinavian Political Studies* 37, no. 3 (2014): 215–38.
13   Mark Blyth, *Great Transformations: Economic Ideas and Institutional Change* (New York: Cambridge University Press, 2002); Pauli Kettunen, *Globalisaatio ja kansallinen me* (Tampere: Vastapaino, 2008); Bob Jessop, *The Future of the Capitalist State* (Cambridge: Cambridge University Press, 2002); David Harvey, *A Brief History of Neoliberalism* (Oxford: Oxford University Press, 2005); Johannes Kananen, *The Nordic Welfare State in Three Eras: From Emancipation to Discipline* (London: Routledge, 2014); Anu Kantola and Johannes Kananen, 'Seize the moment: Financial crisis and the making of the Finnish competition state', *New Political Economy* 18, no. 6 (2013): 811–26; Christian A. Larsen and Jorgen G. Andersen, 'How Economic ideas changed the Danish welfare state: The case of neo-liberal ideas and highly organized social democratic interests', *Governance* 22, no. 2 (2009): 239–61.
14   For a discussion of financialisation and the financial crisis of 2007-2008, see e.g. Melinda Cooper and Martijn Konings, eds, *Rethinking Money, Debt, and Finance after the Crisis* (Durham, NC: Duke University Press, 2015).
15   Clare Bambra, 'Social inequalities in health: The Nordic welfare state in a comparative context', in *Changing Social Equality: The Nordic Welfare Model in the 21st Century*, ed. Jon Kvist, Johan Fritzell, Bjorn Hvinden and Olli Kangas (Bristol: Policy Press, 2011), 143–63; Olli Kangas, 'Välskäri vaiko rauhanneuvottelija? Sosioekonoisia terveyseroja selittävät tekijät Euroopassa, in *Kansallista vai paikallista? Puheenvuoroja sosiaali- ja terveydenhuollosta*, ed. Hennamari Mikkola, Jenni Blomgren and Heikki Hiilamo (Helsinki: Kela), 52–75.
16   See also Nikolas Rose, *The Politics of Life Itself: Biomedicine, Power, and Subjectivity in the Twenty-First Century* (Princeton, NJ: Princeton University Press, 2007).
17   Clarke et al., *Biomedicalization*.

18 These implications will vary according to geographical location and according to traditional conceptualisations of public health – including the ones scrutinised in this volume.

19 Clarke et al., *Biomedicalization*; Rose, *Politics of Life Itself.*

20 See e.g. *Terveysalan kasvustrategia: Terveysalan tutkimus- ja innovaatiotoiminnan kasvustrategia, tiekartta 2016–2018* (Helsinki: Ministry of Employment and the Economy, 2016).

21 Ibid.

22 Mianna Meskus, *Elämän tiede: Tutkimus lääketieteellisestä teknologiasta, vanhemmuudesta ja perimän hallinnasta* (Tampere: Vastapaino, 2009). See also Jaakko Harkko et al., *Preliminary Study of Strengths, Weaknesses and Sustainability of the Nordic Welfare State* (forthcoming).

23 See e.g. Ida Ohlsson Al Fakir, *Nya rum för social medborgarskap. Om vetenskap och politik i 'Zigenarundersökningen' – en socialmedicinsk studie av svenska romer 1962–1965* (Växsjö: Linnaeus University Press, 2015), 300.

24 Hubert Dreyfus and Charles Taylor, *Retrieving Realism* (Cambridge, MA: Harvard University Press, 2015).

25 See also Thomas Kuhn, *The Structure of Scientific Revolutions* (Chicago: University of Chicago Press, 1962).

26 The example is chosen arbitrarily. It could have been whichever object in the human and social sciences: 'the welfare state', 'the economy', 'the unemployed', 'the body', 'the nervous system', etc.

27 Cf. Nikolas Rose, *Politics of Life Itself.*

28 Ibid.; David Armstrong, 'Foucault and the sociology of health and illness: A prismatic reading', in *Foucault, Health and Medicine*, ed. Alan Petersen and Robin Bunton (London: Routledge, 1997); Elianne Riska, *Masculinity and Men's Health: Coronary Heart Disease in Medical and Public Discourse* (Lanham, MD: Rowman & Littlefield, 2006).

Index